THE
CANCER
INDUSTRY

OTHER BOOKS BY RALPH W. MOSS, PHD

Herbs Against Cancer

Alternative Medicine Online

Questioning Chemotherapy

Cancer Therapy

Free Radical: Albert Szent-Gyorgyi
and the Battle Over Vitamin C

Caring
(with Annette Swackhamer, RN)

A Real Choice

An Alternative Approach to Allergies
(with Theron G. Randolph, MD)

The Cancer Syndrome

THE CANCER INDUSTRY

The Classic Exposé
on the Cancer Establishment

by

Ralph W. Moss

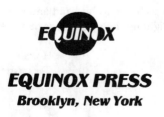

EQUINOX PRESS
Brooklyn, New York

Originally published by Grove Press, Inc.
in 1980 as *The Cancer Syndrome.*

Major revised edition published by Paragon House
in 1989 as *The Cancer Industry.*

ISBN 1-881025-09-8

Library of Congress Catalog Card Number: 96-84574

10 9 8 7 6 5 4 3 2

Manufactured in the United States of America

To Martha

There is nothing more admirable than when two people who
see eye to eye keep house as husband and wife, confounding their
enemies and delighting their friends, as they themselves know best.

Homer
The Odyssey, Book VI

Contents

Acknowledgments

Many individuals contributed to the making of this book. Needless to say, any remaining errors are solely my responsibility. The following people read the original text, or portions of it, and offered valuable comments at various stages: Irwin D. J. Bross, Ph.D., Alan Gaby, M.D., Joseph Gold, M.D., Virginia Livingston-Wheeler, M.D., Linus Pauling, Ph.D., Alec Pruchnicki, M.D., Charles Russell, Ph.D., Barbara Solomon, M.D., and Jonathan Wright, M.D.

My friends and family members contributed their help and support, especially my parents and my children. My agent, Ruth Hagy Brod, and editor, Kent Carroll, performed above and beyond what was required of them. I wish to express my appreciation to those who worked on the production of the original Grove Press book, including Claudia Menza, Reginald Gay, and Diane Root.

Many workers and scientists in the cancer field, especially former colleagues at Memorial Sloan-Kettering Cancer Center, shared their knowledge, ideas, and theories freely. Among those colleagues was a friend and teacher, Dr. Kanematsu Sugiura, who died while the book was going to press. I am also indebted to the hundreds of cancer patients I have known. Esther Moore, who died tragically at forty-four, embodied the courage of these patients: "If death is coming, then death, come on with it, but let me meet you at the door, dammit, on my feet!"

Chapter 8, "The Laetrile Controversy," was first prepared for Louis Lasagna, ed., *Controversies in Therapeutics* (Philadelphia: W. B. Saunders and Co., 1980). My thanks to Dr. Lasagna and his publisher for permission to reprint it here. Thanks to Herman Goodman for bringing this manuscript to the attention of its first publisher.

The following are some of the individuals who helped me in the preparation of the revised 1989 version: Elaine Boies, Dean Burk, Ph.D., Lawrence Burton, Ph.D., Stanislaw R. Burzynski, M.D., Ph.D., Peter Barry Chowka, Marcus Cohen, Michael L. Culbert, Harris L. Coulter, Ph.D., Robert DeBragga, the Hon. Mike Driscoll, Joseph Gold, M.D., Gar Hildenbrand, Robert G. Houston, Beatrice Trum Hunter, John T. Johnson, Avis Lang, Patrick M. McGrady, Jr., Robert Marx, Pamela Maurath, Linus Pauling, Ph.D., Irwin Peck, Alec Pruchnicki, M.D., Emanuel Revici, M.D., my editor Ken Stuart, Le Trombetta, Jim Turner, Patricia Spain Ward, Denise and Frank Wiewel, and Ronald G. Wolin.

This 1996 updated edition is once again dedicated to my wife, Martha, this time on the occasion of our thirty-second wedding anniversary.

1996 Update

The year 1996 marks the twenty-fifth anniversary of President Nixon's "war on cancer." During this time, the federal government has spent over $25 billion on cancer research, while the American Cancer Society (ACS) and various other private organizations have spent a nearly equal sum. When this war was launched in 1971, leading scientists promised Congress a cure in time for the Bicentennial. That didn't happen, and almost everyone agrees that overall the results of the war on cancer have been meagre. Something is terribly wrong, and this book attempts to tell why.

In a sense, I started researching this book soon after I was hired at Memorial Sloan-Kettering Cancer Center as science writer (later assistant director of public affairs) in 1974. I began writing in earnest after I was fired in 1977 for opposing their coverup of positive data on the drug laetrile, an incident described in chapter 9 of this book. I had, in the words of the *New York Times*, acted in a manner that conflicted with my "most basic job responsibilities" (November 24, 1977). In other words, I refused to collaborate in falsifying data.

The book (initially called *The Cancer Syndrome*) was published in 1980 and went through six printings and various editions, was featured on '60 Minutes,' and serialized in newspapers and magazines, here and abroad. Then, between 1987 and 1990 I updated and expanded it into the present volume. There have been many requests for a new edition. In studying the text, I find that it would be difficult to simply update it, without taking into account fundamental changes in today's situation. And that would be a new book. Rather than trying to unweave the web, I have made only minor textual changes, but have decided to provide the reader with this extended preface (and several notes at the ends of chapters) to explain how things have fundamentally changed.

First, however, you should understand the following facts:

• Despite a few bright spots, the statistics on cancer incidence and mortality continue to be gloomy. The number of Americans developing cancer rises each year and now approaches 1.4 million; this does not even count the 800,000 cases per year of superficial skin cancer. An estimated 554,740 Americans will die of cancer in 1996. Even the ACS acknowledges that "there has been a steady rise in the cancer mortality rate in the US in the last half century" (*1996 Facts and Figures*). In 1930, the age-adjusted death rate was 143 per 100,000 of the general population; by 1992 it had climbed to 172. In fact, 40 percent of all Americans will develop life-threatening cancer.

• Progress in the war on cancer has been agonizingly slow. Much of the progress we hear about was actually achieved before 1971. Out of the hundreds of thousands of compounds screened, only a handful have been found to be really effective in extending life. More often than not, they simply shrink the tumors. But in most cases, such shrinkages have not been proven to correlate with increased survival of patients (see my 1995 book *Questioning Chemotherapy*).

• *The FDA has still not approved any non-toxic agents as treatments for cancer. NCI has still not conducted a single fair and competent study of any alternative cancer therapy.* In fact, it recently cancelled a small clinical trial of Burzynski's antineoplastons. A completed trial of hydrazine sulfate was marred by serious irregularities.

• The persecution of alternative doctors continues. On May 6, 1992, Jonathan Wright, M.D. was raided by FDA agents accompanied by armed King County, Washington sheriffs. Glenn Warner, M.D., an oncologist who uses a mixture of both conventional and alternative treatments had his medical license taken away. And Stanislaw R. Burzynski, M.D., Ph.D.—whose story is told in chapter 14 of this book— has been indicted on 75 counts of fraud for providing his medicines, antineoplastons, to cancer patients. He faces up to 300 years in prison for following the dictates of his conscience and his medical oath.

Given all this, you might conclude that things are even worse than is indicated in this book. Yet that is not the case. In fact, on the whole, the situation for alternative medicine is more promising than it has been for many years. How can that be? Because when we look at things in perspective, the forces of repression are losing ground, while interest in alternative medicine is growing. Since around 1992, there has been a shift in the public's perception of this area.

The key is that the federal government has changed its stance.

Because of this, media interest has been unleashed and die-hard opponents are increasingly isolated as out of step with current realities. Amazingly, even the ACS has (for the moment, at least) stopped distributing its notorious "unproven methods" sheets and is rethinking its whole negative approach. The NCI remains highly derogatory, but that too could change in the next few years.

How did this happen? And what does it portend for the future? That is what I want to write about in this new preface.

The OTA Report

The most momentous week in the modern history of cancer alternatives began on July 15, 1985. As will be described in this book, it was during a few fateful days that two of the leading alternative cancer clinics in North America—that of Dr. Burzynski of Houston, Texas and of Lawrence Burton, Ph.D. of Freeport, Bahamas—were raided by government agents. Burzynski's papers and records were seized by the FDA, never to be returned. Burton suffered an even more frightening ordeal: his Immunoaugmentative Therapy (IAT) clinic was physically padlocked by Bahamian authorities, acting at the behest of US health authorities. (For more on Burton and IAT, see chapter 12.) Burzynski and his patients fought it out in the courts, which provided some legal relief. But Burton's patients took their struggle directly to Congress, which turned out to be an even more effective strategy.

The Congress they encountered in 1985 was hardly friendly towards alternative cancer treatments. But Congressmen get cancer, too, and were fascinated to hear their constituents' stories of the unusual treatment in Freeport. Also, Congress's confidence in the "war on cancer" was waning. As the years rolled by, the elusive cure never materialized. By 1985, Congress was in the mood for change.

Burzynski never stopped treating patients. But the IAT clinic remained shut for months, disrupting a treatment that many believed was saving their lives. In face-to-face encounters, constituents made a compelling case to Congressmen to help reopen the clinic.

Rep. Guy Molinari (R-NY) was one of these representatives. A reporter at the *Staten Island Advance* wrote an illuminating series on the closure. (Her husband was a Burton patient.) Intrigued, Molinari flew down to Freeport. In January, 1986 he held tumultuous public hearings in lower Manhattan. Shortly thereafter, the Burton clinic reopened.

But matters didn't end there. On June 27, 1986, Molinari and 23 other Members of Congress formally requested that the Congressional Office of Technology Assessment (OTA) carry out a study of Dr.

Burton's treatment. Similar requests were received from Senator James Abdnor (R-SD) and Congressman Matthew J. Rinaldo (R-NJ). An additional 14 members of the House and Senate subsequently endorsed Molinari's original letter, bringing the total number to 40. Most of these were also inspired by constituents taking the treatment.

In his letter to Dr. John H. Gibbons, director of the OTA, Molinari and his colleagues requested a "comprehensive evaluation" of the Bahama-based treatment. "While there has been much controversy revolving around the efficacy of IAT, the truth of the matter is no one at this time can say with assuredness whether IAT works or not," they said. "The result of OTA's investigation may open a new door and possible avenue of hope for thousands of terminally-ill cancer patients."

Later that summer, Rep. John D. Dingell (D-MI), then the powerful chairman of the House Committee on Energy and Commerce, also wrote to Gibbons, requesting a report on alternative cancer treatments in general. "Some [alternative treatments] are offered by respected members of the medical community," he wrote, "and others by what many would term charlatans. Many of these treatments may be without benefit, some may actually be harmful, and some, probably a small number, may have value. However, there is a general lack of objective information..." (letter of August 12, 1986). Dingell asked that his own request be merged with Molinari's and that OTA use the Burton–IAT treatment as a "case study of the general issues involved."

In September, this project was approved by OTA's oversight body, the Technology Assessment Board (TAB), of which Dingell himself was a member. OTA promised the case study on IAT by late 1987 and a final report on alternative treatments by the summer of 1988.

The OTA (which was dismantled by Congress in 1995) had an excellent reputation for objectivity. It had been established in 1972 to provide political leaders with clear, objective, and unbiased information on technical issues. Over the years, it had conducted many controversial studies, but this was to be their most controversial ever. Most members of the alternative cancer community were guardedly optimistic about the choice of OTA to conduct such a study. They foresaw a possibility that OTA would expose a cancer coverup, the way that a respected Justice Department attorney, Benedict Fitzgerald, had done for a similar Congressional investigation in 1953.

The OTA had also carried out a number of other studies that augured well, including one on the question of controlled clinical trials that ended with a call for a "greater emphasis on cancer prevention"

(OTA-BP-H-22, August 1983). The author of those words was Hellen Gelband, who was now appointed Project Director of OTA's study on unconventional cancer treatments.

OTA began by appointing an 18-member Advisory Panel for the project. Rosemary Stevens, Ph.D., a historian of science at the University of Pennsylvania who had worked with Gelband on the previous study, was appointed its chair. It was a non-controversial choice. But the panel itself was an odd amalgam, hopeless entangled in ancient antagonisms. On the one hand, there were strong defenders of alternative methods such as Gar Hildenbrand, then vice president of the Gerson Institute, and John Fink, author of *Third Opinion,* and a leader of the International Association of Cancer Victors and Friends.

They were cheek by jowl with long-time opponents of such methods such as Robert C. Eyerly, M.D., a leader of the ACS's Unproven Methods Committee. Also present was Grace Powers Monaco, then the president of Emprise, Inc., a company which had earned the enmity of many in the alternative field for attempting to create a totally one-sided database on unconventional cancer treatments. Barrie Cassileth, Ph.D., a psychologist from the University of Pennsylvania, was another panelist. She had carried out, but then failed to publish, a study on Burton's patients which advocates said proved that they lived longer than the norm. Dr. Herbert Oettgen of Sloan-Kettering Institute, who had a marginal interest in alternative medicine, was also included.

At the same time, the OTA staff systematically excluded those who could have truly balanced the vehemently anti-alternative forces on the panel: articulate critics of the cancer establishment, such as research analyst Robert G. Houston or journalist Peter Barry Chowka. It also went out of its way to downgrade the importance of this advisory council. The board was there simply as "a giver of general advice, a source of contacts...and a quality control mechanism," but could not "sign off on reports, provide minority opinions, or come to a consensus" ("Facts Concerning OTA's Study of Unorthodox Cancer Treatments," September 9, 1987). In any case, consensus under the circumstances would have been impossible, and it seemed like a gratuitous putdown.

Almost immediately, problems also arose between the OTA staff members who were writing the report (principally Ms. Gelband and her assistants) and the alternative medical community. The alternative people saw themselves as a beleaguered minority, who needed to use public pressure of various kinds even to get a fair hearing. The OTA staff saw themselves as dedicated public servants, trying to conduct a difficult study under pressure from both sides, but particularly from advocates of methods that, on the face of it, were dubious and strange.

So for the first year there was a notable lack of progress towards either designing the IAT study or writing the broader report. At the first meeting of the Advisory Panel in July, 1987 (almost a year after beginning) the OTA staff was still outlining its plans for the study.

"The meeting was notable for bringing the unconventional treatment supporters together with the mainstream in a neutral forum," the staff later reported. "Discussion was generally non-confrontational and informative." But "no clear direction for the report as a whole emerged." This was to remain true for several years.

In that same year (1987), Dr. Burton submitted to OTA a case study of 11 patients who had been treated at his clinic for a deadly form of cancer called mesothelioma. This small study claimed that patients treated with IAT lived three to four times the national average of conventionally-treated patients. Some were in fact long-term survivors.

This was important news, for mesothelioma is almost uniformly and rapidly fatal. But OTA never even commented on these findings. And two years later, its sister agency, the NCI, was still demanding that Burton present them with a "best case" series, as if they had never heard of his mesothelioma paper. These were the sorts of experiences that intensified Burton's already well-established paranoia. But in this case he wasn't alone in his misgivings. Burton's supporters forcefully reminded the OTA staff that it was their Congressionally mandated task to compile exactly such retrospective analyses.

But by this time, Burton's mood and health were slipping, fed by his disappointments. By December, 1987, many people feared that another coverup was in the making. At that juncture, a handful of activists, led by Clinton Miller, long-time lobbyist for the National Health Federation, took actions that almost scuttled the whole report process. They released information to influential reporter Jack Anderson that Dr. Roger C. Herdman, head of OTA's health and life sciences division, had previously been employed as Sloan-Kettering's vice president.

"Sloan-Kettering is the enemy of non-traditional cancer therapies," they were quoted as saying. "It is unthinkable that OTA would place a necessarily biased former vice president of Sloan-Kettering in charge of this study and expect anyone to give it credibility" (*Washington Post*, 12/13/87).

The group also charged that Dr. Herdman owned $75,000 worth

of stock in Oncogene Science, Inc., which had interests in the cancer diagnostics marketplace. They also reported that his boss, Dr. Gibbons, owned stock in Genentech Clinical Partners (*Washington Times,* December 22, 1987). (They might have added that Lewis Thomas, M.D., the president of Memorial Sloan-Kettering, was on the advisory panel of the OTA.)

Both scientists denied that this represented a conflict. In fact, there was no evidence that they had committed any crime or that their previous associations or investments had anything more than a marginal connection to the present study. The alternative community's dealings with Dr. Herdman and Dr. Gibbons had always been satisfactory. (Dr. Gibbons became Pres. Clinton's science policy advisor.) Busy as he was, Dr. Herdman was quite accessible and always gave a fair hearing to complaints. Because of this, I joined a group of activists who hurriedly sent a telegram of apology to Dr. Herdman for this and other insults directed at him personally. The report survived the storm.

The most serious problems stemmed from relations with the lower-level staff members, who were actually writing the report. There was simply no reservoir of trust between them and the subjects of their inquiry. The staff writers routinely downplayed or even suppressed information that was at all favorable towards alternative treatments. The most egregious example involved Patricia Spain Ward, Ph.D., campus historian of the University of Illinois Medical Center, Chicago, who had been hired as a contractor by the OTA. Dr. Ward was perceived as a skeptic about alternative medicine because she had written a negative paper on Andrew Ivy, M.D., proponent of the unconventional drug Krebiozen, who had once been president of her medical school.

But Dr. Ward took the assignment because she was concerned about the lack of adequate evaluation of such treatments. She thought that OTA "with its sterling reputation for courage and fairness, would again capture the gratitude of the nation by producing a truly disinterested, unbiased treatment in the troubled realm of unconventional cancer treatment." By 1987, she reflected, "hostility and distrust so thoroughly pervaded both sides of this chasm...that only an agency of OTA's standing could hope to bridge it" (*Speech to OTA Advisory Board,* March 9, 1990).

In good faith, Dr. Ward prepared reports for the office on three controversial treatments—the Gerson diet, the Hoxsey herbal treatment, and the more conventional immune stimulant, BCG. She herself was surprised to find that there was considerable scientific support for the potential benefit of all three of these treatments. But the OTA staff apparently had a different sort of conclusion in mind, and refused to circulate these reports to its own Advisory Council members. In a letter to Ward, they claimed these were too positive in tone. Under protest from board members, the reports were finally released.

Yet internal reports that were downright hostile to alternatives were circulated to panel members unimpeded. The attempted suppression of Ward's reports was a defining moment. Not surprisingly, hostility towards the staff, and between various board members, broke out into the open at the advisory panel meeting of September 28, 1988.

The staff had circulated a partial draft of the final report to the advisors but "had asked the panel not to circulate this draft to others." As it turned out, they later complained, "it was widely copied and circulated, and a large number of observers at the panel meeting had copies."

One of these was Robert G. Houston, a long-time critic of the cancer establishment, and this gave him the chance to write a stinging rebuttal, *Objections to a Cover-up: The OTA Report on Alternative Therapies.* This he distributed at the meeting, much to the consternation of OTA staff members. (The public was allowed to attend, but not address, that meeting.) In fact, throughout this entire OTA struggle, Houston played an important role as both research analyst and strategist for the alternative side. He produced two other short but brilliant works: *Misinformation from OTA on Unconventional Cancer Treatments* and *Repression and Reform in the Evaluation of Alternative Cancer Therapies,* which was published by a patients' rights organization, Project Cure, Inc.

The OTA staff later complained that "the tense atmosphere and combative nature of many of the observers and panel members strained the discussion" at this 1988 meeting. "There was a great deal of criticism of the draft, largely from the panel members on the unconventional side." But from the perspective of some panel members such as Hildenbrand and Fink, this first draft could have been written by any group of not particularly well-informed quackbusters, not objective government investigators.

After these events, Michael Evers, J.D., president of Project Cure, who was himself an OTA contractor on the legal dimensions of the problem, invited 16 leaders of the alternative cancer movement to a private conference dubbed the *Coolfont Conclave: The Turning Point.* This was held at a Berkeley Springs, WV conference center from August 26 to

29, 1988.

Evers called this emergency meeting in response to growing alarm that OTA's report was turning into an unprecedented disaster for the alternative cancer movement. The meeting discussed the first draft in detail, with a chapter-by-chapter analysis. It identified what it perceived as its major flaws and then elicited proposals for improving it. (Several pro-alternative OTA panel members and consultants were in attendance.) It also analyzed the various policy options that had been presented by OTA at the July 28 meeting and discussed a "comprehensive plan of action for a grass roots campaign and lobbying of Congress."

The mood at the meeting was upbeat and militant and a decision was made to vigorously fight against any attempt by OTA to suppress alternative treatments, IAT in particular. It was at this meeting that I decided to launch a newsletter to cover developments in the field of cancer politics, especially OTA. And, in fact, the first issue of *The Cancer Chronicles* came out less than a year later.

After the Coolfont meeting, publicity on the developing fiasco intensified. Gar Hildenbrand, John Fink, Frank Wiewel, and I made numerous television and talk radio appearances on the topic; there were mail-in campaigns directed at OTA itself, at Members of Congress, and especially at its parent body, the Technology Assessment Board. Throughout the following year, in fact, Congress continued to feel pressure on this issue, and to pass that pressure along to OTA. The final report revealed that more than half of all Congressmen telephoned or wrote to OTA expressing concern about the study.

One glaring omission from the draft report was any progress in actually testing IAT. In July, 1989, representatives of Dr. Burton met with the OTA in Washington; on August 29, 1989 there was a follow-up meeting in Freeport, Bahamas between Dr. Burton himself, his representatives, and OTA's "IAT Working Group" (who were mainly mainstream academic scientists). Burton was in a conciliatory mood and agreed to test IAT in patients with Dukes' C and Dukes' D colon cancer. This would have been a difficult patient population, at best.

The Burton side proposed a three-stage evaluation process: a review of his center's clinical records; a "pre-trial" of patients who were already coming to the clinic; followed by a full-scale randomized controlled trial in the U.S., to be performed in accordance with all of FDA's stringent requirements for new drug approval.

The most innovative part of the proposal was the so-called "pretrial." Its purpose was, according to one of Burton's representatives, "to provide the necessary evidence to cut through the massive governmental red tape now required for New Drug Approval." NCI would not need to recruit the patients for this trial, but could simply perform before and after evaluations of patients, such as CAT scans in order to verify their diagnoses. OTA could then simply observe and record what happened to patients who took the treatment. Did they live longer? Did they feel better? Did their tumors shrink? This is what is known as a field study or outcomes research, and is one way of assessing the value of a treatment.

Then on October 20, Dr. Herdman sent Dr. Burton a ten-page "General Description of a Clinical Trial of IAT Agreed Upon by Dr. Burton and OTA." This draft caused consternation in Freeport, and confirmed Burton's worst fears. Among other things, it contained no mention of the "pre-trial," which had been Burton's own contribution.

"I have not agreed to much of what you have chosen to include in your report," Burton replied angrily on November 17, 1989. "Your report reflects little more than an outline to obtain negative results." Congress had asked OTA to develop a statistical analysis of IAT's efficacy, utilizing existing data and to develop a clinical protocol of the treatment. Yet, after three-and-a-half years, OTA had failed on both counts and now sent him this deficient outline.

In its proposal, OTA wrote that "no single clinical trial can produce an answer to the question 'Is IAT a safe and effective treatment for any type of cancer?' " This was technically true, if only because FDA routinely requires at least *two* well-controlled trials. It seemed like a disingenuous objection.

"NCI trials produce answers about other substances," I pointed out in *The Cancer Chronicles* at the time. "IAT is a biological treatment, susceptible to clinical trials. Given enough patients, the answer could be forthcoming. Yet OTA precludes in advance the effectiveness of any clinical trial, thus turning its back on the scientific method."

OTA next said, "Clearly, what we would like to know is whether IAT produces any clinical benefit to one of the main types of cancer patient for whom it is commonly prescribed, and, in particular, whether it may improve the chances of survival."

Fair enough: improved survival is certainly one of the most important parameters and everyone wants to find a cure for a statistically important cancer. (In *Questioning Chemotherapy,* I argue that life extension has not been proven for the vast majority of instances in which chemotherapy is employed.) But OTA then added that it "approached the task of an IAT clinical trial design with the aim of maximizing the likelihood of getting a clear answer to a narrower question, but one that is of obvious importance: does IAT shrink tumors?"

That was sheer legerdemain: by 1988 it was abundantly clear that IAT did not conspicuously shrink many tumors, but, if anything, stabilized patients' immune systems and increased their quality survival time. As Burton himself told '60 Minutes,' IAT *controlled,* but didn't cure, cancer. "I don't think there is a cure," he told reporter Harry Reasoner. "There's no such thing. We'd rather talk about a control. The patients control their own cancer…(in) a symbiotic relationship. The body is living with the cancer."

The destructive onslaught against cancerous (as well as normal) cells is chemotherapy's game. For decades, in fact, new chemotherapeutic agents had been screened for merit by seeing whether or not they shrank tumors. By suddenly insisting that IAT *shrink tumors* in any prospective trial, OTA was dooming the test to almost certain failure. (And this from the people who "wrote the book" on the problems of clinical trials in cancer!) The OTA staff also seemed to be preparing a fallback position for themselves, just in case the treatment actually showed some benefit in a clinical trial. For then, if the patients lived longer, or reported higher performance scores, OTA could always say, "But their tumors didn't disappear. So the treatment was a failure.")

OTA added that "smaller and still worthwhile effects on survival would probably require the study of a much larger number of patients." But in that case, how was it ever going to be possible to evaluate the claims of a treatment that helped patients live longer?

Also, Congress had set no limit on the size or cost of the IAT trial. (And in fact OTA spent $500,000 to prepare its written report.)

Here, too, it seemed that OTA was preparing a fallback position: "Sure, the treatment *seemed* to work, but only for a negligible group. Our conclusion is…that more tests are needed."

OTA's third claim was that "in the proposed clinical trial, it is important that patients with a relatively common cancer, and one for which treatment options are limited, be the focus of attention." This was so that "an important public health problem will be addressed."

Again, one could hardly argue with this. But because of the extension of chemotherapy's use to just about every type of cancer (Dukes' C colon cancer was just then joining the ranks), it was considered "unethical" to give unconventional treatments to most patients.

Also, the great success stories of chemotherapy were always in relatively obscure types of cancer. Childhood leukemia constitutes less than two percent of all cancers and many of chemotherapy's other successes were in diseases so rare that many clinicians had never even seen a single case (Burkitt's lymphoma, choriocarcinoma, etc.)

Why should IAT be held to more demanding standards than chemotherapy? Was there to be a level playing field, or not?

It did not escape Dr. Burton's attention that this particular precondition precluded a study of mesothelioma, his most obvious success.

But by now it was widely believed that OTA had no intention of actually doing a trial of IAT. OTA had, the staff wrote, "completed its formal part in the process...." The "trial's realization" depended on Burton and "members of the U.S. cancer research community," principally NCI, many of whose members were hostile to Burton for his vociferous attacks on the cancer establishment. But, Dr. Herdman warned, NCI "will have its own procedures and criteria for deciding on the priority to be given funding of this study."

In other words, OTA handed the Burton problem over to the tender mercies of NCI. Not surprisingly, no such clinical trial ever took place and the world still awaits hard data on the efficacy of this treatment. NCI simply had other priorities.

By 1990, the report inched towards closure. In late February, interested members of the public received copies of the 560-page final draft. (After nearly four years of work, the OTA gave critics, such as myself, little more than a week to prepare their remarks.)

"In its present form," I wrote in an emergency issue of *The Cancer Chronicles,* this report "will wreak tremendous damage on the movement, with the public, the media and especially on Capitol Hill."

The report digressed into all sorts of arcane directions, but found no room for Sloan-Kettering's studies on laetrile between 1972 and 1975 (see chapter 9). Similarly, it devoted two whole pages to the comments of a pair of doctors hostile to Burzynski, but then merely reported as a fact that "Burzynski wrote a rebuttal of their report, contesting their reading of the clinical data." None of his rebuttal points were even hinted at. (See chapter 14 for a detailed discussion.)

The final report was due out on May 30, 1990. But the OTA Advisory Panel, to its credit, convinced the staff to open the morning session of its third and final meeting to public comment. Fifteen people, most of them critics, were given five minutes each to speak.

"The cancer alternative movement is facing one of the greatest challenges in its history," I wrote in the *Chronicles*. The purpose of the report is "to bury this growing movement under a mountain of falsehoods. It is unworthy of the agency from which it comes or of the Congress, which commissioned it. If released in anything like this form, the report would set back the cause of non-toxic therapies and freedom of choice for years." That was because "every time you complain to your Congressmen about suppression and coverup, s/he may throw the OTA's 'proof' in your face."

Alarmed, I called for an "effective and militant campaign against this report," including an intensive day of lobbying on Capitol Hill on March 8, 1990. I ended with this emotional appeal to cancer patients:

"To you we say: if you are aroused and well-organized you can do anything. You can stop vicious reports; you can foil the medical-industrial complex; you can change the face of American medicine. Don't doubt your strength....Don't be discouraged by this report but unleash your tremendous anger and direct it at all those who would deny you your freedom of choice...."

Gar Hildenbrand, who was both an Advisory Panel member and an outspoken activist, called on supporters of the Gerson diet and cancer patients in general to practice civil disobedience outside the meeting. "On March 9th," he wrote, "hundreds of people with cancer, people recovering from cancer, and worried well people will walk into the streets. In the early morning, at the Office of Technology Assessment, cancer patients will lie down in front of the doors to tell Congress: 'You allow this system to go unchallenged OVER MY DEAD BODY.'"

As planned, on the day before the meeting, March 8, scores of people gathered for a day of lobbying. I was among them. In general, Congressmen and their aides were sympathetic to their complaints. But there were ominous signs, as well. A bomb threat was phoned in to the hotel where most of the report critics had gathered. The caller ranted about quacks and con men. Michael Evers, who was coordinating the lobbying efforts, asked the FBI to investigate, but they never caught the perpetrator. Happily, no bomb went off and the FBI concluded that the caller was a crank.

On the following morning we arrived at OTA headquarters to find a squad of tactical police with night sticks, Plexiglas shields, and several waiting paddy wagons. This seemed provocative, since it was understood that any protest would be entirely non-violent. The staff later complained about the "hostile atmosphere" at this final meeting with "shouted personal attacks on the integrity of the project staff." It omitted all mention of the police presence outside.

With the exception of a representative from NCI, each of the 15 speeches that day was highly critical of OTA. Each was bracketed and occasionally interrupted by resounding applause from the assembled cancer patients, who had come in response to a call to attend from various alternative organizations, including *The Cancer Chronicles.*

Seymour M. Brenner, M.D., a radiologist from Brooklyn, New York, spoke first. He told how he saw between 100 and 150 patients per day. "After 39 years, he said, "I have seen no significant progress" in the treatment of cancer. In 1988, he had offered, he said, "to do a research program into the investigation of alternative methods," using standard safeguards. But the FDA commissioner told him he would first have to do five year's worth of laboratory and animal work.

"I see millions of people dying in five years," he told the commissioner. "I see hundreds of billions of dollars being spent in five years." Brenner wanted his medical colleagues to be told, "If you have a patient who is considered hopeless, with an established diagnosis of cancer, refer them to [an impartial] panel." This panel would then decide if the patient was indeed advanced enough to be given last-ditch alternative treatments.

It is noteworthy that Brenner does not practice any unconventional treatments himself. In fact, his peers regard him as one of the top four radiologists in Brooklyn, according to the independent *Castle Connolly* guide to the best doctors in New York City. But he was honest enough to admit that he knew of at least ten cancer survivors who had been treated with alternative methods (principally that of Dr. Emannuel Revici) and who "would have died under my supervision."

"I am tired of watching people come to my office and plead for their lives and I have nothing to offer them," an impassioned Brenner told the OTA. "I'm frustrated and I'm angry and I'm depressed when I see a 27-year-old woman who says, 'Don't let me die,' and I have to let her die." The OTA panel seemed stunned by his words.

The next speaker was journalist Peter Barry Chowka. "The only victory now in sight," Chowka said, "is one of public relations over the reality that has become a medical Vietnam." People by the millions were discontented with conventional medicine and turning towards alternatives, he reminded them. "The OTA report does not adequately address the urgency of this context." He compared it unfavorably to the 1953 report from attorney Benedict Fitzgerald. By contrast, Fitzgerald had concluded that there was indeed a coverup of promising alternative cancer treatments.

Attorney Michael Evers told the panel that the draft report was "a travesty. Its authors have violated every known rule of fairness and impartiality." He also showed how subtly OTA could twist the facts.

Richard Jaffe, Dr. Burzynski's attorney, pointed out the various biases against his client in the report. For instance, OTA had relied on an old NCI report on the failure of antineoplastons to cure a certain type of mouse leukemia. But OTA failed to note that Burzynski himself had warned NCI that his treatment does *not* work against leukemia.

Virginia Livingston-Wheeler, M.D, the only major alternative practitioner to speak that day, called the report "quite extensive, but not always accurate. Seldom accurate...My work was not covered...." (Dr. Livingston herself died of a heart attack on a trip to Europe that summer. She was 84 years old. On Livingston, see chapter 13.)

In my own remarks to the panel, I said, "This report...was supposed to investigate a coverup. Instead, it has become part of that coverup. In its present form it will set back the study of non-toxic cancer treatments for years to come."

I recounted my own experiences at Sloan-Kettering with Dr. Kanematsu Sugiura and his work on laetrile (see chapter 9). "Now, where are the Sugiura studies in your report? Where are they?" I demanded, angrily. "The OTA report was supposed to contain all the information that could be found, rather than a selective culling. But it's gone! It's as covered up today as it was in 1975.

"I'm not afraid of you," I concluded, "and I'm not afraid of what you're doing. You'll continue with this? Fine. We'll continue to fight you. If you're smart, you'll save the reputation of OTA and radically revise this report."

This meeting strengthened the hand of those on the OTA advisory board who wanted a more balanced presentation. In September, 1990—four years after its start—OTA finally released *Unconventional Cancer Treatments* (GPO #052-003-01203-3). And, indeed, to almost everyone's surprise, the final report did contain some major revisions, all of them giving it greater balance. As I wrote in the *Chronicles*, "although the report still contains many examples of bias, double standard, error and innuendo, it is an improvement over earlier versions. About half the misrepresentations are now corrected." My conclusion was that "the final OTA report is something we can live with."

The staff had finally discovered about 200 scientific papers supporting the use of alternative cancer treatments. The Summary, Options, and Recommendations had been completely rewritten by the panel chair. In essence, the final report underlined the potential importance of these treatments and called for their fair and adequate testing.

In his foreword, Dr. Gibbons added that "while mainstream medicine can improve the prospects for long-term survival for about half of the approximately one million Americans diagnosed with cancer each year, the rest will die of their disease within a few years."

For thousands, he said, "mainstream medicine's role in cancer treatment is not sufficient." Gibbons remarked that "the debate concerning unconventional treatments is passionate, often bitter and vituperative, and highly polarized." Echoing Rep. Dingell's original letter to him, he wrote that "if history in this area is predictive, some few unconventional treatments may be adopted into mainstream practice in the years ahead, others will fade from the scene, and new ones will arise." That someone in authority thought that conventional treatments were deficient and that at least a few alternative treatments might eventually be "adopted into mainstream practice" was new.

Specifically, OTA made a series of recommendations to NCI. The main ones were: obtain good information about unconventional cancer treatments; use up-to-date screening methods; facilitate "best case" reviews of unconventionally treated patients; establish a reporting system for remissions with such treatments; and provide funding "large enough to provide for a fair test" of innovative methods.

Out of all these, however, NCI only accepted the idea of "best case review," and drew up some guidelines to help those intending to prepare such summaries. But it rejected out of hand all other OTA recommendations. For example, OTA recommended that information on alternative treatments disseminated by NCI be evaluated for adequacy and quality. NCI replied that it already had a program of telephone monitoring in place. Regarding OTA's proposal for a registry of remarkable remissions, NCI responded that "maintaining a population-based registry would be difficult, if not impossible." But OTA never suggested a "population-based registry," just a simple database of those who seemed to be helped by such methods.

OTA also reminded NCI officials that it was their "mandated responsibility to pursue information and facilitate examination of widely used 'unconventional cancer treatments' for therapeutic potential."

NCI's arrogant response was that it "has funded a grant to develop a comprehensive database on 'unconventional' cancer treatments." This was an apparent reference to the Emprise, Inc. grant, which had been given to a group of self-proclaimed enemies of "health fraud," headed by Grace Monaco, a lawyer who had helped Aetna develop its RICO racketeering suit against Dr. Burzynski. (Emprise, Inc. went out of business soon after NCI, under public pressure, decided not to extend its grants.)

NCI likewise rejected OTA's proposal for a balanced panel to fund evaluations of alternative therapies. NCI said that "the preferred solution is to encourage the proponents of 'unconventional treatments' to interact directly with {NCI's] staff." For those who had tried that route in the past, this was a bitter joke indeed.

One should understand that by 1990 NCI was being attacked on many sides for its bureaucratic policies and its refusal to consider new directions in the war on cancer. As the 20th anniversary of the war on cancer loomed (December 23, 1991), there was a drumbeat of criticism. At the behest of the late Congressman Ted Weiss (D-NY), the General Accounting Office (GAO) had conducted a study, which concluded that "there has been no progress" in preventing breast cancer. *Science* magazine, usually a strong supporter of mainstream research, also concluded that the war on cancer was a "saga of substantial investments...but little success."

University of Illinois medical school professor Samuel S. Epstein, M.D. and I co-authored a series of guest editorials in the *Chicago Tribune, Los Angeles Times* and *USA Today*, pointing out, for example, that "Last year, the congressional Office of Technology Assessment reported on some 200 papers supporting such innovative therapies and recommended that the cancer institute actively investigate them. It refused" (*Chicago Tribune*, December 12, 1991).

But NCI had circled the wagons. Science analyst Robert G. Houston's prescient comment at the time was that "Congress may have to force the NCI legislatively to expend a portion of its budget on novel therapies reported to work."

In fact, what was about to happen was even more amazing than any of us could have fantasized. An old Chinese adage suggests that when a rock blocks the path, the most prudent course is to walk around it. In the following year, a path was found around the NCI boulder.

The Office of Alternative Medicine

One of the original signers of Rep. Guy Molinari's letter to the OTA had been Iowa Democrat Berkley Bedell. Bedell was a character straight out of Horatio Alger: as a teenager, he had saved fifty dollars from his paper route money to start a small fishing tackle company.

Berkley & Co. became one of the largest such manufacturing companies in the world. He did this without ever taking a partner or a loan.

Not surprisingly, Bedell was chosen as the nation's first Small Business Person of the Year and in 1974 was elected to Congress. As a measure of his popularity he ran as a liberal Democrat in a solidly Republican part of Iowa and was overwhelmingly elected six times. In fact, he would probably be there today, if he hadn't gone fishing at the Quantico, Virginia Marine Corps Base one day and contracted a severe case of tick-borne Lyme disease.

In 1987, Bedell was forced to retire from Congress because of ill health. After three series of intravenous antibiotics at the Walter Reed Army Hospital his disease had still not been brought under control. By 1990, in fact, he had severe, Lyme-related arthritis in his knees and other joints.

In desperation, he turned to alternative medicine. He heard about a farm-based treatment that consisted of administering a specially prepared kind of milk product. It was whey made from the colostrum (first milk) of a cow whose udders had first been injected with a sample of Bedell's own blood. The treatment had been thought up by a Minnesota farmer named Herbert Saunders. But, odd as it seemed, it had some scientific plausibility. It was related to a promising medical treatment called *transfer factor,* which had been discovered by Dr. Henry S. Lawrence at New York University in the 1950s but had then languished in obscurity (*J Clin Invest* 1954;33:951).

"After I drank a teaspoon of this whey every one-and-a-half hours for a few weeks," Bedell later told his former Congressional colleagues, "my symptoms of Lyme disappeared and I no longer suffer from that disease." There was some publicity on his case and not surprisingly Bedell found himself besieged by calls from others suffering from this often intractable disease. (Herb Saunders in under indictment for practicing medicine without a license and his treatment is no longer available.)

"Unfortunately," Berkley added, whimsically, "little Miss Muffett is not available to testify that the curds and whey which she was eating are safe" (*Hearings Before Appropriations Subcommittee,* June 24, 1993). Following this Lyme disease episode, Bedell was further diagnosed with an unrelated prostate cancer. After receiving thoroughly conventional treatment, he had signs that the disease was returning. He therefore treated himself with a non-toxic agent known as 714X, invented by a Franco-Canadian microscopist named Gaston Naessens. Bedell ascribed his own recovery of good health to this particular treatment.

Bedell's remarkable progress toward good health made a deep impression on many of his colleagues, especially Sen. Tom Harkin, a fellow Iowa Democrat, who served 12 years with him on Capitol Hill.

In the year or so following the OTA Report, it became painfully obvious to observant members of Congress that NCI had no intention of carrying out the various recommendations of the report. The cancer institute seemed mired in its own prejudices against anything that smacked of the unconventional.

Because of the terms of the National Cancer Act, passed by Congress in 1971 to find a way around the massive bureaucracy of NIH, NCI was semi-autonomous and politically privileged. The director of the NCI didn't report to the director of the NIH, as had formerly been the case, but to a cancer advisory board and a three-person President's Cancer Panel, which reported directly to the chief executive. NCI had long since created its own vast bureaucracy, more stultifying in fact than the one at NIH.

As fate would have it, Sen. Harkin happened to be chairman of the Appropriations Subcommittee that oversaw the $10 billion-a-year NIH budget. Understandably, he also had a few friends at NIH who wanted to please him. And what would please him most would be to get to the bottom of some of the amazing stories Berkley was now telling him.

Bedell and Harkin drafted a piece of legislation, which Bedell then intensively lobbied for among his former colleagues. Broadly speaking, the idea was to rectify the problems that had been revealed by the OTA Report.

And so on November 22, 1991, a fateful day, Congress passed Sen. Harkin's bill, mandating the formation of an "Office for the Study of Unconventional Medical Practices" within NIH. The office simply bypassed the NCI roadblock, for the time being, at least. Some NIH officials were not exactly thrilled when they woke up the next morning to discover an office of "quackery" plunked down in their midst. For some, it was as if the Roman Curia had capriciously sanctioned in the basement of the Vatican an office for the propagation of atheism!

The office was given a small budget of $2.2 million that first year— less than a thousandth of the overall NIH appropriation. "Though just a drop in the bucket by federal budget standards," wrote the *Congressional Quarterly*, "the office is a symbol of the new visibility being won by medical treatments that haven't gained mainstream approval" (1/31/92).

The acting director of the office was Stephen Groft, D. Pharm. He appointed an ad hoc advisory board and called its first public meeting for June 17-18, 1992. Unlike OTA, the NIH warmly welcomed all those interested in alternative medicine to come and present their views. Jay Moskowitz, Ph.D., deputy director of the NIH, opened the meeting. His friendliness towards the initiative was palpable.

As at OTA two years earlier, I spoke at this meeting.

"We come here with an open mind—yet history teaches us to be wary," I began. I admitted that "one would have to be made of stone not to recognize the importance of this development. Yet we have to pinch ourselves—to stop and ask 'What exactly is going on here?' After all, NIH has never been a friend of non-toxic and nutritional treatments." I proceeded to recount many of the misdeeds of NCI over the years. What I underestimated was the extent to which these were the misdeeds of NCI, which often acted quite independently of the parent body. One simply could not equate the two agencies.

I concluded, "If NIH is now serious about launching a new era of cooperation, then we will enthusiastically work with them towards our common goal, the conquest of cancer."

Margaret Mason, "Body and Soul" columnist for the *Washington Post* was present, as were many others from the mainstream media. "Something wonderful happened—and a quiet grass-roots revolution in health care was official recognized—last week on the sixth floor of government Building C in Bethesda" (June 26, 1992).

After the success of this first meeting, NIH convened an even larger gathering at the Westfields International Conference Center in Chantilly, VA. NIH actually paid the way for over 100 practitioners and defenders of alternative medicine to discuss the future of such topics as ethnomedicine, natural products, pharmacological treatments and nutrition/lifestyle changes. Such a gathering had never occurred before, much less under the government's aegis.

There were also broad and productive discussions of methodology, information dissemination and peer review—three days of intense idea sharing and debate. Brian Berman, MD, a doctor at the University of Maryland who had studied homeopathy in England, was appointed by NIH to chair the overall conclave. Frank Wiewel and I were asked to co-chair the Panel on Pharmacological and Biological Treatments. NIH's Dr. Jay Moskowitz gave the keynote address. "The era of quacks and quackbusters has come to an end," he told the enthusiastic gathering. There were now "opportunities for rewarding breakthroughs" by exploring alternatives. He declared that "the alternative and establishment communities are converging."

But Moskowitz went further. He said, "Not all alternative medical practices are amenable to traditional scientific evaluation, and some may require development of new methods to evaluate their efficacy and safety." This opened the door to "field investigations" of such treatments, to find out what the outcome really is when people go to nonconventional clinics for treatment. In effect, this was Dr. Burton's "pretrial" suggestion, but sanctioned by a top leader of the government's biomedical community. This approach may seem common sensical to the lay reader, but was revolutionary at NIH, where an almost religious belief in randomized clinical trials (RCTs) prevails.

There was widespread discontent with the negative and cumbersome name of the office. Soon afterwards, it was changed to the catchier but rather provocative Office of Alternative Medicine, or OAM. (In 1996, there is talk of changing it again, this time to the Office of Complementary and Alternative Medicine.)

On this instance, the eloquent Ms. Mason wrote, "The momentum is there. Hundreds of men and women—kindred health-care professionals—have found each other. There is no turning back" (*Washington Post,* October 2, 1992). The media suddenly discovered that not all alternative practitioners were kooks or quacks. There followed hundreds of stories, including a five-day series on the "Eye on America" segment of the *CBS Evening News with Dan Rather.* Rather's series was appropriately titled "New Age—New Rage."

Newsweek, which had lambasted laetrile in 1977, suddenly realized that "the medical establishment has for years shunned so-called alternative medicine and insurance companies have refused to pay for it, while federal officials have harassed its practitioners." Now faced with spiraling health care costs, *Newsweek* reported that "the federal government can no longer afford to be so smug. They are now "serious about unconventional therapy" (July 13, 1992).

The Los Angeles Times joined in with a lengthy piece, "Scrutinizing Alternative Paths to Health" (September 29, 1992). Even the staid *The New York Times* ran several guardedly favorable articles on the "mainstreaming of alternative medicine." *The Sunday Times* carried a report from Pulitzer Prize-winner Natalie Angier allowing that NIH, "long a stern protector of the most rigorous brand of science," was "about to start venturing into the realm of alternative medicine" (December 10, 1992).

Predictably, however, some people were not pleased. One could hear cries of opposition, much of it ultimately originating from a core of determined "quackbusters" affiliated with the National Coalition Against

Health Fraud. One prominent opponent of such methods, Victor Herbert, M.D., complained to *Internal Medicine News and Cardiology News* that the new office was a "rip-off of the public of $2 million...," and "a way created by con artists to promote cons as a legitimate therapy" (December, 1992).

In the following month, he elaborated in a *New England Journal of Medicine* book review, claiming that "a deceived Congress, at the urging of a misguided former congressman" forced the NIH to "waste $2 million in 1992 and 1993 in an attempt to validate 'alternative therapies.'" In addition, Congress had required NIH to include on its [ad hoc advisory, ed.] committee "a number of persons who make their living promoting health cons..." (December 17, 1992).

But, despite the grumbling about "governance by horoscope," the establishment of the OAM marked an irreversible turning point in the attitude of the media and much of the public toward alternative medicine. Before OAM, media attention tended to be sensationalistic, unreliable, or even downright nasty. After 1992, coverage was not only more intense but of a generally higher quality. (To jump ahead for a moment: by the end of 1995, OAM was receiving between 15 to 25 media inquiries *per day*. About three quarters of the stories generated by these inquiries were of a positive nature.)

On October 24, 1992, NIH appointed Joseph Jacobs, M.D. to be the first full-time director of the office. Dr. Jacobs, at 46, was the immediate past president of the Association of American Indian Physicians. He had grown up on a St. Regis Mohawk reservation in New York State and received his bachelor's degree from Columbia, an M.D. from Yale University School of Medicine and a M.B.A. from the Wharton School of Business.

One problem was that members of the Ad Hoc Advisory Committee (of whom I was one) were never consulted about the appointment of the director, and there were objections to this fact. Dr. Jacobs may have mistaken this as opposition to his appointment.

In addition, Dr. Jacobs seemed conventional in his medical orientation, and had never really studied or practiced any form of alternative treatment. He sharply disagreed with this assessment, however. "I have had some critics in the alternative medical community who feel that my lack of identity in that community did not qualify me for this job," he later said. "My response to that characterization is that I feel I was born into alternative medicine since my mother was a full-blooded Mohawk from Canada and upstate New York who frequently availed herself of traditional herbal medicines for me and my siblings when the need arose" (*Appropriations Subcommittee Hearings,* June 24, 1993).

Harkin as well as Bedell and some of the other advisors were insistent that the first order of business was for OAM to send out teams of investigators to bring back reports on potentially useful alternative treatments, especially for cancer. This sort of field work happened to be the way that Bedell himself organized the very successful research branch of his own small company. Don't sit around, he told his staff. Go find out what's happening in the field.

But Jacobs, and many at NIH, saw things differently. Science, they inferred, was not fishing tackle! There were complicated issues of methodology as well as medical ethics that had to be considered. For example, the repercussions of NIH statements could be vast. What would happen if OAM did validate a particular treatment? What should be done with that information? Would a report from OAM on an apparently successful cancer treatment lead to its acceptance—or to public pandemonium, with further scorn from the medical establishment? These, by the way, are still live issues. Needless to say, they roiled many a meeting over the next several years.

But, if only for political reasons, some field work had to be done. So in early 1993, Jacobs and his deputy Daniel Eskinazi, D.D.S., accompanied at times by a number of ad hoc advisors, paid site visits to a few unconventional therapists. They went to see Dr. Burzynski, for example. They later visited Charles Simone, M.D. and the 96-year-old Emmanuel Revici, M.D. in New York, and I accompanied them. I came away from these meetings profoundly disturbed by the lack of enthusiasm or support (financial and otherwise) from Dr. Jacobs for such studies.

In fact, over the next few months, my own interactions with Dr. Jacobs deteriorated. He vehemently rejected the line of argument you will read in this book, that there is an economic dimension to the "establishment's" opposition to alternative cancer treatments. After these arguments it became increasingly difficult for me to reach the director or other members of the staff, nor did I particularly want to. What had started out as a very warm and collegial relationship had suddenly turned ice cold. And what I heard from other staff members was not reassuring. Although Jacobs had an M.B.A. from a major business school, I heard repeated complaints of disorganization.

A major problem was that NIH, without the knowledge or approval of the ad hoc board, had given $750,000 of OAM's first money to NCI to conduct a trial on antineoplastons. Jay Moskowitz had done this, thinking (he said) that the board would be pleased to see the money spent in such a productive way. But then it became Dr. Jacobs' problem. No one seemed able to discover exactly what had happened to this money. To me, this was a travesty. I felt that OAM should protect its fledgling autonomy and keep control of all such studies in its own hands. (NCI later announced that it would fund a clinical trial on antineoplastons at Memorial Sloan-Kettering, which I regarded as the "killing field" of alternative cancer treatments. In 1995, excoriating Dr. Burzynski, the NCI and Sloan-Kettering cancelled this small trial, without producing any evaluable results.)

To summarize, the major controversies were as follows:

Should the emphasis of the OAM be on conducting site visits to promising clinics or on funding small "requests for applications" (RFAs) from a variety of institutions, most of them academic. Senator Harkin and the subcommittee's ranking member Arlen Specter (R-PA) agreed with Bedell's field investigation strategy, and had in fact sent Jacobs authorization to hire five full-time field investigators. Yet OAM never acted on that request.

Should OAM focus on killer diseases, like cancer and AIDS, or on more peripheral issues and illnesses?

Should OAM work *with* agencies like the NCI or *through* them?

Should OAM seek FDA approval for testing compounds or methods, even if such approval were not legally necessary?

The office badly needed a chartered, permanent Alternative Medicine Program Advisory Council (AMPAC). But this was delayed by red tape within the new Clinton Administration. Therefore, the office endured a rocky period, during which the authority of the Ad Hoc committee was cancelled, even before the permanent council had been appointed.

During this time, Dr. Jacobs ran the office virtually without any structured input from the alternative community. Because of his orthodox background, he did not have many contacts in the field, but seemed uneasy with many of the advisors he had inherited. The main continuity was provided by the 20 or so co-chairs of the panels from the Chantilly conclave. A subcommittee had been charged by Dr. Groft with producing an extended report on the meeting. They continued to meet by phone and in person. And indeed, in late 1994 this report was finished and published by the Government Printing Office as a 372-page survey of the field, entitled *Alternative Medicine: Expanding Medical Horizons* (NIH Publication No. 94-066). It is an excellent introduction to the field and a blueprint of research opportunities.

But relations among the co-chairs could be difficult, especially since they had no statutory authority. For instance, on February 4, 1993 there was a two-hour phone conference of the 20 co-chairs of Chantilly panels. It was an extremely fractious and contentious meeting. It seemed to me at the time that the OAM staff was trying to ramrod proposals through without adequate input from outside advisors. Frank Wiewel, Gar Hildenbrand, and I struggled hard, but were completely outvoted on a number of key issues pertaining to the direction of research. The selection of participants for this meeting excluded Berkley Bedell, who usually spoke with authority on such occasions.

Disaffection among those who had originally formed the office reached such a height that on June 24, 1993 Sen. Harkin held public hearings of his Appropriations Subcommittee to find out what exactly what going on at the office. Other attendees at these hearings included Senators Barbara A. Mikulski (D-MD), Slade Gorton (R-WA), Harry Reid (D-NV), and Claiborne Pell (D-RI). Some physicians and patients also spoke, such as David Eisenberg, M.D. and Charles Simone, M.D. But the centerpiece of the meeting was the testimony of Mr. Bedell and Dr. Jacobs and their exchanges with Senator Harkin.

After much hesitation, Berkley Bedell had decided it was necessary to go public with his smoldering concerns about the direction of OAM. With Jacobs sitting there, Bedell told the subcommittee:

"In my opinion, for this office to be successful in carrying out the investigations called for in this legislation, one of the requirements will be a director who is willing to stand up to these powerful forces. I am sorry to tell you that in my opinion our current director has not yet shown that commitment. I hope this will change. I believe it must" (*Special Hearing, Appropriations Subcommittee,* June 24, 1993).

These were fighting words, even though Bedell had stopped just short of calling for Jacobs's resignation. Jacobs responded as best as he could, and one couldn't help but sympathize with the difficult job he had taken on. But on some issues he sounded like a temporizing bureaucrat:

"Important issues such as determining the scope of the assignment and determining the magnitude of the solutions need to be addressed prior to initiating a major initiative," was one such reply.

The plain-spoken Harkin could not hide his frustration or anger. "I see no reason you can't...start pushing [the NCI director] a little bit, to get this process moving a little bit faster. You see, I'm faced with a problem here. I'd like to put more money into the office, but you're telling me you can't even hire scientific investigators...and you give money to NCI that goes into a black hole some place and you never see it again and nothing happens....Maybe I should shut the whole thing down?" In closing, Harkin told Jacobs, "We've had enough time. You will hear from me."

But aside from a growing hostility between Jacobs and certain ad hoc advisors, nothing of substance happened. In November, 1993 I wrote a *Cancer Chronicles* editorial, "Please, Senator Harkin!" Until that point, I had been fairly muted in my own criticism of Jacobs and the office. I now heard a rumor from a government employee that Jacobs was planning to remove my name and that of Bedell, Hildenbrand and Wiewel from the list of nominees for the advisory council.

I decided to pull out the stops.

"The Office of Alternative Medicine is adrift," I publicly wrote Senator Harkin. "There is no longer an advisory board. Please help get this [Program] Advisory Council approved....Please act now to revitalize the OAM, or it may soon exist in name alone."

From Jacobs' point of view, a group of outside meddlers were trying to tell him how to run his office. From our point of view, the office belonged to the people, and especially of those who had fought against overwhelming odds for the fair evaluation of alternative methods.

But Jacobs overreached when he tried to eliminate his critics from the board. For it was he, and not what he called the "gang of four," who were about to leave the scene. On May 17, 1994, HHS Secretary Donna Shalala finally made her appointments to the eighteen-member panel, with terms randomly assigned from one to four years. The proposed board included all four of the disputed members. And immediately thereafter, Dr. Jacobs informed colleagues that he was resigning effective the end of September, 1994. As *Science* magazine noted, Jacobs' decision to leave was precipitated by his objection to having certain individuals included on the permanent advisory board to his office (July 15, 1994).

In a follow-up article, *Science* confirmed that Jacobs had indeed fought to keep us off the permanent board and then, when he came to believe "that the top NIH staff would go along with demands from Harkin's office and include on the list of candidate advisors [the] four activists picked by Harkin," he resigned (September 30, 1994).

"Jacobs ran afoul of the activists who lobbied to create the alternative medicine program," said *Science* (ibid.). The magazine quoted me as saying that Jacobs had "acrimonious dealing" with some board members "over priorities of research." These advisors, *Science* explained, "wanted Jacobs to devote more time and money to investigating controversial therapies...a topic that Jacobs included under duress in the first round of research awards.

"Moss argues [that] the NIH office has chosen to research 'soft' topics less likely to offend the biomedical establishment."

This was followed by a long article in the *New York Times*. Natalie Angier reported on the "acrimony and disgruntlement" in the new office. She quoted me as saying, "I'm happy about his resignation. He seemed very uncomfortable with the job, and I wasn't happy with the direction of the office. I see it from the point of view of NIH wanting to do things the way NIH usually does."

But the fight was not over. Jacobs used the occasion of the second major story in *Science* (September 30, 1994) to go out with a blast at Senator Harkin and what he now called "the Harkinites." He claimed we four were guilty of "pressuring his office, promoting certain therapies, and...attempting an end run around objective science."

Science also claimed that "Jacobs' fears that the office would be forced to conduct field studies have been borne out." An interesting choice of words—were field studies something to be "feared"?

There followed an interregnum period, in which an Acting Director, Alan Trachtenberg, M.D., a long-time NIH employee, managed to keep the office together under extremely trying circumstances. Then, in February, 1995 NIH announced the appointment of a new permanent director, Lt. Col. Wayne Jonas, M.D. Dr. Jonas was head of the fellowship training program at the Walter Reed Institute of Research in Washington, D.C. He is considered an expert on research methodology, but also had long-term interests in various alternative medicine techniques, such as homeopathy, electroacupuncture, nutrition, qigong, and even radionics.

In *The Cancer Chronicles*, I noted that most people in the alternative community were genuinely happy with the appointment, which was approved by Harold Varmus, M.D., NIH Director, and his new Deputy Director, Ruth L. Kirschstein, M.D., who had taken a personal interest in the direction of the office.

However, in print I myself greeted Dr. Jonas's appointment with what I called "guarded enthusiasm." Why guarded? I liked Dr. Jonas personally, but having just been through a bruising struggle with Dr. Jacobs, I wondered aloud "if Wayne will be able to do what his predecessors were unable to do." I did call on the alternative community to give him "all the support they can muster" to fight against the enemies of the office. (I was thinking of the quackbusters, whose attacks had steeped up around this time.) In effect, I declared a personal moratorium on criticism, since I felt that Dr. Jonas deserved a chance to salvage the office and implement his own vision of its future in coordination with the new Council.

In my opinion, this has been a wise policy. Bedell still feels the office has essentially failed to carry out its mandate to do field research. But no one doubts that Jonas has done a brilliant job at rescuing and reorganizing the office, articulating a coherent set of priorities, and establishing extremely cordial relationships with both the conventional and the alternative medical communities. He now has the support of virtually all members of the Advisory Council. It has been an amazing turnaround.

Of course, that does not mean that all problems have been resolved—far from it. But at least that most valuable of all assets, trust, has been established, and there is a coherent strategy for doing both the kind of field research Bedell and others want and the more academic studies favored by many members of the board.

One answer has been to fund centers of alternative medicine at leading medical centers in the country (a program that began before Jonas came aboard). At this writing, such centers have been initiated at Columbia-Presbyterian, Harvard University, Stanford University, and the University of Maryland, to name a few. NIH has even given a grant to Bastyr University, a fully accredited naturopathic institution in Seattle. And at the University of Texas a special center has been created to study alternative treatments specifically for cancer.

In 1992, the OAM received $2.2 million. In 1996, the initial problems resolved, Congress awarded the office an unprecedented $7.5 million. This came at a time of severe budget cuts. This fact alone is an indication of the faith that the Congress and the American public place in the enormous potential of alternative treatments. And with growing national recognition of the failure of the conventional war on cancer, hopes will increasingly turn towards those techniques that have been scorned as "unproven" by an ossified cancer establishment.

It is my dream that this small office, which grew out of the political struggle, can fulfill a huge mission. The NCI has simply abrogated its responsibility to vigorously investigate all new leads in the fight against cancer. Responsibility for this huge area has fallen on the shoulders of this tiny office, which can make history if it can validate even a single new approach to the cancer problem. It deserves the vigorous and enthusiastic support of the Congress and of all citizens who want to see an end to the scourge of cancer.

Underlying Problems

But all will not be clear sailing. Unfortunately, the fact that the government is finally encouraging a serious study of alternative methods does not render the main conclusions of this book invalid. Before alternative medicine can receive a fair testing, or be accepted, certain major obstacles have to be overcome. The biggest of these, in my opinion, is the entrenched opposition of the "medical-industrial complex."

Monopoly is a long-standing problem. As early as the 1950s and 1960s, five major drug companies, which the Federal Trade Commission described as a cartel, were convicted of fixing the prices of then-new antibiotics. Since 1989 there has been an unprecedented wave of mergers: SmithKline and Beecham; Bristol-Myers and Squibb; Glaxo and Wellcome; Pharmacia and Upjohn. In early 1996, Sandoz and Ciba-Geigy announced that they were "rushing into each others' arms" (*Wall Street Journal*, 3/7/96) to create a giant with a market value of over $60 billion.

Such mega-mergers have turned the pharmaceutical industry "upside down in the past three years" (*ibid.*). Each of the top ten companies now has annual sales of between six and twelve billion dollars. These mergers raise the specter of even greater monopoly, patent abuse, and the stifling of innovation—all things that are disastrous to that spirit of open inquiry in which medicine thrives.

The immediate result of the mergers of the 1990s may be layoffs and other cost-cutting measures, raising their profitability in the short run. But they do not solve the industry's underlying problem, which many analysts identify quite simply as *too few good ideas*.

Role of the FDA

Congress's response to such problems has been anemic, at best. It was the antibiotics scandal that led to the famous hearings on the drug industry of Sen. Estes Kefauver's Antitrust and Monopoly Subcommittee. Yet ironically, what emerged from those hearings was not an assault on monopoly, but the safety and efficacy provisions of the FDA. These were feared by the drug industry at the time, but turned out to be in their interest, since they actually "raised the barrier of entry to new competitors and, over the long run, strengthened the position of the largest companies," (Robert Teitelman, *Profits of Science*. NY: Basic Books, 1994).

At first sight, the FDA *appears* to have an adversarial relationship with the drug industry. After all, FDA regulates them, tells them what they can and cannot do. But in truth, the major impact of FDA regulation is not to hamper industry giants, but to bar the entry of smaller competitors into their fields.

Structurally, the FDA mirrors the industry it regulates: it is "highly centralized, hierarchical, full of pharmacologists, biochemists, chemists, physicians" (Teitelman, *op.cit.*) And the FDA, as a branch of the executive, has a powerful enforcement arm, which can make those whom it generally regards as its true adversaries (small drug and food supplement makers, health entrepreneurs, and alternative practitioners of all kinds) bend to its might-makes-right argument, as in its infamous armed raid on Jonathan Wright, M.D. on May 6, 1992.

FDA's general mandate is to limit risk to the public; the drug industry's goal is to limit competition. But their common strategy is the same: a stifling of innovation, especially when it originates from outside the members of the Pharmaceutical Manufacturers' Association, the "club." This convergence delivers rewards for insiders.

"Both manufacturers and regulators were thus designed not for great leaps of thought but for careful progress," said Teitelman. "The combination of increased regulation and pricing freedom gave the big companies a weapon against smaller competitors...," this astute business journalist added. "By lowering regulatory barriers, the club would have invited many small competitors to play."

Or as an economist wrote, "The sources of innovation are declining. With the cost of developing a new drug soaring, research is a game smaller companies cannot afford to play" (*Business Week*, February 21, 1977). And there are few blockbusters in the pipeline.

New ideas are limited to a relatively small pool of conventional thinkers. Drug executives are distressed by "the sinking realization that their research pipelines—the lifeblood of the industry—are drying up." Some say privately that "the industry is running out of ideas" (*Wall Street Journal, op.cit.*).

Are they surprised? The industry has spent decades discouraging radical innovation in medicine, branding them as "unproven" or even "quack" ideas. Now they are surprised that they have nothing radically new to offer for the treatment of cancer and other diseases. One might think that at such a juncture the industry would turn to alternative medicine, which is certainly rich in ideas. But that is difficult given the mindset they have helped to foster.

But sometimes they do go hunting the fields of alternative practices.

In May, 1995, for example, the Swedish giant, Pharmacia, Inc. invited Helen Coley Nauts to come to Lund to lecture on her father's treatment, Coley's toxins (see chapter 7). She gave a brilliant speech and one can only hope that something positive will come of this. But predictable problems arise when pharmaceutical companies try to fit such treatments into the standard new drug development process.

Drug companies are not charities. They exist to serve their employees and stockholders, who invest their money in order to obtain good returns. They incur extraordinary expenses in researching, developing, and marketing new products. Much of this goes to fulfilling the regulatory requirements of the FDA. In return, the government gives them 17-year legal monopolies called patents, as a way of recouping these costs.

But one cannot patent Coley's toxins. These are naturally occurring byproducts of common bacteria. Someone I know recently produced 1,000 cubic centimeters of the toxins for $1,000—enough to treat many patients for months at a time. With mass production, even such prices could plummet. Coley's toxins could become virtually free!

The problem with Coley's toxins are emblematic of those of alternative treatments in general: often, they are natural products which one can buy by the carload. But the drug industry is predicated on enormous costs and even greater returns. Nature does not always cooperate in this scheme. And so there is an economic imperative to "improve" on nature's formulas, to create what the current NCI director Richard Klausner, M.D. calls "non-natural natural products."

Unfortunately, none of NCI's clever modifications ever seems to produce an agent that works as well as the original product. Recombinant tumor necrosis factor (TNF) simply cannot hold a candle to Coley's all-natural formula of one hundred years ago.

And academic scientists have a collateral problem: how do they build a reputation for brilliance by rediscovering the work of some neglected or maligned scientist, who may have died decades ago? Can you investigate quackery without being suspected of it yourself?

And so, as we approach the Third Millennium, we are faced with an enormous paradox. The drug companies are awash with cash, inhabit architecturally stunning facilities, and wield astounding hardware; but they are beggars when it comes to new ideas. Alternative medicine has many brilliant ideas, but has few resources allocated to their development. (OAM's budget is still less than 1/1000th of the NIH total.)

How can this be resolved? In the end, the public could decide the issue by voting, not just at the ballot box, but with its feet and pocketbooks. Since the first edition of this book, we have witnessed an enormous shift in public acceptance of alternative treatments. A 1993 survey by the ACS estimated that 9 percent of cancer patients already use complementary therapies, but this rose to 14 percent in the higher-income and more influential groups (Kennedy, BJ. *J Cancer Educ* 1993;8:129-131). Other reports put the figure much higher—as high as 50 or 60 percent (McGinnis, LS. *Cancer* 1991;67:1788-1792; and Hauser, SP. *Curr Opin Oncol* 1993;5:646-654).

In 1994, a conventional oncologist at New York Hospital polled her breast cancer patients and found that 30 percent had consulted unconventional therapists and 25 percent were already using some form of alternative treatment (OAM, *Workshop on the Collection of Data,* Bethesda, MD, 1994).

Only about five percent of these patients abandon conventional medicine to pursue such treatments, as most patients want to combine both kinds of approaches.

And this is a worldwide trend. In Holland, Poland, and England between 16 and 25 percent of cancer patients admit to using complementary treatments (Van der Zouwe, N. *Ned Tijdschr Geneeskd* 1994; 138:300-306; Pawlicki, M, et al. *Pol Tyg Lek* 1991;46:922-923; Downer, SM. *BMJ* 1994;9309:86-89).

In South Australia 46 percent of children with cancer were receiving complementary, as well as conventional, treatment (Sawyer, MG, et al. *Med J Aust* 1994;160:323-324). In Germany, the figure reached 53 percent (Morant, R, et al. *Schweiz Med Wochenschr* 1991;121:1029-1034), and so on.

This is the background to the rise of the U.S. Office of Alternative Medicine. This development truly has the feel of an irresistible force, an idea whose time has come. The Congress of the United States has put its seal of approval on this trend. Appropriations for it almost certainly will continue to grow.

Yet at the same time, the pharmaceutical industry appears to present an immovable object in its path. For how can the "medical-industry complex" cope with this emerging new world of patient empowerment, with its emphasis on low-cost prevention, good nutrition, improved life style, and natural medicine?

Perhaps the next turning point will be passage of the Access to Medical Practices Act (S-1035), which was drafted by Berkley Bedell, and introduced into the Senate by another one of his many admirers, Sen.

Tom Daschle (D-SD). Co-sponsors include many of those who had already gravitated towards the OAM, including not just Sen. Harkin, but such influential legislators as Senators Abraham, Dole, Grassley, Hatch, Hatfield, Pell, Reid, Simon, and Simpson. This landmark bill would "permit an individual to be treated by a health care practitioner with any method of medical treatment such individual requests." This is a modest proposal indeed! For it represents a daring "freedom of choice" salvo, at a time when many other health reform schemes threaten to greatly restrict patients' rights. Behind its seemingly innocuous words lies a revolutionary concept, a fact not lost on the bill's opponents, who include the FDA, and some self-proclaimed "consumer protection" organizations.

Passage of this bill could bring the whole question of medical freedom of choice to the fore. Passage will not be easy. Nevertheless, even if it takes a years, with sufficient public pressure, it could certainly pass. It will then make dispensing alternative treatments legal, while placing the persecutors of alternative doctors outside the law.

The Cancer Industry is an angry book, and it often generates anger in those who read it. Many readers wonder, what can be done? There is no quick fix. But by educating your own doctors, political representatives, journalists, and opinion-makers of all kinds, any individual can make an important contribution to the resolution of the issues raised in this work.

One in three Americans, and two-thirds of America's families are slated to face cancer. There is no time to waste.

—Ralph W. Moss, Ph.D.

« 1 »

The Crisis of
Credibility

Twenty years ago, there was tremendous optimism about curing cancer. America had put a man on the moon, and it was natural to ask whether the nation which could achieve that once-proverbial impossibility couldn't also conquer humanity's most dreaded disease.

Congress had appointed a blue-ribbon National Panel of Consultants on the Conquest of Cancer whose purpose, in the words of Senator Ralph Yarborough (D.-Tex.), was to "recommend to Congress and to the American people what must be done to achieve cures for the major forms of cancer by 1976. . . ."

In his forward to the consultants' final report, Senator Yarborough put the case for an all-out war on cancer bluntly:

> Cancer is a disease which can be conquered. Our advances in the field of cancer research have brought us to the verge of important and exciting developments in the early detection and control of this dread disease . . . (Yarborough, 1970).

At the same time, forces close to the American Cancer Society, calling themselves the Citizens' Committee for the Conquest of Cancer, began a skillful public-relations campaign aimed at passage of a "war on cancer" act. In full-page ads, the Citizens' Committee cried out:

MR. NIXON: YOU CAN CURE CANCER

If prayers are heard in Heaven, this prayer is heard the most: "Dear God, please. Not cancer."
Still, more than 318,000 Americans died of cancer last year.
This year, Mr. President, you have it in your power to begin to end this curse (*New York Times,* December 9, 1969).

R. Lee Clark of Houston's M. D. Anderson Hospital and Tumor Institute declared unequivocally that "with a billion dollars a year for ten years we could lick cancer" (Edson, 1974)

On December 23, 1971, after much political jockeying, President Nixon signed into law the National Cancer Act, thus launching a full-scale assault on the dread disease. Congress had designated the act "a national crusade to be accomplished by 1976 in commemoration of the 200th anniversary of our country. . . ." (Rosenbaum, 1977). Nixon called for "the same kind of concentrated effort that split the atom and took man to the moon." This was Richard Nixon's Christmas present to the nation.

From the start, all this talk about curing cancer in time for the Bicentennial was good public relations, but terrible science. Curing cancer was just not like sending a man to the moon. Landing on the moon—or sending Voyager 2 to Uranus—is basically an engineering feat. Not enough was known about cancer to be able to predict its cure.

Writing for a business audience in 1970, Jerry E. Bishop, the *Wall Street Journal*'s science writer, spelled out the dilemma and the reason for the deception:

It is highly unlikely that any group of experts can promise that cures for major forms of cancer will be achieved within five years even if appropriations for cancer research were unlimited. To do so could raise high hopes among the public and result in a disenchantment, as 1976 rolled around, that might do considerable harm to public support of cancer research in the long run. Yet without such dramatic promises, public enthusiasm for a major "assault" on cancer that the researchers have longed for may be more difficult to arouse (August 26, 1970).

4

Thus, in Bishop's view, the "war on cancer," with its inflated rhetoric and promises, was a clever way to prime the public for a war it might not otherwise support. Not surprisingly, soon after the war was launched, it was in trouble. "Will the war ever get started?" *Science* magazine asked two years later (September 7, 1973). "President Nixon's war on cancer . . . appears to be stalled in low gear, plagued by an increasingly bitter three-way battle for control of the $500 million of federal funds. . . . ," wrote the *Wall Street Journal* (July 28, 1973).

The administrators of the war drew up incredibly complicated 1,000-page battle plans including an elaborate radial chart entitled "National Cancer Program Strategy" that will undoubtedly live on as a classic example of bureaucratic obscurity (National Cancer Institute, 1975).

No sooner had the plan been drafted than it came under sharp criticism from scientists within the cancer field itself. The basic assumption of the plan seemed to be that cancer could, in fact, be controlled by existing means. This corresponded to the political needs of President Nixon and the American Cancer Society, but simply didn't correspond to the scientific reality.

"There are many types of cancer for which today's technologies simply do not work," said a National Academy of Sciences panel headed by the president of Memorial Sloan-Kettering Cancer Center. "What is most urgently needed for problems of this kind is an abundance of new ideas, and these are most likely to emerge from the imagination and intuition of individual scientists. It is much less likely that the administrators of large programs . . . at the center of a highly centralized bureaucracy can generate the kinds of ideas that are needed" (*Wall Street Journal*, July 23, 1973).

By 1974 the public, which had enthusiastically hoped a cure for cancer was in the offing, was beginning to feel it had been betrayed. The cancer war was Nixon's "other war," and when Nixon resigned over Watergate, this only fueled public suspicion of a double-cross.

"The Cancer Rip-Off" was science writer Lee Edson's summary of the situation, less than three years after the war had been launched (Edson, 1974).

"We don't know how to attack cancer, much less conquer it, because we don't understand enough about how it works and what causes it," said Rockefeller University's Dr. Norton Zinder, who had been asked by the National Cancer Advisory Board (a body of laypersons and professionals established by Nixon) to head a committee to look into the NCI's virus program, upon which most hopes were then pitched (ibid.).

Zinder's committee found that the virologists had made the assumption

5

that human cancer was indeed caused by a virus. But, said the review committee, which included top scientists from Sloan-Kettering, the National Cancer Institute, New York University, and the University of Colorado, "these assumptions were wrong. There wasn't enough knowledge to mount such a narrowly targeted program" (ibid.).

The committee also found some peculiar financial transactions within the multimillion-dollar program. They wrote: "It is in large part an in-house operation and those who run it are also often recipients of large amounts of the money they disperse" (ibid.). Private companies clustered around the National Institutes of Health in Bethesda, Maryland, were charging the government 144 percent overhead, plus a 9 percent profit to perform virus research.

In early 1975 criticism of the program began to make headlines. Nobel laureate James Watson declared at a cancer symposium at the Massachusetts Institute of Technology that the American public had been sold a "nasty bill of goods about cancer" (*New York Times,* March 9, 1975). It was a "soporific orgy," which produced no "promising leads," as it claimed, but "only delaying actions" (Rosenbaum, 1977). Watson reputedly summed up the entire situation in four well-chosen words: "A bunch of shit!" (ibid.).

A few weeks later, Dr. Charles C. Edwards, who had resigned in January 1975 as Secretary of Health of the U.S. Department of Health, Education and Welfare, wrote in an article that the war on cancer was politically motivated and based on the dubious premise that cancer could, "like the surface of the moon, be conquered if we will simply spend enough money to get the job done" (*New York Times,* March 22, 1975).

As the Bicentennial approached, the leaders of the cancer war frantically attempted to come up with some bona fide achievements that would placate an increasingly restless public. "All of us receive a multitude of inquiries on what the National Cancer Program is doing to help people," wrote Frank J. Rauscher, Jr., Ph.D., director of the program (and of the National Cancer Institute). "In short, 'What are we doing with the taxpayer's money?'"

To answer that question, Rauscher issued a list of accomplishments. With no false modesty, the young virologist, who had been called "Nixon's protégé" (*Medical World News,* May 26, 1972), declared, "In every sense, these advances are remarkable and have already saved many lives" (National Cancer Institute, 1976a).

First on the list was a combination of drugs used after surgery to decrease the recurrence rate of breast cancer. The method was brand new at the time and virtually unproven, but Rauscher called it "a great and justifiable cause for optimism."

Several months earlier, however, this treatment method had been sharply criticized in *Science* magazine as one whose "significance has been greatly exaggerated" (March 12, 1976). And Mary E. Costanza, a doctor at Tufts-New England Medical Center Hospitals in Boston, has warned that "all in all, there is reason to be skeptical as well as optimistic about the effects of long-term chemoprophylaxis against breast cancer" (*New England Journal of Medicine*, November 20, 1975).

Second on Rauscher's list was "a study of the treatment of breast cancer with less radical surgery" that had shown "it may be as effective as radical surgery."

Far from being an accomplishment of the war on cancer, the use of limited surgery in breast cancer had long been the position of mavericks in the cancer field, who had had to buck the establishment to get their position heard (see chapter 3).

The report went on to repeat many of the claims that had been made for surgery, radiation, and chemotherapy over the years. It included such inspired achievements as "a communication network [that] has been developed . . . to provide cancer information to health professionals" and "toll-free telephone services . . . established at each Center." It also stated that "scientists within and outside the National Cancer Program have found again that fluoridation of drinking water does not contribute to a cancer burden for people"—a claim sharply contested by unorthodox scientists such as Dean Burk, Ph.D., and John Yiamouyiannis, Ph.D. (*Congressional Record*, December 16, 1975).

What the report didn't say was what millions of people had been led to expect: that the National Cancer Program had found a cure for even one major type of human cancer.

Not long after this, Dr. Rauscher stepped down as head of the cancer program.

By 1979—ten years after the promised quick cure—the beginning of the end still did not appear to be in sight. "A medical Vietnam" is how Food and Drug Administrator Donald Kennedy, Ph.D., succinctly described the war on cancer. In June 1979 Kennedy resigned his post to return to academe. His inability to ban saccharin and the unorthodox cancer therapy laetrile were two of the main reasons given for his rather sudden departure (*New York Times*, October 6, 1979).

"We have been simplistic," said Dr. Arthur Upton, who succeeded Rauscher as head of the National Cancer Institute. "I think we're wrong to expect a cure to come soon" (*Wall Street Journal*, October 24, 1978).

There's a "crisis of credibility," said Dr. Theodore Cooper, the former assistant director of the Department of Health, Education and Welfare (ibid.).

In 1985 *Forbes* wrote about "the baffling standoff in cancer research. . . . Cancer researchers have made enormous strides in learning about the mechanisms that relate to cancer," the magazine suggested. "But the long-awaited cure for cancer is as far away as ever" (July 15, 1985).

"Just how serious are we about winning the war on cancer?" An article in *Hippocrates* wondered in January/February 1989.

The reason for this crisis is the tremendous gap between the promises and claims of cancer orthodoxy and the grim reality. No amount of cheerful optimism has been able to obscure the obvious fact that we are not winning the war on cancer.

Every day more than 1,350 people die of cancer in the United States. Over 500,000 a year. One every 63 seconds.

Over one million Americans a year discover that they have a malignancy. These are the most serious cases. If we add to this over 500,000 cases of skin cancer and about 40,000 cases of carcinoma-in-situ (limited to one small site) of the uterine cervix, over one and a half million of us will be treated for cancer each year (American Cancer Society, 1989).*

At the present rate 30 percent of us will contract cancer. One in five will die in this chronic epidemic. There has been a slow but steady increase in the age-adjusted death rate from the disease since 1950 (Bailer and Smith, 1986).

While public spokespersons give us assurances and declarations about cancer, it is obvious that, even after two decades of intensive work, little is really known about the disease in any fundamental sense. What exactly is cancer? Scientists can describe certain features common to cancer cells. For example, they are strangely misshapen and immature. They can invade neighboring tissues. They can break free from a tumorous growth, float through the blood or the lymph system, and set up new colonies (called metastases) in other vital organs.

According to the American Cancer Society (ACS), "Cancer is a large group of diseases characterized by uncontrolled growth and spread of abnormal cells" (ACS, 1988). Yet even so basic a summation does not find universal acceptance. Not only do many unorthodox doctors contest this definition, but the chancellor of Memorial Sloan-Kettering Cancer Center told the author that he believed cancer to be a single disease and that some "as

*Skin cancer (basal cell carcinoma) and carcinoma of the uterine cervix are generally so readily curable through surgery and radiation that they are not included in the official cancer statistics.

8

yet unidentified pathological mechanism is involved in all varieties of cancer" (MSKCC *Center News*, March 1975).

Thomas recently reaffirmed that belief:

> It's beginning to seem almost certain that cancer will turn out to be not a hundred different diseases but a single, very profound disturbance, set off by the same (in principle, at least) common perturbance of the genetic information carried by all living cells (Thomas, 1986).

One ACS-published textbook stated that "to date no single definition of cancer is universally acceptable" (Rubin, 1971:18). A dozen years later an updated edition affirmed, "Various definitions of cancer have been put forth over the years. None is an all-encompassing or entirely satisfactory conception. . . ." (Rubin, 1983:20).

While basic discoveries in genetics and virology have brought us closer to an understanding, there is no unanimity among scientists on some basic facts of cancer. "The exact cause of cancer remains undetermined," Dr. Philip Rubin has concluded (ibid.).

But if cancer is a biological puzzle, it is even more a social, economic, and political one. The newspapers, magazines, radio, and television are filled daily with a welter of confusing and conflicting stories about it.

We are told that great strides are being made in the conquest of the disease—and then we are told that the incidence of cancer is on the rise. We are told that chemicals cause cancer—but then that animal tests prove nothing and human data are inconclusive. We are told to examine our bodies for changes in every wart, mole, and growth—and then we are told that we are suffering from "cancer phobia." We are told that we must be protected from cancer quackery—and then we learn that twenty states legalized a supposedly quack remedy.

Why is there such confusion, controversy, emotion, and bitterness associated with the question of cancer? The main reason appears to be that cancer exacts an enormous toll, yet our medical and political leaders continue to pursue losing strategies.

The emotional toll of cancer is incalculable. Most cancer victims suffer the agony of a painful, disabling, and socially stigmatized disease (Sontag, 1977). They live in fear of the disease—an unknown terror—and of death. They live in fear of the orthodox treatments: surgery, irradiation, and poisonous chemotherapy. Men fear castration, physical or chemical. Women fear the loss of their sexuality, their breasts, and their womb. These are the bitter human facts about cancer.

Despite much easy talk about cures, victims are rarely free of the fear that someday the cancer will return. "Five-year survival" is a conventional milestone for cancer patients, and a realistic goal for doctors. Anyone who survives five years after diagnosis is probably in the clear. But the doubts and fears remain in the back of a cancer patient's mind—often for a lifetime. This emotional background lends all disputes in cancer a particular urgency. Each side in such a controversy believes the other side is raising false hopes, causing needless despair, or even performing murder by proxy.

Equally important is the financial burden of the disease, which has become truly staggering in recent years. The 1979 *ACS Cancer Facts & Figures* cited an undated *Consumer Reports* estimate that the average cost of cancer was $20,000 for the medical services alone. Samuel S. Epstein estimated a cost range of $5,000–30,000 (Epstein, 1978).*

Such figures, although considerable, seem to understate the true economic impact of cancer. A survey of cancer patients in the New York Metropolitan area in 1971–72 showed that the range of total costs was $5,000–50,000. The average at that time was $21,718. Twenty percent spent over $30,000 (Cancer Care, 1973:21). As the authors of this study indicated, however, "the point regarding costs is that they exceed family income" (ibid.). The median cost of the illness ($19,054) was *two and one-third times* the family's median income.

This situation has only worsened in recent years. A day in a cancer hospital in the late 1970s cost up to $600, according to Robert M. Heyssel, executive vice president and director of Johns Hopkins Hospital. He added an important point: "Each new medical or scientific breakthrough improves the quality and the outcome of care, but in most instances the cost of care rises proportionately" (*New York Times,* July 16, 1979).

In the late 1970s, medical inflation outstripped the overall rate of price rises. In fact, according to some economists, medical costs were *doubling* every five years (*Time,* May 28, 1979).

Direct treatment costs for cancer in the 1970s were about $20 billion a year. Today the cost, both to the individual and to society in general, is considerably greater. A study by the National Center for Health Statistics put overall medical costs for cancer at $71.5 billion for 1985. $21.8 billion of this was for direct costs; $8.6 billion for so-called morbidity costs (the

---

*"There is surprisingly little information in detail about the costs of long-term illness," according to Cancer Care, Inc. (1973). The American Cancer Society adds that "the cost of cancer treatment varies so widely from case to case that it is difficult to cite any typical figure" (ACS, 1979).

cost of lost productivity), and $41.2 billion for mortality costs. Cancer accounts for 10 percent of the total cost of disease in the U.S., and its share of the total cost of premature death from all causes is 18 percent (ACS, 1988).

Estimate for the average cost of terminal breast cancer is usually in the $60–65,000 range (Thomas, 1988).

In 1982 Bloom and colleagues studied 301 childhood cancer patients. Their *total annual* cost from the disease was nearly $30,000 per year. Approximately half was spent for hospital treatment, with the other half for ambulatory care and out-of-pocket expenses (Cancer Care, 1988).

At that rate, if a child receives treatment for three and a half years, the actual cost could be around $100,000. And costs are going up.

These frightening figures can have an impact on the patient's treatment and theoretically on his or her survival. A study in the *New England Journal of Medicine* reported that the choice of lung-cancer treatment was often determined by the social and economic status of the patients. Patients who were either not insured privately and/or unmarried often did not opt for expensive chemotherapy. Yet in the case of lung cancer, as the authors point out, this made little difference in the outcome of their illness: "Despite the fact that privately insured and married patients were more aggressively treated, they did not survive longer after diagnosis" (Greenberg et al., 1988).

Short of some simple, economical cure, any "breakthroughs" could greatly increase the cost. What would happen, for instance, if an experimental drug treatment currently priced at $50,000 per patient turned out to be an effective anticancer agent? Who can put a lid on such expenditures without being accused of cruelty?

But the direct expenses of cancer are only about half of the total cost to society. Adding the *indirect* costs, such as loss of earning power due to premature disability, the expense to society of research into the disease, or the billions spent on regulating industry, produced a total of around $40 billion in 1978 (Epstein, 1978).

As stated the National Center for Health Statistics figured the total cost of cancer at $71.5 billion (NCI, 1987). At that time the direct cost of all illness in the U.S. was $371.4 billion (ibid.). Direct costs are $500 billion, and continue to increase at twice the rate of inflation (*The Economist*, December 17, 1988). If indirect costs have continued to rise at the same rate, then the total cost of cancer in 1991 will be over $100 billion.

The logical corollary of this massive expenditure, however, is that *someone* is receiving much of the money that the cancer victim disburses. Cancer care is not a charity; it is a business—big business.

To begin with, cancer patients pay 50 million visits to their physicians each year (Applezweig, 1978). In his or her frantic search for help, a cancer patient may bounce from one specialist to another, from an internist to a surgeon to a radiologist and, finally, to a practioner of innovative medicine. Although no one consciously planned it that way, cancer generates a great deal of business for the medical profession.

If each new cancer patient undergoes only one surgical operation (the average at Memorial Sloan-Kettering Cancer Center), this means that America's surgeons perform almost a million cancer operations each year. This does not include the many thousands of operations for skin cancer or benign growths, nor the biopsies, which exceed the number of large-scale operations.

Another source of revenue for doctors and hospitals is the use of radiation in the diagnosis and treatment of cancer. In 1979 there were 270,000 X-ray units in the United States, 120,000 of them in the hands of medical doctors or related health professionals—the rest belonging mainly to dentists (*New York Times*, July 4, 1979). In 1973 it was estimated that there were 3,000 telecobalt units, 300–400 linear accelerators, and 35–50 cyclotrons treating cancer patients throughout the world (Richards, 1972).

According to some experts, 70 percent of all cancer patients receive X-ray therapy each year (*New York Times*, July 4, 1979). Today that figure would mean nearly 750,000 individuals.

It is impossible to give an accurate cost figure for these treatments, which vary widely from hospital to hospital. Since each patient usually receives a *series* of X-ray treatments, the financial impact of this form of therapy is apparent.

Hospitals find radiation equipment to be a worthwhile investment. Memorial Sloan-Kettering, for example, spent $4.5 million to replace all its radiation machinery a decade ago (MSKCC *Center News*, July/August 1977). Over 1,000 hospitals rushed to install CAT (computerized axial tomography) scanners during the first several years of their availability, at a cost of $700,000 or more per machine. (*Time*, October 29, 1979). Each CAT scan cost the patient between $220 and $400, according to a survey of New York hospitals (see also *Medical World News*, June 14, 1976, and *New York Times*, May 15, 1988).

Magnetic resonance imaging (MRI) devices, which emerged in the 1980s, cost up to $2 million each, but are a "medical godsend" to General Electric, Diasonics, Siemens, Philips, and Picker International, which manufacture the machines, and to the physicians who own and operate them (*New York Times*, May 15, 1988). A turning point came in 1985, when the U.S. government decided to cover many MRI tests under Medicare insurance (Standard & Poor's, 1988).

Physicians buy partnership shares in these facilities and then send their patients to be scanned there. In many cases a doctor can earn 25 to 100 percent or more per year on an investment of $5,000 to $100,000. These investments are generally only open to doctors. The more patients he sends, the more money his center earns.

"The arrangements are wrong because they produce a terrible conflict of interest for a doctor," Arnold Relman, M.D., editor of the *New England Journal of Medicine*, told the *Wall Street Journal* (Waldhoz and Bogdanich, 1989).

For example, physicians who bought partnership shares for $25,000 each in 1986 in an Elizabeth, New Jersey, scanner, received $10,000 profit per share in six months. That amounts to an annualized return of 80 percent, after just two years of operation. The venture's prospectus projects a total profit, after ten years, of nearly $250,000 per share (ibid.).

Despite their high cost, by 1987 there were already 1,322 MRIs installed worldwide (Standard & Poor's, 1989); 481 of the U.S. units were investor-owned. And there are more to come. On New York's Long Island, for instance, there are already 14 MRIs, although the state health planning agency says that only six are needed. In the greater Los Angeles area there are 50, and that is expected to triple by 1991 as a result of a "rampant entrepreneurial spirit," according to UCLA professor Dr. Robert Lufkin (Waldhoz and Bogdanich, 1989).

Greed has also affected the mammography field. Physician-investors in Mammography Plus, a breast-cancer detection center in Los Gatos, California, are sent periodic pep talks: they were told in a quarterly letter that 20 percent of their fellow investors ordered only five or fewer mammograms, another 20 percent referred six to ten patients, while 18 percent ordered thirty or more (ibid.).

"One physican has referred 115 patients during the first quarter," the letter from two of the doctor-investors enthused. "A fine example for us all to follow" (ibid.).

Not that the big centers are not fighting back. Upscale Memorial Sloan-Kettering has fielded a posh, designer-decorated mammogram van, undercutting independent operators by offering examinations for only $60 instead of the usual $125 or $200 paid in a hospital or a doctor's office. A Wall Street health-care analyst commented:

> Ancillary care is where the bucks are, it's that simple. Expensive high-tech services like magnetic resonance imaging, mammogram vans, and various types of chemotherapy are not only highly profitable, but for a big cancer center like Memorial, they help breed a kind of consumer loyalty. And with

lean years looming ahead, establishing a broad and devoted patient base is a very important concern right now (Goodell, 1989).

Memorial officials speak proudly of "our particular brand of cancer care," and there is even talk about opening Memorial franchises around the country—what has been called the "McDonalding of cancer care" (ibid).

Another high-tech, high-cost entry in the cancer war is positron emission tomography (PET), which brings with it supposedly sharper images and a $5 million price tag (Standard & Poor's, 1988). PET is being touted as "the greatest thing since penicillin," although most doctors believe it is no better than cheaper tests. The price of a single PET scan is $1800 (*Wall Street Journal*, April 3, 1989).

But the biggest bonanza of all may turn out to be a space-age device called a proton beam accelerator. This three-story-high machine, being installed at Loma Linda University Medical Center near Los Angeles, shoots protons at tumors. Protons are supposedly more accurate than other forms of radiation. In some rare types of cancer (e.g., malignancies at the base of the brain), prototypes of the Loma Linda machines have greatly increased the customary cure rate. But these appear to be the rare exceptions. For instance, the device is helpless against metatasized cancers, which account for two-thirds of all malignancies.

"There's some usefulness, no doubt about it," said Y. Joe Kwon, a radiation oncologist in Victorville, California. "It won't make a major impact on the cure rate for all cancers. It will make a little dent, but it will cost a lot to make that dent" (*Wall Street Journal*, March 17, 1989).

"It's a great physics project, but some of the medical claims are lunatic," says Joseph Imperato, a radiation oncologist and assistant professor at the Northwestern University Medical School (ibid.).

The money involved is astronomical.

"It's the most complicated machine ever used in a hospital setting by far," enthused the director of the Loma Linda project, James Slater, M.D. With a price tag of $40 million—$20 million for the machine and $20 million for its unique building—it is also the most expensive.

Loma Linda will attempt to treat 100 patients a day, operating around the clock if the demand is high enough. Although the price schedule is not yet known, the cost for treating cervical cancer will be somewhere between $13,000 and $23,000.

A San Diego company, hired by Loma Linda to market the device, predicts there will be approximately twenty proton beam accelerators in the United States within the next five to ten years, and a similar number in

Europe. Dr. Slater predicts that there will eventually be 100 such devices in the United States, with the cost falling to $10 million for each machine (ibid.). At that rate, the national cost will add up to a billion dollars—not counting another billion or so for installation.

An unexpected source of income is new forms of breast surgery. A study at the Long Island Jewish Medical Center found that when doctors remove only the lump instead of the whole breast, the cost is 37 percent more. The increased cost is largely the result of additional radiation treatments required after the lumpectomy. Of about 500,000 patients who undergo breast cancer surgery in the United States each year, about 100,000 are now having lumpectomies. But according to Dr. Eric Munoz, by 1990 between 40 and 50 percent of all patients might eventually be treated in this way (*New York Times*, November 25, 1986).

Drugs, too, have begun to assume importance in the cancer field. Although still modest by Wall Street standards, their sales are climbing steadily and form an important part of the cost of cancer for many patients (see chapter 5). The cost of drugs has skyrocketed in the 1980s. From 1981 through 1986 the price of prescription drugs soared 79 percent, while the consumer price index as a whole advanced only 28 percent. In 1987 alone the cost of drugs rose 8 percent and general medical expenses 5.8 percent, while the overall price increase was only 4.4 percent, according to the Bureau of Labor Statistics (*New York Times*, February 9, 1988).

"The drug companies evidently feel that they can get away with whatever the market will bear," said Representative Henry A. Waxman, the California Democrat who chairs the House health and environment subcommittee (ibid.).

To give some examples: A *single* injection of TPA, Genentech's anti-blood-clot medicine, costs $2,200. A year's worth of Factor VIII (produced by Armour), which speeds blood clotting, costs $25,000. AZT, a drug used in the treatment of AIDS, is $8,000 per year.

The cost of AZT led to civil disobedience in late January 1988, when nineteen people were arrested outside a distribution center of Burroughs Wellcome in California. The company responded by reducing the average cost from $10,000 to $8,000. (The firm will reportedly sell $130 million worth of the drug in 1988, with profits—after R&D expenses—of $20 million.) (*New York Times*, February 9, 1988).

Cancer drugs traditionally lag behind readily marketed substances such as clotting factors, but not by much. In 1986, according to *Business Week*, $450 million was being spent annually on cancer chemotherapy. But by the early 1990s, several biological products—the result of intense work on gene-splicing proteins and targeted antibodies—may *each* rival that entire market.

The drug companies are now spending about $200 million a year to develop these biological response modifiers (September 22, 1986).

Alpha interferon became the "first cancer drug of the new era" when it was approved by the FDA in 1986 for the treatment of a rare form of blood cancer called hairy-cell leukemia. Another biological that has made headlines is interleukin-2, promoted by President Reagan's surgeon at NCI, Steven A. Rosenberg. According to *Business Week,* interleukin (or IL-2, as it is commonly called) is "complex, expensive and toxic in its present form."

Just how expensive is highlighted by the activities of Biotherapeutics, Inc., a treatment center that offers state-of-the-art biological treatments for those who are willing and able to pay. The clinic, located in Franklin, Tennessee, was founded in 1985 by former NCI scientist, Robert K. Oldham, M.D. In the first year Oldham received over 1,000 requests for treatment and offered 120 persons experimental cancer treatment that had not yet gotten FDA approval—at fees of up to $35,000 apiece (ibid.). Even when and if IL-2 is approved for general use, it is not likely to be much cheaper. That is because it is patented and its price set by Immunex, a $78 million Seattle company, which has licensed it to Hoffmann–La Roche for clinical testing (ibid.). Other new drugs that promise to be very costly are gamma interferon, tumor necrosis factor, monoclonal antibodies, and colony stimulating factor. Ironically, these increased costs are often the result of the Orphan Drug Act of 1983, which was supposed to be a boon to consumers by encouraging the drug companies to develop treatments for relatively rare diseases. "Lawmakers little envisioned, however, that drugs would fetch such high prices . . . ," according to a front-page story in the *New York Times* (February 9, 1988).

Another reason for soaring medical costs is the increased use of in-office medical diagnostics. When SmithKline Beckman was looking for a proper advertising symbol with which to sell physicians on their new diagnostic equipment, they settled on a goose with a golden egg.

Cancer diagnosis is a huge medical business, fanned by the public's fear of the disease and forty years of publicity by the American Cancer Society. In 1974 more than 56 million women over the age of seventeen had Pap smears in the United States—and this for only one, relatively minor type of cancer (*Science,* July 13, 1979).

In a country where the medical system already consumes 11 percent of the gross national product, diagnostics have become one of the most lucrative parts of the system. It is seen as the physician's way of narrowing the irksome gap between his/her average yearly income ($80,300 in 1986) and that of the surgeons ($162,400). "We are only at the dawn of a push to turn great numbers of American physicians into hidden capitalists," said Uwe E. Reinhardt, a Princeton University professor who specializes in medical-cost issues (*New York Times*, May 15, 1988).

"It's a win-win-win-win situation," enthused Dr. Andrew P. Morley, chairman of the American Academy of Family Physicians. Cancer physicians use a great many diagnostic procedures, and the cancer victim and the insurance companies must pay for them. "At least a third if not more than half of what we do is of no benefit," said UCLA Professor of Medicine Robert H. Brook, "or of such marginal benefit that I think we could reach agreement in society that insurance should not pay for it" (ibid.).

One of the biggest cost generators remains the CAT (or CT) scan, a device that has become quite commonplace in doctor's clinics. It is expensive—but how necessary? Some critics say not very. "I find one person with a treatable lesion for every thousand CT scans I do, and the CT scans cost $300 each . . . ," said Dr. William B. Schwartz, a professor of medicine at the Tufts University School of Medicine. MRI scans cost $500–$1000 per hour examination (Waldhoz and Bogdanich, 1989.) Schwartz asks "at what point we can do more good by spending the money on, say, preventive medicine or the environment" (*New York Times*, May 15, 1988).

So great has fear of cancer's economic cost become that a new industry has sprung into existence: cancer insurance.

"Insurance salesmen are now marketing cancer insurance door-to-door in the vicinity of Three Mile Island," according to Sam Allalouf, public-relations director for Cancer Care, Inc. (*New York Times*, July 16, 1979).

Such insurance often provides coverage which simply duplicates that of Blue Cross or the other major plans—or fails to provide needed coverage. In 1978 the attorney general of Ohio conducted an investigation of an insurance company that billed itself a "pioneer and world's leader in the field of cancer expense insurance." The policies, he said, paid the cancer victim only while he was hospitalized ($100 per day). This appears to be a liberal payment; however, most patients spend an average of only fourteen days a year in the hospital. Most treatment today is provided on an out-patient basis.

As one indication of the profit to be made in the field: this insurance company paid out only 40 percent of the premiums it collected in Ohio, compared to 90 percent paid out by Blue Cross.

By the late 1980s health insurance companies and agencies had become major players in the cancer field. By setting reimbursement policies on various therapies, the insurance companies are "making decisions about the medical care of patients," according to an article by three Boston physicians, including Emil Frei 3d, M.D., in the *New England Journal of Medicine* (Antman, 1988).

The cost of treatment has become so great that cancer without insurance generally means second-rate care and almost certain bankruptcy. Thirty-seven million Americans are currently without such coverage.

But for those who do have insurance, there are problems as well. Insurers will generally pay for standard care—surgery, radiation, and chemotherapy—even when it holds out little hope of a cure. But they generally refuse to pay for experimental treatments.

At first this nonpayment clause was applied selectively to unorthodox practitioners; the cost of experimental toxic chemotherapy was usually borne by the federal research establishment. In the late 1980s, however, "funding for the costs of patient care has largely been deleted from research budgets" (ibid.). The insurance companies then balked at paying for these expenses since they too involved the experimental and unproven—even when administered at the most orthodox cancer centers.

The companies have been erratic. "Because the insurance industry is a decentralized industry," Mary McCabe, a clinical trial specialist at the NCI's Cancer Therapy Evaluation Program, explained, "reimbursement for a specific therapy is made in some areas of the country with some insurance carriers but in other places for that same therapy, it is not," (*Infectious Disease News*, January, 1989). She noted:

> In the past, they [i.e., insurers] inconsistently or infrequently invoked that exclusion, and they have paid. But, certainly, with the heavy financial pressures on insurance carriers, this exclusionary process has been one way of tightening the belt—to not pay for a patient's care if it relates directly to an investigational therapy (ibid.).

"Most patients assume that they are covered by health insurance for the costs of an investigational therapy . . . ," wrote Frei and his colleagues. "They are surprised and frequently angry to discover that the insurer will not cover these costs" (Altman et al., 1987).

Patients have not been the only ones to get angry. Orthodox physicians balked loudly when their own money and favorite projects were at risk— even though in the past some cancer bureaucrats had eagerly cooperated in the attempts of insurance companies to cut off payments to unconventional therapists, such as Dr. Lawrence Burton (chapter 12) and Dr. Stanislaw Burzynski (chapter 14). They were, in effect, hoist with their own petard.

At the beginning of 1989 an ad hoc committee—organized by the NCI and involving physicians, the drug industry, and cancer support associations—drafted a consensus protest letter to the insurance companies.

The presence of the drug industry in this meeting is significant. One proposed solution to the problem is that pharmaceutical companies pay the cost of clinical research; they, after all, will be the ultimate beneficiaries of any positive results. Frei and colleagues veto this proposal, however, because they consider it "a major financial disincentive to investment in this industry . . ." (ibid.).

If NCI-sponsored scientists are being hurt, one can imagine the effect of insurance companies' refusal to pay unconventional clinics. In fact, many of the tribulations of Drs. Burton, Burzynski, and other alternative practitioners stem from the hostile opposition of the major insurance carriers.

The current crisis in cancer cries out for new solutions. The public is confused, frightened, restless, and skeptical of the old, inadequate ways of treating the disease. The growing personal and national cost of cancer—the incredible tragedy and suffering, plus the staggering financial waste of it all—make new directions not just a dream, but a necessity.

« 2 »

The "Proven" Methods

Officially, however, all is well with the cancer war. Publications of the cancer establishment continue to exude optimism about the current ways of managing the disease.

Cancer is not just treatable, but *curable*. In fact, it has been called "one of the most curable of the major diseases in the country" (ACS publication cited in Greenberg, 1975). "Many cancers can be cured," we are assured, "if detected early and treated promptly" (ACS, 1988).

What exactly does the American Cancer Society mean by "cure"? In general parlance, as in the dictionary, a cure is a restoration to health or a sound condition—the elimination of a disease.

For years, however, the American Cancer Society maintained a peculiar definition of a cancer cure as a five-year survival after diagnosis. Asked by a *New York Times* reporter for his definition of the word, a baffled ACS vice president admitted, "I've never gone to a dictionary to look up a definition of cure. We really do not know what we mean by cure because there is a great difference between cure and long-term survival" (*New York Times*, April 17, 1979). The chancellor of Memorial Sloan-Kettering Cancer Center, Lewis Thomas, M.D., agreed; he "rarely hears the term 'cure' when doctors talk among themselves," he told the same reporter.

In recent years, however, the ACS definition of cure has become even hazier. For example, among the 2 million cured cancer victims in the United

21

States the ACS once included individuals who "still have evidence of cancer" (ACS, 1979). And while most people can be considered cured after five years, some patients can be declared cured after only *one* or perhaps three years (ACS, 1988).

This peculiar bookkeeping of cure rates has led to some bizarre situations. A man who is treated for cancer and survives five years is entered in the record book as a cure. What happens, if he has a recurrence of this cancer sometime later? What happens if he dies? He will then be in the paradoxical situation of having been officially cured of cancer, and dying of it at the same time.

This Alice-in-Wonderland logic may actually help to overstate the number of people being permanently freed of the disease, and to exaggerate the benefit of the so-called proven methods of treatment.

The bottom line for a cancer therapy is how many people it actually saves. By the ACS's own statistics, about 40 percent of Americans who get cancer this year will be alive five years after diagnosis. While this is up from about 33 percent ten years ago, it still leaves more than half the cancer population beyond the reach of conventional methods. In addition, the methods of measuring cancer statistics are highly disputed (see p. 23).

Two interpretations of this anomaly are possible. First, one might say there is something wrong with the currently employed "proven" methods of treatment. This the cancer establishment will not say, since it has helped promote these methods for many years and is committed to them.

The difficulty, says the American Cancer Society, lies with people themselves. They need education to trust in these methods; and in the fight against cancer the best weapons are an annual checkup and a check, according to the famous slogan.

If people would avail themselves of the current methods of dealing with the illness through earlier diagnosis and treatment, the Society claims, 174,000 cancer victims could be saved each year.

But there are serious questions about the safety and efficacy of some of these diagnostic techniques. After many years of trying, there is still no chemical test that can detect the presence of cancer in the body, and "it will apparently be many years before a biochemical assay for cancer will be in use" (Maugh and Marx, 1975:94), a statement that has turned out to be a realistic prediction. The establishment must therefore rely on less certain methods for detection, whose value is in doubt.

For over forty years the Society has been associated with the Pap smear test for cancer, a prime means of diagnosing cervical and uterine cancer.

The rate of death from this type of cancer has indeed plummeted since the 1940s. For years the ACS lauded the Pap test as the *cause* of this decline. However, some observers have claimed that the Pap test had little to do with this trend:

> The mortality rate from cervical cancer was already dropping in this country in the late 1940s, before screening became popular, and the critics suggest that Pap smears have made little or no contribution to the continuing decline (*Science*, July 13, 1979).

In 1979 the ACS quietly dropped its recommendation that women receive an *annual* Pap test and insisted only on a *regular* one (ibid.). It now recommends that a person take the test annually until three consecutive tests are negative, and then less frequently (ACS, 1988).

Why then has the Pap test been so widely utilized in the United States? According to two scientists from New York University and Yale University School of Medicine, the answer is primarily economic. As they told *Science:*

> The annual Pap smear has become so entrenched in this country partly because it has been so heavily promoted and partly because so much of the cost is borne by the private individual. In England and Canada, where the governments bear practically all the costs, annual tests are not recommended, at least for low-risk women (*Science*, July 13, 1979).

The Pap smear may indeed be, as the magazine suggests, "an idea whose time has gone."

No less questionable—or controversial—has been the use of X rays to detect breast cancer: mammography. The American Cancer Society initially promoted the procedure as a safe and simple way to detect breast tumors early and thus allow women to undergo mastectomies before their cancers had metastasized.

Three hundred thousand women were enrolled in a joint ACS-NCI (National Cancer Institute) program at twenty-seven breast cancer detection centers in 1972 and given an average of two rads of radiation per examination (*New York Times*, March 28, 1976).

Criticism of this project started almost immediately within the NCI. Dr. John C. Bailar III, editor of the *Journal* of the National Cancer Institute, went public with these criticisms in January 1976 when he wrote:

There is a body of information that the benefits to women under the age of fifty may not be as great as was thought when the project was started (ibid.).

There is a possibility, Bailar added, that the procedure would cause as many deaths through the carcinogenic effect of radiation as it would save through early diagnosis.

As the controversy heated up in 1976, it was revealed that the hundreds of thousands of women enrolled in the program were never told the risk they faced from the procedure (ibid.). Young women faced the greatest danger. In the thirty-five- to fifty-year-old age group, each mammogram increased the subject's chance of contracting breast cancer by 1 percent, according to Dr. Frank Rauscher, then director of the National Cancer Institute (*New York Times*, August 23, 1976).

The NCI appointed a committee of experts, headed by Dr. Lester Breslow of UCLA, to recommend a way out of the dilemma. The Breslow report recommended that the agency discontinue the routine use of X-ray screening for breast cancer in symptom-free women under the age of fifty (*New York Times*, July 15, 1976). An "extremely reluctant" American Cancer Society deferred to this decision, which was a direct slap in the face to their early-detection strategy.*

In the 1970s the NCI recommended mammography in symptom-free women only when they (1) age fifty or over, (2) age thirty-five to forty-nine and had had cancer in one breast, and (3) age forty to forty-nine whose mother and/or sister had had the disease (Cancer Information Service, 1977).

The question of breast cancer detection is urgent: one out of ten women in the United States will develop this disease sometime in her lifetime (ACS, 1988:20). When tumors are found in a very early stage, they are largely curable through surgery and other means. In advanced stages the prognosis is very poor. A great deal is therefore at stake in early detection.

The ACS has a strategy for detecting breast cancer, which it calls its "three-part, personal plan of action," including a clinical breast exam, breast self-examination, and mammography. This seems perfectly reasonable, yet each has generated sharp controversy within the medical profession and among the public.

Many doctors perform clinical breast examinations on their patients and teach their patients to do so as well. The Cancer Society suggests that all women over twenty conduct a breast self-examination (BSE) every month.

*In the midst of the debate, Kodak took out full-page ads in scientific journals entitled "About breast cancer and X-rays: A hopeful message from industry on a sober topic" (see *Science*, July 2, 1976). Kodak is a major manufacturer of mammography film.

THE "PROVEN" METHODS

"BSE can detect suspicious lumps or call attention to fibrocystic breast tissue" writes an ACS vice president (Laszlo, 1987:142).
Yet in April 1987 the U.S. Preventive Services Task Force questioned
that recommendation. They stated that there is little scientific evidence that
self-examination is accurate and no prospective data showing that it saves
lives (Thomas, 1988).
In fact, most self-detected lesions are quite large and therefore have a
poor prognosis. "The medical care system is saying to the woman, 'Find
your own incurable disease and then we'll treat it,' " according to radiologist Myron Moskowitz, M.D. (ibid.).
Many doctors are unskilled at finding small lesions. In fact, a study
done by the Breast Cancer Detection Demonstration Project in the 1970s
found that only 8 percent of breast cancers were found through physicians'
clinical examinations alone. Ninety percent were seen on mammograms,
which are X-ray examinations of the soft tissues of the breast. The ACS
believes that women over fifty and those with family histories of breast
tumors and, naturally, those who have found suspicious lumps should all
have mammograms. Few would disagree with this. But they go further and
recommend that *asymptomatic women in their forties* should have mammograms every one to two years.
This is the nub of the controversy. The National Cancer Institute, the
American College of Radiology, and the AMA agree with them. But the
American College of Physicians, the American College of Obstetricians and
Gynecologists, the U.S. Preventive Services Task Force, and the Canadian
Task Force on the Periodic Health Examination all disagree (ibid.).
A controversial study done by Dr. David M. Eddy, head of Duke
University's Center for Health Policy Research, and published in the *New
England Journal of Medicine* included a cost/benefit analysis of mammog-
raphy. It concluded that if 25 percent of the nation's women aged 40 to 49
were screened annually from 1987 to the year 2000, it would save 373 lives
a year but would cost approximately $402 million to do so (Eddy, 1987).
In an accompanying editorial, Dr. John C. Bailar, then head of epidemiology and biostatistics at McGill University in Montreal, concluded:
"Routine screening of this age group should be discontinued" (Bailar, 1987).
Then there is the question of the risk from radiation. "A very small
amount of radiation is used in performing mammograms, but the benefit
seems to far outweigh the risk," says Laszlo. It is certainly true that the
amount of radiation involved has decreased over the last decade, from about
1.5 or 2 rads in the 1970s (*U.S. News and World Report*, May 14, 1979) to
0.2–0.4 rads per breast today with new machines and fast paper (Strong,
1989).

But that doesn't mean that all risk has been removed. As radiologist Philip Rubin, M.D., wrote in his ACS-sponsored textbook, ". . . tumor induction information for extremely low doses . . . has been difficult to obtain [and] . . . is a subject of great debate" (Rubin, 1983).

According to Eddy, the risk of radiation-induced cancer through such a mass screening program is about one in 25,000. This seems small until one considers that there are 18 million women in the U.S. between the ages of 40 and 49.

Cost, quality, and availability are other problems. Mammograms average $150 per study, "which alone makes it inaccessible for many low-income people" (Laszlo, 1987.) Four states have mandated that insurance companies pay for the procedure, but in most others it is not covered.

Cheaper tests are sometimes available, but their quality is often questionable, as it takes a skilled radiologist to read the X rays. Bad mammography can even be dangerous, due to faulty equipment or misdiagnoses. According to a report in *Medical World News,*

> Screening mammography is a growth industry these days. Facilities are popping up in shopping malls, and mobile mammogaphy vans are cruising some city streets. Nonradiologists—particularly obstetricians and gynecologists—are setting up their own shops and funneling patients into them (Thomas, 1988).

And despite increased and earlier detection, breast cancer is still on the rise. There will be an estimated 142,000 new cases in 1989—seven thousand more than the year before (ACS, 1989). The breast cancer death rate went up 3 percent in the thirty years between 1953–55 and 1983–85. No one knows why. Cancer remains an unpredictable disease.

Although real progress has been made in diagnosis through devices such as magnetic resonance imaging (MRI), no current method of cancer detection is likely to dramatically decrease the death rate from the disease. In fact, there are many instances in which patients have followed the ACS's advice, gotten checkups, received approved therapy early in the course of their illness, and still died.

From 1976 to 1978, the public had a dramatic illustration of the unpredictability of the "proven" methods of diagnosis and treatment. Senator Hubert H. Humphrey (D.-Minn.) was treated for bladder cancer and died in full view of the media.

Humphrey did not die because he lacked knowledge about the disease.

He was, in fact, one of the staunchest supporters of orthodox cancer research on Capitol Hill (Prescott, 1976).

Nor did he fail to get early diagnosis. Doctors found tiny, apparently nonmalignant growths, no bigger than pinheads, on his bladder in 1966. By 1973, however, Senator Humphrey had cancer of the bladder. This was treated, with apparent success, by X-ray therapy. He then underwent urologic examinations every six months. In May 1976 Humphrey's physician, Dr. Dabney Jarman, declared that he found no reason to prescribe further treatment for the condition (*New York Times*, May 6, 1976). A few months later the cancer was back with a vengeance.

On October 6, 1976, Senator Humphrey was operated on by a team of doctors at Memorial Hospital, the treatment wing of Memorial Sloan-Kettering. His surgeon, Willard Whitmore, appeared before the press and television cameras at a crowded news conference and declared, "As far as we are concerned, the Senator is cured" (*New York Times*, October 8, 1976). He added that 70 percent of patients who undergo this operation have no recurrence of their cancer (ibid.). Merely as a preventive measure, to "wipe out any microscopic colonies of cancer cells that may be hidden somewhere in the body" (ibid.), his doctors began treatment with experimental drugs. Within about a year, Senator Humphrey was dead. In that short time he had withered from a vigorous middle-aged man to an old, balding, and feeble cancer victim. Humphrey himself blamed chemotherapy for at least contributing to his demise, calling it "bottled death" and refusing in the end to return to Memorial Hospital for more drug treatments (*New York Daily News*, January 14, 1978).

Humphrey was certainly not alone in his experience with orthodox therapy.

In Humphrey's case, as in many others, the orthodox strategy of early detection and early treatment with surgery, radiation, and chemotherapy proved ineffective. Many cancer patients have their cancers detected in an early stage, receive proper treatment and skillful care—and yet they still die. Such cases are soon forgotten, however, in the deluge of favorable publicity over such successful treatments as those of Ronald Reagan.

Years of cultivating the press had made the American Cancer Society virtually sacrosanct. From 1945 to 1975 one could search in vain for an incisive, critical article on the Society or its methods. Then, in the mid-1970s, criticism suddenly burst into the open about the whole topic of cancer. The "war on cancer" had made the leading organizations visible and vulnerable.

In 1975, as part of the trend, Daniel S. Greenberg, a well-known Washington reporter, published an article titled "A Critical Look at Cancer

Coverage" (Daniel Greenberg, 1975). The piece, which appeared in the respected *Columbia Journalism Review*, was widely reprinted and quoted. Studying government figures and talking to cancer therapists and researchers, Greenberg found that the cancer picture was in fact very discouraging: it is "a far gloomier picture than has been generally conveyed to a hopeful public by our leading cancer research institutions and by the American Cancer Society." Greenberg noted that

> Today's patient, who is supposedly the beneficiary of the burgeoning of cancer research that began in the early 1950s, has approximately the same chance of surviving for at least five years as a patient whose illness was diagnosed before any of that research took place (ibid.).

By surveying the then most recent National Cancer Institute figures, published in 1972, Greenberg found that the cancer survival rates for most types of cancer had largely remained static from the 1950s on. What improvement was noted from 1930 to 1950 was probably the result of better support systems and nursing care in the hospitals surveyed rather than true improvements in cancer therapy.

By adding some more recent data supplied by NCI, Greenberg contended that the survival rates for some kinds of cancer had actually *declined* in recent years. The one-year survival for cancer of the colon, for example, had been 68 percent in the period 1965–69; it fell to 65 percent in 1970–71, according to government figures. Why the decline? Some experts told Greenberg it was because of the more vigorous application of proven methods like toxic chemotherapy, which sometimes kills those patients on whom it is used.

Orthodox cancer literature has stressed the dramatic breakthroughs in the treatment of leukemia and other childhood diseases. Undoubtedly, dramatic improvement has been made in this area. But Greenberg found that "the official statistics do not support the optimistic claims" emanating from cancer center public-relations offices. The survival rates for all kinds of leukemia, for example, although "apparently improving as a result of new chemotherapies, remain tragically low." The median survival time in government statistics on leukemia victims is still measured in *months*, not years (see chapter 5).

A cancer statistician cautioned Greenberg to take all cure statistics on relatively rare diseases, such as leukemia, with a dose of skepticism:

> When you're dealing with such small numbers [he said] it is easy for a small amount of misdiagnosis to produce a big change in the survival statis-

tics. I wouldn't be surprised if they're curing a lot of leukemia that never existed (ibid.).

Another scientist told him that the high cure rates in general are based on inept diagnoses. Some regional hospitals, he said, list people with undiagnosed lumps and bumps as cancer cases. These often turn out to have been noncancerous. Nonetheless, such cases go into the records as cancer patients, and when they survive five years they are officially "cured" of a disease they never had.

"Actually," this researcher told Greenberg, "there has been little improvement since 1945."

There are many ways to arrange statistics to make them look favorable to a particular method.

Clinicians can select their cases, for example, and choose only those patients they feel have the best chances of survival. In *The Savage Cell*, Pat McGrady, Sr., remarked on this phenomenon:

> If one examines closely enough the cases operated upon by a surgeon enjoying an extraordinarily high cure rate, he is almost certain to find that the surgeon has refused to operate on many patients with only a fair-to-middling chance of cure. The cure rates by other surgeons of equal skill may be low because of the number of long-shot gambles they take in trying to cure patients of doubtful curability (McGrady, Sr., 1964:310).

Most clinicians would like to have a high cure rate: such statistics can be instrumental in determining the allocation of federal grants, promotions, or the procurement of future patients. The temptation is always present for one doctor or an entire center to arrange its statistics in such a way as to exaggerate the progress actually being made.

Research-oriented institutions, for example, may carefully select patients for clinical trials of new agents. In pilot research projects, doctors generally want to show high cure rates and long survival figures. Patients in such studies may be given the best possible backup care in order to increase their chances of survival.

"Clinical researchers don't like to treat dying patients," a scientist told Greenberg bluntly. "Poor risks can be sent elsewhere to die."

At the 1975 ACS Science Writers' Seminar, then NCI director Frank Rauscher responded to Greenberg's charges: Greenberg's figures, while accurate, were out-of-date and did not reflect the progress of the war on cancer. ACS president Dr. George P. Rosemond even predicted that by 1978 "we will have reached the potential saving of one in two cancer victims" (*New York Times*, March 22, 1975). But when updated figures did appear, the new statistics did not support this argument.

The National Cancer Institute program issued "Cancer Patient Survival Report No. 5" in 1976. It was the most complete compilation of data on cancer survival made up to that point. By and large, the government report confirmed many of Greenberg's contentions and threw additional light on the frequent failure of orthodox therapy.

Although survival rates for six of the ten most common forms of cancer had improved since the early 1960s, the average improvement was minuscule. Large numbers of people were still dying of all types of cancer, despite adequate treatment with the so-called proven methods of therapy.

In no common form of cancer were there any real "breakthroughs" between 1950 and 1973 (see Figure 1). For example, in that period the five-year survival rate (so-called cure rate) among whites increased 4 percentage points for breast cancer, 9 for bladder, 3 for colon, 2 for lung, and 1 for pancreas. The rate for stomach cancer remained static. It went down 2 percentage points for cancer of the cervix (NCI, 1976b).

In almost every case, the 1967–73 five-year survival rate for blacks was far less than for whites: 30 percentage points less for cancer of the corpus uteri; 29 points for cancer of the bladder, and so forth. NCI ascribed these differences to "socioeconomic factors not yet identified in detail."

In Greenberg's report the "cure" rate for pancreatic cancer was 1 percent—in other words, 99 out of 100 were dead five years after diagnosis. For lung cancer it was 9 percent; for colon—the most common cancer in males—it was 46 percent among whites, 35 percent among blacks.

Aside from these less-than-encouraging survival figures for most common cancers, the 315-page report also yielded many examples of a decline in survival for the less common tumors. For example, the one-, five-, and ten-year survival rates for lip cancer declined several percentage points in the latest figures. For pancreatic cancer the one-year survival rate had been 17 percent for whites in 1950–54. This dropped to 10 percent in 1960–64 and climbed back to 14 percent in 1970–73, still several points below the 1950–54 figure, however. This decline coincided with the increased use of chemotherapy in the treatment of this malignancy: in 1950–53 only 2 percent of these patients had received chemotherapy, but in the 1970s over 20 percent received it (ibid.:131).

There is even some doubt that these official figures, unpromising as they seem, really tell the whole truth. They may actually make the "proven" methods appear more successful than they actually are.

To begin with, these government statistics are based on results gath-

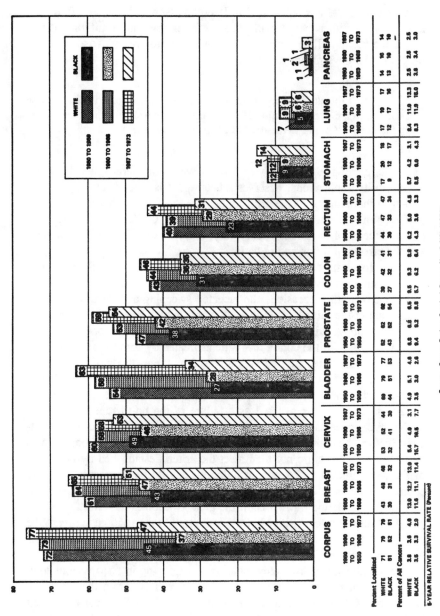

FIGURE I

Five-Year Relative Survival Rates (Percent) For Ten Common Types of Cancer

ered from four "tumor registries" in Berkeley, New Orleans, Hartford, and Iowa City. Together they provide data on fewer than half a million patients out of the many millions who had cancer during the period 1950–73. The editors of the government study concede:

> It is difficult if not impossible to assess whether data contributed by these registries are a true reflection of cancer patient survival throughout the United States (*HEW News*, Bethesda, Md., September 19, 1977).

There is an alternative view on the value of therapy which, while radical in its implications, deserves a hearing. It is most frequently associated with the name of Dr. Hardin Jones. Dr. Jones, who died in 1978, was professor of medical physics at the University of California, Berkeley, assistant director of its Donner Laboratory, and an expert on statistics, aging, and the effects of drugs and radiation.

Dr. Jones spoke at the Eleventh Annual Science Writers' Seminar held by the American Cancer Society in New Orleans in March 1969. On this and numerous other occasions, he repeated sweeping and disturbing observations about the failure of orthodox therapy, which he had first elaborated in a New York Academy of Sciences presentation in 1956 (Jones, 1956).

First, he said, the notion that patients treated by conventional therapies live longer than untreated victims "is biased by the methods of defining the groups." Thus, Jones claimed, if a person in the untreated category dies at any time while he or she is being studied, this is recorded as a death in the control group, and is registered as a failure of the no-treatment approach. If, however, patients in the treated category die during the course of treatment (before the course is completed), their cases are rejected from the data since "these patients do not then meet the criteria established by definition of the term 'treated.' " A patient dying on day 89 of a prescribed 90-day course of chemotherapy would be dropped from the list of treated patients. The longer the period of treatment, the greater becomes the error.

"With this effect stripped out," Jones said to the 1969 gathering, "the common malignancies show a remarkably similar rate of demise, whether treated or untreated."

Second, said the Berkeley radiologist, beginning in 1940 various low-grade kinds of malignancies were redefined as cancer. From that date, the proportion of "cancer" cases being cured increased rapidly, "corresponding to the fraction of questionable diagnoses included."

Third, Jones's research showed no relationship between the intensity of treatment and survival rates. Radical surgery, for instance, did not seem to be more successful than more limited operations that removed only the tumor and small amounts of normal tissue.

Fourth, there is no proof that early detection affects survival. "Serious attempts to relate prompt treatment with chance of cure have been unsuccessful."

Jones concluded that

> evidence for benefit from cancer therapy has depended on systematic biometric errors. . . . The possibility exists that treatment makes the average situation worse (ibid.).

To reporters Jones once stated that, in his opinion, "radical surgery does more harm than good," and as for radiation treatment, "most of the time it makes not the slightest difference whether the machine is turned on or not" (*Santa Ana* [Calif.] *Register*, January 19, 1974).

Though Jones's arguments certainly seem to contradict universally held beliefs on the value of therapy, little research refutes his position. In fact, from 1956 (when he first propounded his views) to 1978 only three studies tested the validity of his conclusions. All three upheld his theory (Houston and Null, 1978).*

It is also obvious that orthodox treatments have not been able to stop the rise in cancer mortality: there has been a steady increase in the cancer death rate in the United States in this century. Cancer accounted for one in 27 deaths in 1900, one in 16 in 1920, one in 12 in 1930, one in nine in 1940, one in seven in 1950, one in six in 1960–70, and one in five in 1988 (ACS, 1988).

It might appear that the reason for this increase is simply that we are living longer and that cancer is a disease of old and middle age. But this is not the only reason for the increase: these figures are *age-adjusted,* and have already taken into account the shift in seniority among the population.

In fact, people appear to be getting cancer earlier than ever before. Pediatrician Ronald Glasser notes that during the Christmas holidays of 1975, "of the twenty-three children admitted to the largest pediatric ward of the University of Minnesota Hospitals in a single day, eighteen had cancer." After noting that the cancer "death rate has been going up continuously," he adds:

*See also articles by G. H. Green in *Australian and New Zealand Journal of Obstetrics and Gynecology* (vol. 10, 1970) and by B. Zumoff, H. Hart, and L. Hellman in *Annals of Internal Medicine* (vol. 64, 1966).

As alarming as these figures are, they are still misleading. The cancers we are seeing today did not begin yesterday or the day before, but twenty, thirty and even forty years ago. Scientists now agree that most adult malignancies have their beginning in childhood. . . . (Glasser, 1979).

Thus, the overall picture is not a bright one, despite the sugary optimism of the official pronouncements. Evaluating progress and success in the war on cancer depends on statistics. How many people are dying? How many are actually being saved? These questions are central to the political debate on cancer. NCI's appropriation in 1988 was almost $1.5 billion. The agency is requesting nearly $2.2 billion for 1990 (NCI, 1988). But Congress and the voting public respond best to graphs and charts showing improvement. Statistics hold the key.

For years boosters of the cancer war controlled this terrain, claiming great progress in fighting the disease, with dramatic numbers to back them up. Almost without exception, the media echoed these claims.

"A Quiet New Optimism," "More Lives Retrieved," "Research: Finally Striking It Rich," were typical headlines of the early and mid-eighties (*U.S. News and World Report,* August 20, 1984).

Ten years ago the standard figure for cancer "cures" (generally interpreted as five-year, disease-free survival) was around one-third (ACS, 1979). In the intervening decade, however, the cancer establishment upped its claims. At this writing it is standard practice to claim that almost half of all cancer patients are being cured. "Forty-nine percent will be alive five years after diagnosis," according to the American Cancer Society (ACS, 1988). At first blush this seems like a remarkable improvement.

Upon closer examination, however, this enormous increase in cancer survival is little more than a statistical artifact, designed to improve the image of the cancer warriors in the eyes of Congress and the public. The problem was well put in a 1987 article in *Scientific American:*

> Three out of ten U.S. residents will, at present rates, be diagnosed as having cancer. This depressing statistic creates a demand for good news, a demand that the National Cancer Institute, which must sell its program to Congress every year, and the charities that support research and care are eager to meet. As a rule the good news comes as an announcement that the five-year survival rate for one or another form of cancer has increased (*Scientific American,* June 1987:29).

Are we making progress or failing? To find out, we must take a closer look at the figures themselves.

Statisticians have devised various methods to judge progress over the years. The three main ways are:

1. The number of people contracting the disease per year.
2. The number of people dying each year.
3. The number of people surviving for a set length of time.

The most central issue in the case of cancer would seem to be the death rate. If people continue to die at a high rate, then no matter what anyone says, we still have a major problem. And here there is no doubt: the death figures are rising.

This information is printed in the American Cancer Society's useful annual survey, *Cancer Facts and Figures*. In 1962, for instance, there were approximately 278,000 deaths from cancer in the United States. By 1982 there were more than 433,000. In 1988 the estimated figure was 494,000. By 1989 America for the first time had over half a million deaths (and a million new cases). In thirty years the number of victims has nearly doubled. While lung cancer accounts for much of this rise, deaths from brain cancer and multiple myeloma have also shown a "surprisingly sharp increase" (*New York Times*, March 18, 1988).

On this count alone, a naive observer might say we are losing the war. Statisticians point out, however, that such figures can be deceiving. The "graying of America" has brought with it an increase in overall cancer mortality. More people are living long enough to die of cancer. In addition, the population as a whole has increased during this time.

Adjusting the statistics to take these changes into account yields the more reliable age-adjusted figures. Even when this is done, however, the *age-adjusted cancer mortality figures show a 8.7 percent increase* in deaths from the disease in the 20-year period between 1962 and 1982—from 170.0 to 185.0 per 100,000 Americans (Bailar and Smith, 1986).

Another measurement of progress is the incidence of the disease. Here, too, there has been a significant increase. From 1973 to 1981 the crude incidence rate for all neoplasms combined rose by 13 percent (ibid.). When age-adjusted, the rise in cancer incidence is 8.5 percent.

That leaves the third category, the "cures," or five-year survivals. Here, too, at first glance there has been little improvement. According to Bailar and Smith, the absolute five-year survival among whites in 1973 was 38.5 percent; five years later, in 1978, it had only reached 40.1 percent.

The cancer warriors were clearly disturbed by such unimpressive figures. They therefore found a more impressive set of figures to bring before

FIGURE 2

Trends in Survival by Site of Cancer, by Race

Cases Diagnosed in 1960–63, 1970–73, 1974–76, 1977–78, 1979–84

Site	White					Black				
	Relative 5-Year Survival					Relative 5-Year Survival				
	1960–63[1]	1970–73[1]	1974–76[2]	1977–78[2]	1979–84[2]	1960–63[1]	1970–73[1]	1974–76[2]	1977–78[2]	1979–84[2]
All Sites	39%	43%	50%	50%	50%	27%	31%	38%	38%	37%
Oral Cavity & Pharynx	45	43	54	53	54	—	—	35	35	31
Esophagus	4	4	5	6	7	1	4	4	2	5
Stomach	11	13	14	15	16*	8	13	15	16	17
Colon	43	49	50	52	54*	34	37	45	44	49
Rectum	38	45	48	50	52*	27	30	40	40	34
Liver	2	3	4	3	3	—	—	1	1	5
Pancreas	1	2	3	2	3	1	2	2	3	5
Larynx	53	62	66	69	66	5	7	58	59	55
Lung & Bronchus	8	10	12	13	13*	—	—	11	10	11
Melanoma of Skin	60	68	78	81	80*	—	—	62##	—	61*
Breast (females)	63	68	74	75	75*	46	51	62	62	62
Cervix Uteri	58	64	69	69	67	47	61	61	63	59
Corpus Uteri	73	81	89	87	83*	31	44	61	58	52*
Ovary	32	36	36	37	37*	32	32	41	40	36
Prostate Gland	50	63	67	70	73*	35	55	56	64	60*
Testis	63	72	78	86	91*	—	—	77#	—	82#

Urinary Bladder	53	61	73	75	77*	24	36	47	53	57*
Kidney & Renal Pelvis	37	46	51	50	51	38	44	49	54	53
Brain & Nervous System	18	20	22	23	23	19	19	27	24	31
Thyroid Gland	83	86	92	92	93	—	—	88	92	95
Hodgkin's Disease	40	67	71	73	74*	—	—	67*	79*	69
Non-Hodgkin's Lymphoma	31	41	47	48	49*	—	—	47	46	49
Multiple Myeloma	12	19	24	24	24	—	—	28	30	29
Leukemia	14	22	34	37	32	—	—	30	31	27

Source: Surveillance and Operations Research Branch, National Cancer Institute. All figures are rounded off.

[1] Rates are based on End Results Group data from a series of hospital registries and one population-based registry.

[2] Rates are from the SEER Program. They are based on data from population-based registries in Connecticut, New Mexico, Utah, Iowa, Hawaii, Atlanta, Detroit, Seattle-Puget Sound and San Francisco-Oakland. Rates are based on follow-up of patients through 1985.

*The difference in rates between 1974–76 and 1979–84 is statistically significant (p<.05).

#The standard error of the survival rate is between 5 and 10 percentage points.

##The standard error of the survival rate is greater than 10 percentage points.

— Valid survival rate could not be calculated.

Congress: a variant on the five-year survival statistic called the *relative survival rate*. According to cancer officials, relative survival rate is "considered a more accurate yardstick" for measuring cancer progress (ACS, 1988).

Relative survival rates take into account the "expected mortality figures." Put simply, this means that if a person hadn't died of cancer he might have been run over by a truck, and that must be factored into the equation. With the use of this rubber yardstick, *49.2 percent* of today's cancer patients will be alive five years after diagnosis. This is where the "fifty percent cured" claim comes from. Heady from this paper success, the NCI and the National Cancer Advisory Board (NCAB) have called for *doubling* this alleged cure rate by the year 2000. Such a vast improvement, we are told, will mean the saving of hundreds of thousands of lives (ibid.).

The way this "increase" played in the press can be seen from a story in the normally sober *U.S. News and World Report:* "Overall cancer survival, now almost 50 percent for all patients, has jumped almost 5 percentage points since 1981. . . . Much of that progress is due to better combinations of surgery, drugs and radiation," according to Dr. Vincent DeVita, Jr., then director of the National Cancer Institute (August 25, 1985).

On May 8, 1986, these euphoric claims of great progress came undone. Dr. John C. Bailar III, a former editor of the *Journal of the National Cancer Institute,* published a special article in the *New England Journal of Medicine.* Bailar, then a researcher at the Department of Biostatistics of the Harvard School of Public Health, and his colleague, Elaine M. Smith of the University of Iowa Medical Center, delivered a devastating critique of NCI's number juggling.*

There was no disagreement over the Bailar-Smith figures (as opposed to their interpretation), since they came from the most up-to-date data available from NCI's SEER program.

The authors set out to assess the "overall progress against cancer during the years 1950 to 1982." Their conclusion was that these years were associated with "increases in the number of deaths from cancer, in the crude cancer-related mortality rate, in the age-adjusted mortality rate, and in the age-adjusted incidence rates." On the other hand, the "reported survival rates" also increased. Apparently more people were getting cancer and more people were dying of it—even on an age-adjusted basis—yet more people were surviving longer. How to explain this paradox?

*Bailar has since become head of epidemiology and biostatistics at McGill University, Montreal.

Bailar and Smith indicated several flaws in the way NCI reported statistical progress. For one thing, NCI generally reports whites-only figures. Nonwhites (the term employed by Bailar and Smith, since several racial groups are included) are kept in a separate category, untallied with the main group.

"A study of cancer rates over several decades shows that the cancer incidence rate for blacks is higher than for whites, and that the death rate is also higher" (ACS, 1988). *The black male cancer death rate has gone up an extraordinary 77 percent over a 30-year period.* Survival rates are also worse. The presence of these black people would depress the statistics. NCI's solution is to list them in separate (but equal) charts, and then to present the white charts as the norm. By the time this reaches the public, blacks have been all but forgotten in the general euphoria over the alleged 49.2 percent cures.

For example, in his 1990 budget request for $2.195 billion, Dr. DeVita wrote, "In 1971, only 35 percent of patients were cured of cancer . . . today half of all cancer patients can be cured" (NCI, 1988). By sliding from actual cures in 1971 to potential cures today, DeVita begs the questions raised above.

U.S. News, picking up the cue, tells us that "overall cancer survival" is "now almost 50 percent for all patients" (August 26, 1985). What this really amounts to, however, is a questionable way of tallying the survival of *white* patients only. This point is omitted from the story, and is revealed only in a footnote to an earlier article (August 20, 1984).

A second peculiarity is that lung cancer is sometimes omitted from the statistics. The reason is that the main cause of this increase, cigarette smoking, is unrelated to anything NCI has done in the area of treatment.

NCI frustration with smokers is understandable; what is not understandable is how they can skew their figures in this way.

Bailar and Smith cogently remark, "Reasons for such an omission have not been clearly stated, although it conveniently reverses the overall rise in mortality from cancer." In fact, the rise in lung cancer, according to the two authors, can be seen as "the best illustration" of their contention that "despite great effort over many years, research on cancer treatment has failed to deal effectively with the cancer problem." NCI does not take it that way. It treats lung cancer as a kind of aberration. When they exclude lung cancer, the overall age-adjusted mortality from cancer since 1980 shifts from an 8 percent increase to a 13 percent decrease!

Yet if one is to exclude cancers whose mortality rates have increased for reasons unrelated to treatment, one should in fairness also exclude those whose rates have been *decreasing* for similar reasons. These include cancer of the stomach and of the cervix. When this is done, the age-adjusted mortality shifts from 130.1 in 1950 to 128.9 in 1980—a change of less than 1 percent. "It is difficult to claim success in the war against cancer on the basis of these figures" (Bailar and Smith, 1986).

Third, NCI's use of relative survival rates resulted in an instant increase in the cancer survival statistics by about eight or nine percentage points! Take, for instance, the eleven-point "gain" in five-year survival of breast cancer patients (from 63 percent to 74 percent) from the sixties to the seventies. Very impressive. But what the cancer warriors do not generally tell us is that eight or nine out of those eleven points are an artifact of the big changeover in statistical methods at the cancer institute.

This changeover makes historical comparisons extremely difficult. For instance, even if we were to grant the accuracy of a current five-year relative survival rate for cancer patients of nearly 50 percent, would this really represent a 16 or 17 percentage-point increase since the late 1970s? Hardly. To compare the old absolute survival rates with the new relative survival rates is, quite simply, to compare apples with oranges. NCI has switched rulers. The *relative* survival rate in 1973 was 46.8 percent. Thus, even with all the fiddling mentioned above, *there has only been an increase of a few percentage points among the white population.*

And this is where the role of early diagnosis comes in. Science writer Robert Houston definitively explained the way this has warped the recent statistics:

> There is a lot of evidence that new techniques indeed are able to diagnose cancer earlier on an average of about one-half year. What does this do? It converts what used to be a . . . four-and-one-half-year survival rate to a five-year survival rate. Nothing has changed on the survival graphs except the points they choose to measure from! Naturally, the earlier the detection, the longer the survival from that point; you have not affected the curve whatsoever (Houston, 1987b).

Evaluating NCI's professed goal of halving the cancer mortality rate by the year 2000, Bailar and Smith produced an interesting chart. It showed that cancer deaths would have to take a "precipitous and unprecedented" nosedive in order for this to happen. "We do not believe that hopes for such a change are realistic," they wrote (Bailar and Smith, 1986).

"The main conclusion we draw," the two researchers wrote toward the end of this devastating critique, "is that some 35 years of intense effort focused largely on improving treatment must be judged a qualified failure. Results have not been what they were intended and expected to be" (ibid.).

Not surprisingly, the Bailar/Smith article was greeted with loud attacks on the authors. NCI director Vincent De Vita said Bailar had "departed with reality" (*Science*, April 24, 1987) and Dr. John Durant, president of the American Society of Clinical Oncology (ASCO), called Bailar "the great nay sayer of our time" (*New York Times*, May 8, 1986). There was little in the way of substantive refutation, however.

The Bailar/Smith article was followed by a second devastating blow. In 1987 the United States General Accounting Office (GAO) looked into the problem and issued a report charging that biases in NCI's reporting methods "artificially inflate the amount of 'true' progress." It pointed out that survival rates tell nothing about life expectancy or the quality of life of the victims. "Using survival rates alone to reach conclusions about general progress is therefore inappropriate," it concluded (U.S. General Accounting Office, 1987).

Dr. Vincent DeVita, Jr., called the report "offensive," and the head of the National Cancer Advisory Board, Dr. David Korn, called it a "shabby polemic" (*Time*, April 27, 1987).

Polemics aside, however, the whole policy of measuring progress by highly questionable cure rates has come under attack. Dr. Bailar is not alone in believing that conventional efforts to cure cancer, over a thirty-year period, have proven ineffective. "Those efforts have not paid off," he said bluntly. "I am not convinced they ever will, and I think it's high time to start getting serious about prevention" (*New York Times*, May 8, 1986).

It is certainly no coincidence that the new director of the National Cancer Institute, Dr. Samuel Broder, has called for a redirection of cancer policy toward prevention, early diagnosis, and swift application of new treatments (*Wall Street Journal*, December 27, 1988). These are high-minded goals. Whether Dr. Broder (who helped develop the toxic drug AZT) will buck the trend of a toxic-drug-oriented medical system remains to be seen, however.

In the early eighties some journalists were already asking, "Has the Fight Against Cancer Been Oversold?" (*U.S. News & World Report*, July 13, 1981). "Where's that Promised Cancer Cure?" (*Science News*, vol. 119, January 3, 1981). By 1986 this became "What Ever Happened to the War on Cancer?" (*Discover*, March 1986).

Finally, in 1988, with Dr. DeVita's departure, they began to talk about the war in the past tense! Reporting on "Stop Cancer," Armand Hammer's one-time, four-year attempt to raise an extra billion dollars for research, the *New York Times* commented:

> In the early 1970s, President Nixon declared another major effort to cure cancer. The "war on cancer," *as it was called*, greatly increased the cancer

institute's budget. It was criticized by some experts as raising false hopes that the disease could be eradicated through heavy spending. Death rates from most major forms of cancer have improved little if at all over the last 15 years.

In view of this, members of the National Cancer Advisory Board have expressed fears that the Hammer campaign *might come to the same end* as the Nixon campaign, and that public support will suffer as a result (December 13, 1988, emphasis added).

The whole history of the war on cancer can be read in these few well-chosen words.

When the war on cancer began to falter, the Bethesda warriors resorted to some questionable statistical strategems. When these were exposed, the key players shuffled their seats and a new war was proposed.

In the 1970s America's undeclared war in Vietnam ended in spectacular defeat. In the 1980s its highly touted war against cancer simply disappeared into the night.

The chief cancer warriors, who for two decades enjoyed the uncritical support of the major media, were never held accountable for the billions and billions of dollars spent on cancer research and treatment nor for a cancer death rate now pushing half a million American victims a year.

The question thus inevitably arises: If the current methods of treating cancer are so inadequate, how and why are they considered proven cures?

« 3 »

Surgery

The most common method of treating cancer is with the knife. Surgery has been practiced since the dawn of medical history to remove malignancies.

There is no doubt that in certain circumstances surgery is a highly effective and indispensable method of dealing with cancer. For example, in 1975 the five-year survival rate of patients with skin cancer, treated surgically, was 85 percent, for breast cancer 60 percent, for colon cancer 40 percent, and 70 percent for cancer of the uterus (Maugh and Marx, 1975). (For changes in survival rates see chapter 2.)

Overall, most of the cancer patients who are cured today are cured because of surgery. Without denying this fact, however, it is important to take a serious look at cancer surgery. For the results of surgery are still so uncertain, and carry with them so many drawbacks, that new approaches are clearly necessary.

Cancer surgery, in general, was not in favor in the ancient world. Hippocrates (c. 460–c. 370 B.C.), who knew cancer well and even coined the term *carcinoma,* urged doctors, "Above all, do no harm." Among his Aphorisms, number 38 states: "It is better not to apply any treatment in cases of occult cancer; for, if treated, the patients die quickly; but if not treated, they hold out for a long time" (cited in Shimkin, 1977:24).

To Hippocrates, as to most ancient physicians, cancer was caused by

43

an excess of "black bile." Cancer was thus seen as what we would call a *systemic* ailment, caused by an imbalance of natural elements within the body, rather than as a local problem.

The Roman medical encyclopedist Celsus (1st century A.D.) remarked that an advanced cancer is "irritated by treatment; and the more so the more vigorous it is." He continues:

> Some have used caustic medicaments, some the cautery, some excision with a scalpel; but no medicament has ever given relief; the parts cauterized are excited immediately to an increase until they cause death (ibid.).

The best course, he suggests is to use *mild* treatments:

> After excision, even when a scar has formed, nonetheless the disease has returned and caused death; while at the same time the majority of patients, though no violent measures are applied in the attempt to remove the tumor, but only mild applications in order to soothe it, attain to a ripe old age in spite of it (ibid.:26).

This principle remained in force for over a thousand years. For example, the Cordova physician Abul Qasim (A.D. 1013–1106) writes that surgery was acceptable in the earliest stages of the disease. "But when it is of long standing and large you should leave it alone. For I myself have never been able to cure any such, nor have I seen anyone else succeed before me" (ibid.:39).

There were two groups of healers who *did* attempt to treat cancer, however. The first were the folk healers and traveling medicine salesmen who provided some sort of medical service for the mass of impoverished serfs or city dwellers who could never afford a physician.

Then there were the surgeons. From the twelfth century on, the church-affiliated physicians abandoned surgery entirely to the lower-class barbers. These gentlemen would consent to remove cancerous growths, with much blood and very little success (ibid.:32).

It is interesting to note that surgery entered the modern world as a very disreputable procedure, little better in the eyes of the medical ortho-doxy than the herbalists and quacks with whom it competed for the same lower-class clientele. Surgeons could not write prescriptions, for example, without the countersignature of a physician, nor could they perform operations except in the presence of a licensed physician.

From the start there was tension between the surgeons and other healers, particularly the folk healers. According to a sixteenth-century document, the surgeons "mind only their own lucres [money]" and

> sued, troubled and vexed divers honest men and women who without taking anything for their pains and skill had ministered to poor people for neighborhood, for God's sake and for charity. . . . [They] would undertake no case unless they knew they would be rewarded with a greater sum or reward than the case extended to . . . (Clark, 1964).

It is hard for us to realize just how ghastly surgery was until the mid-nineteenth century. According to one modern description:

> The surgeon stropped his knife upon his boots. As he operated, he breathed and coughed into the incision, exposed also to the dust in the room and the particles falling from his beard and hair. The patient was strapped to the table and held down by attendants as the knife cut his quivering flesh or a saw hacked off his bones amid fearful shrieks of pain (Morris, 1977).

The predominant attitude toward what is now the standard treatment was generally disapproving and hostile.* Paracelsus (1493–1541), the extraordinary Renaissance physician, is quoted as having said:

> It should be forbidden and severely punished to remove cancer by cutting, burning, cautery and other fiendish tortures. It is from nature that the disease arises and from nature comes the cure, not from the physicians (Issels, 1975).

How, then, did medicine arrive at the current situation, in which these same treatments are considered orthodox?

Surgery rose from quackery to respectability in the nineteenth century mainly because of two great discoveries: anesthesia and asepsis.

Ether anesthesia was originally a carnival sideshow sensation. With

---

*Even less reputable was the use of chemicals to treat cancer. In the Renaissance, arsenic and metals were common ingredients in such "cures." Some metals apparently have an anticancer effect, and recently a form of platinum has been used in the treatment of cancer at major cancer centers (MSKCC, 1976). Nevertheless, in their first appearance hundreds of years ago they "were abandoned because of their toxic effect, only to reappear in secret nostrums" (Issels, 1975).

great difficulty a number of innovators attempted to promote its acceptance in surgery in the 1840s, but with little success. It was only after the Civil War that ether became a standard procedure in American hospitals (Collins, 1966). Once it did so, however, it made longer and more complicated operations possible and relatively painless.

Asepsis, the attempt to eliminate germs in the operating room, had an equally stormy history, including fierce opposition from the surgeons themselves (Shryock, 1962; Thompson, 1949). Nevertheless, once it was introduced, it made cancer operations and other surgery far less likely to end in death from infection, then a common occurrence.

These two developments in surgery coincided with several other trends that tended to increase the incidence of surgery. First, from at least 1900 on (and probably throughout the nineteenth century), cancer was increasing in frequency. This created a growing need for the services that surgeons provided. Second, there was the general tendency in the nineteenth century to use surgery freely as a kind of magic weapon to cure a variety of ills.

This was particularly so in the treatment of women. In the nineteenth century, for example, hysterectomy (removal of the uterus) was even employed to treat women's "emotional problems," on the theory that the seat of a woman's emotions was her womb (Ehrenreich and English, 1973).

Once the technique of hysterectomy had been perfected, and anesthesia and asepsis were available, it was logical that surgeons would employ the knife to remove tumors. Hippocratic restraint was thrown out the window in the nineteenth century's enthusiasm for surgical progress.

This rapid rise of cancer surgery is well illustrated by the early history of what is now Memorial Sloan-Kettering Cancer Center in New York.

The spiritual founder of Memorial Sloan-Kettering was a famous nineteenth-century "woman's doctor," J. Marion Sims. Sims received only a cursory medical training in the South before turning his hand to surgery. An enterprising young man, he resolved to extend the boundaries of surgery in the antebellum era. To do so, he gathered a group of slave women, upon whom he performed experimental operations in a kind of makeshift hospital behind his house.

These operations, says his sympathetic biographer H. Seale Harris, M.D., were "little short of murderous." Some of these slave women received as many as thirty operations in a four-year period. This was the era before ether or antiseptics. Sims claimed to have kept the women comfortable with opium (Seale Harris, 1950).

Sims perfected a new technique for a once-common condition called vesico-vaginal fistula, an abnormal passage between the urinary bladder and the vagina. The doctor then moved to New York City, where his innovation formed the basis of his professional and financial success. He helped to found Women's Hospital, which is still in existence. One of the main functions of the hospital was to allow Sims and his colleagues to perform this operation on large numbers of women, many of them recent immigrants. In addition, Sims developed a select clientele of wealthy ladies.

The correction of vesico-vaginal fistulas thus became, for Sims and his colleagues, a thriving business. "Marion Sims tended to look upon the knife not as the last weapon, but as the first," says Dr. Harris.*

In the 1870's, Sims increasingly turned his attention to cancer. Apparently trying to duplicate the formula he had used successfully with vesico-vaginal fistulas, he began a series of unusually extensive operations on patients at Women's Hospital. Rumors began to spread that Sims was carrying out unnecessary and, in fact, barbaric operations (similar rumors had circulated in Montgomery, Alabama, years before concerning his slave experiments.)

The Lady Managers (trustees) of the hospital became convinced that "the lives of all the patients in the institution were being threatened by . . . mysterious experiments," says Harris. In addition, Sims and his students were said to troop noisily through the wards and treat the women with contempt. Sims was expelled from the hospital, a drastic step taken only in the most serious cases (Seale Harris, 1950; Considine, 1959).

Although he was later reinstated to his position, Sims seems to have remained alienated from the women directors. When the wealthy Astor family, some of whose members were afflicted by cancer, offered $150,000 to Women's Hospital for a cancer wing, the Lady Managers hesitated. Cancer treatment and research were associated, in their minds, with Sims's experiments. Sims had no such hesitation, however, and opened private negotiations with the Astors' lawyer to obtain the money himself.

"A cancer hospital should be built on its own foundations," he wrote the lawyer, "wholly independent of all other hospitals." Consequently, the Astors' donation went to establish the New York Cancer Hospital in 1884, the first private cancer hospital in the United States. (The name was changed to Memorial Hospital in the 1890s, and to Memorial Sloan-Kettering Cancer Center in 1959.) Sims was to have been the first director of this center, but he died before he had a chance to fulfill this goal.

The existence of this and other cancer hospitals greatly increased the prestige of cancer therapy and of cancer surgery in particular. A stable base

---

*Ironically, it is now known that this condition is almost entirely iatrogenic—that is, it is *caused* by faulty procedures on the part of obstetricians and gynecologists. Thus, in a broad sense, Sims and his fellow doctors were unwittingly causing a disease and then curing it (Huffman, 1962; Green, 1971).

of patients provided "teaching material" for the development of new types of operations. Sims had written to the Astors: "Doubtful points of practice can be settled only in the wards of a great hospital."

Over a period of years, patients were persuaded to abandon home care and entrust themselves to a hospital for treatment. After initial resistance, an increasing number of doctors became interested in making cancer a part of their practice.*

As medical techniques in general improved, so too did the scope of cancer surgery. "Talented assistants, blood banks to replace lost blood, a variety of anesthetics, antibiotics, strict antisepsis, tissue replacements, information on the patient's physical and chemical status before, during, and following surgery, and scores of other contributions by physicists, engineers, biologists, and biochemists" aided the aggressive surgeon (McGrady, Sr., 1964:304).

For the treatment of head and neck cancer, for example, ingenious surgeons devised an operation called the commando. This involved removal of the patient's mandible, or jaw. Although the word meant literally "with the mandible," according to one surgeon, it "derived its wide acceptance and popularity from the fact that it brought to mind the slashing attack of the World War I commandos" (Crile, 1974).

For pancreatic cancer, Dr. Allen Oldfather Whipple, president of the American Surgical Association and clinical director at Memorial Hospital, designed the operation that bears his name. The Whipple involved removal of many organs adjacent to the affected gland, on the theory that they might be harboring nests of cancer cells. Yet despite this radical procedure, the survival rate for pancreatic cancer remained persistently low: 5 percent five-year survival for localized pancreatic cancer and 0-3 percent when the disease had already spread (NCI, 1976).

Often unwilling to acknowledge the limitations of their methods, enamored of technology, and hostile to nonsurgical approaches, many surgeons conceived of progress in terms of greater and greater cutting. In 1948, for example, Dr. Alexander Brunschwig devised an operation he called total exenteration. This involved removal of the rectum, the stomach, the urinary bladder, part of the liver, the ureter, all the internal reproductive organs, the pelvic floor and wall, the pancreas, the spleen, the colon, and many of the blood vessels.

Patients were hollowed out in the desperate hope that, by doing so, all

*In the 1890s the New York Cancer Hospital almost became a general hospjtal because of lack of cancer patients and of doctors interested in specializing in this disease (Considine, 1959).

48

remaining cancer could be destroyed. Brunschwig himself called the operation "a brutal and cruel procedure" (*New York Times,* April 8, 1969).

But the ultimate operation was the hemicorporectomy—literally, the removal of half the body. Originated by Theodore Miller (like Brunschwig, a Memorial Hospital surgeon), this operation involved the amputation of everything below the pelvis, in the treatment of advanced bladder or pelvic-region malignancy. Not surprisingly, many patients preferred to die rather than submit to Miller's invention (*New York Times,* November 30, 1969).

Surgery had clearly been taken about as far as it could go. Yet despite the fantastic ingenuity and skill of the surgeons, cancer was still not cured. In fact, as has been shown above, at most one-half of cancer patients undergoing surgery and other "proven" methods lived five years or longer.

Surgery works best on cancers that are detected before they metastasize to other parts of the body and create additional tumors. Once the cancer has spread, surgery is generally useless as a curative procedure, although it may relieve symptoms caused by a large mass pressing against a nerve or organ.

Surgery has come under increasing criticism in recent years for a number of other reasons.

Some doctors and patients hold that much cancer surgery is either unnecessary or excessive in its scope. The fiercest argument has taken place over the question of breast cancer, but the issues raised in this debate appear applicable to other forms of cancer as well.

For years, breast cancer was routinely treated with an operation called the radical mastectomy or the Halsted procedure, after its chief promoter. At the hearings of Senator Edward Kennedy's (D.-Mass.) Subcommittee on Health (of the Committee on Labor and Public Welfare) in May 1976, author and breast cancer victim Rose Kushner summarized the nature of the problem:

> In the United States most of the 90,0000 women who are expected to discover breast cancer in 1976 will be put to sleep without their knowing whether they will wake up with one breast or two. And most of the time, the amputation will be the Halsted radical mastectomy which leaves ugly scars extending into their armpits, and dips and hollows in their chests. Of course, the degree of disfigurement varies with the skill of the surgeon (U.S. Senate, 1976).

In addition, she noted, many women experience an "unattractive and sometimes painful swelling of the affected arm." She might have also men-

49

tioned the pain of the postoperative period, and the psychological and financial costs of the operation.

Yet, even at that time, the operation was considered unnecessary by some of the leading experts in the field. A number of studies suggested that about half of all breast cancer patients could receive much less radical, more sparing treatments without appreciably increasing their risk of a recurrence of the cancer.

The radical mastectomy was *not* routine in England, France, Canada, or the Scandinavian countries. Doctors in these countries regarded it as ineffective and unnecessarily brutal. Questions were raised about the wisdom of the procedure since it was first widely employed and popularized in the 1890s by Dr. William Halsted (1852–1922) of Johns Hopkins University, Baltimore.

The most determined criticism of the Halsted procedure came from George Crile, Jr., M.D., a retired breast surgeon and emeritus consultant in surgery at the Cleveland Clinic. Crile is orthodox in background and training. His father, George Crile, Sr., was in fact one of the most celebrated figures in American surgery. The younger Crile spent many decades treating and researching the causes of breast cancer.

Having started out an enthusiastic partisan of radical surgery he became its most determined foe. Crile's comment on the radical was acerbic: "[It] seems to have been designed to inflict the maximal possible deformity, disfiguration and disability" on the women who receive it, he said, in his popular book *What Women Should Know About the Breast Cancer Controversy* (Crile, 1974).

Crile generally favored the simple removal of the breast and some of the adjoining lymph nodes, but without the extensive mutilation of the Halsted procedure: "If the cancer is so advanced that it cannot be removed by an operation less than radical mastectomy, it has already spread through the system and is incurable by surgery." He also believed that in certain "properly selected cases, equivalent results can be obtained by even simpler operations in which only part of the breast is removed" (ibid.).

By the 1970s, the new breast cancer detection procedures (mammography, thermography, etc.) were detecting tumors so small that they could not even be felt by manual examinations. Presumably, then, they could be located so early that they had not spread. Many of the women with these tumors understandably balked at having their entire breast, muscles, and armpit lymph glands removed. This fueled the demand for the kind of limited operations practiced in much of Europe. Women also objected to being pressured into signing release forms which allowed the surgeon to remove their breast while they were still anesthetized, if their biopsy proved positive. This procedure, common in American hospitals at the time, took the final decision out of the hands of the most interested party, the woman herself. According to Rose Kushner in *Breast Cancer*, there was no appreciable increase in risk or cost in delaying surgery for a few weeks, during which time the patient could make an unpressured decision (Kushner, 1975). Other scientific studies in this country supported Dr. Crile's contention. In a survey conducted by Dr. Maurice S. Fox of the Massachusetts Institute of Technology, patients who received the full-scale radical mastectomy were compared statistically to those who had only had the more limited procedures advocated by Crile and his supporters.

Fox found that the radical, disfiguring, and painful Halsted operation was "no more effective than more conservative, less mutilating treatment."

Dr. Bernard Fisher, a surgeon at the University of Pittsburgh, began a study in 1971 of 1,700 patients at thirty-four medical centers. In this study, patients whose tumors were believed to be confined to the breast were treated either with radical mastectomies or simple breast removal with or without postoperative irradiation. In 1979 he told reporters there was "no difference in survivals . . . between those who underwent radical surgery and those treated more conservatively." (*New York Times,* January 29, 1979).

Because of such studies, and the general impact of the women's movement, the 1980s witnessed massive changes in the treatment of this disease. "The treatment of breast cancer is in rapid flux," said the editor-in-chief of the *New England Journal of Medicine,* "frustrating to those who want absolute guidelines now" (Relman, 1989).

Nevertheless, the trend is obvious—towards more sparing and humane treatments.

Today treatment depends on the extent of the disease and the patient's age. If there is substantial involvement of the lymph nodes, or even wider metastatic spread, then treatment is palliative. When there is no such involvement, or only minor involvement on the affected side, then the most common treatment is the modified radical, i.e., total mastectomy and a removal of the lymph nodes in the affected armpit (axillary node dissection). This operation has largely replaced the conventional radical mastectomy, or Halsted, for the treatment of all primary operable breast cancers (Merck, 1987).

Over the last ten years, however, the trend has been towards even more conservative procedures. Primary operable (Stage I and Stage II) breast carcinomas are now routinely treated by partial mastectomy ("lumpectomy") plus a standard lymph node removal; this is often followed in about three weeks by irradiation of the remaining breast (ibid.).

Such an operation leaves the woman's breast practically intact, and the therapeutic results are quite comparable to the older operations, which could be physically and psychologically devastating (Moss, 1984).

In 1989 a long-simmering controversy over the value of chemotherapy in the early stages of breast cancer flared anew (*Wall Street Journal*, February 22, 1989). The debate centered on four papers that appeared in the *New England Journal of Medicine* of February 23, 1989. When women without lymph node involvement were given chemotherapy after breast surgery, they appeared to experience a small benefit. The problem was that these post-surgical treatments did *not* result in permanent gains:

> All [four studies] find small improvement in disease-free survival but, after follow-up periods of three to four years, no definitive improvement in overall survival—that is, survival with or without disease (Relman, 1989).

This hardly seems like an earth-shattering advance. Yet some specialists immediately called for offering chemotherapy to all women after breast cancer surgery, a position encouraged by the National Cancer Institute.

The controversy over breast cancer surgery has thus been long and extremely bitter.

When Rose Kushner published *Breast Cancer* (now entitled *Alternatives*) in 1975, "the American College of Surgeons censured the book," she recalls, and "the American Cancer Society refused to recommend it. Remember, that was more than four years ago, and a lot has changed. But the medical establishment then thought I was a kook at worst and a pest and an agitator at best" (*New York Times*, October 22, 1979).

Partial mastectomies and even lumpectomies have now become standard practice in most hospitals. The Halsted is only being practiced by older surgeons who cannot adjust to the change. Arthur C. Upton, then director of the National Cancer Institute, even nominated Kushner to serve on the National Cancer Advisory Board, and a Consensus Development Conference on the Treatment of Primary Breast Cancer in June 1979 decided that there should be a time lapse between the biopsy of suspicious breast tissue and any "definitive surgical procedure." They also decreed that the Halsted radical mastectomy should no longer be used as a treatment of choice for local breast cancer (ibid.).

In fact, the minimalists have all but won this important battle. Why, then, did American surgeons cling to the Halsted procedure for so long, making it, in Crile's words, the "central dogma" of all surgical practice in the United States? Crile's answers shed light not only on the breast cancer controversy but on other aspects of the cancer controversy as well.

First, there were historical reasons. The radical mastectomy was an *American* innovation. (Although developed in England in 1867, it was not widely accepted until Halsted adopted it about twenty years later.) The use of the Halsted challenged for the first time the dominance of European physicians and surgeons over American medicine—a dominance that dated from before the American Revolution. The American surgeons were very proud of Johns Hopkins University, with its famous "Big Four" of Halsted, Sir William Osler, William H. Welch, and Howard A. Kelly. Halsted was the chief of surgery and enjoyed an outstanding reputation. According to one history of Johns Hopkins:

> Halsted was a perfectionist and his operations were works of art. His surgery was poetry—poetry of a sort few men understood. . . . When he dealt with cancer he struck for its roots without compromise. When he did a breast [sic] it was a finished piece of work. . . . (Bernheim, 1948).

Halsted's successors, however, were not perfectionists and sought ways to cut corners on his classic operation. "You can usually do with less," said Bertram Bernheim, M.D., a Johns Hopkins surgeon. It was another Hopkins surgeon, John M. T. Finney, first president of the American College of Surgeons (1913), who showed how to adapt the Halsted radical to "mass production" (Bernheim's phrase).

> Where Halsted took four hours to do a cancer of the breast—and skin-grafted every case—Finney knew that that would never do for practical purposes and, using Halsted's main ideas, showed how much the same thing could be accomplished with no skin-grafting and in one-third the time (ibid.).

Yet Bernheim admits that the mass production surgeons' "percentage of cures never were quite so high as Halsted's."

The second reason for the veneration of the Halsted procedure, said Crile was economic. Even when surgeons took shortcuts, the Halsted was a longer, more challenging and difficult operation than the one it replaced. Surgeons, "almost by definition," prefer those procedures which require a maximum of skill over simpler operations because they are more challenging. "And, in a free-enterprise system," he added, "the fee for a larger operation is also larger."

This factor was accentuated by the payment structure in the United States. Group payment plans paid surgeons two to three times as much for performing the Halsted than the simpler operation that left the patient's muscles and glands more or less intact. "The more appalling the mutilation," said George Bernard Shaw, "the more the mutilator is paid" (quoted in Crile, 1974).

When there are a lot of surgeons, who are paid "piecework," there will, ipso facto, be a lot of surgery, critics say. As the late Dr. John H. Knowles once put it, "We have surgical manpower creating its own demand. The more surgeons you have, the more surgery is going to be done, simply because the surgeons are there and they have to make a living" (quoted in ibid.).

Both Crile and Knowles believed that such pressure to perform more complicated and more expensive procedures acted "through the subconscious." It is important to point out that surgeons did not sit around scheming how to mutilate patients for money. Rather, they evolved rationalizations and theories to justify a course of behavior that happened to be in their collective economic interest.

A third reason for the persistence of the Halsted operation was the conservatism of the medical profession—especially the surgical division. It takes many years for a surgeon to perfect a procedure like the radical mastectomy. By this time, not only does part of his livelihood depend on it but he is emotionally attached to it as well. He may have advised it for members of his own family, for friends, and, of course, for many patients. To admit that he was wrong may leave him open to criticism, attack, and possibly even malpractice suits.

Finally, most of the surgical faculty of most American medical schools, Crile said, is made up of practicing surgeons who teach only part-time. This has its good side, certainly, since it helps integrate teaching and practice. But the disadvantage is that the prejudices of today's generation of practitioners is passed on to the next generation almost without change. All these factors created an air of almost religious orthodoxy around the radical mastectomy.

But every orthodoxy must have its heretics. Crile was one of them. For many years he refused to publicize his views about the radical mastectomy, lest he be accused of propagating his beliefs in order to increase his surgical practice. He wrote his book on the subject after he had retired from practice and after numerous magazine articles had already appeared doubting the wisdom of the Halsted operation. Nevertheless, members of the surgical staffs of two Cleveland community hospitals saw fit to write to the Academy of Medicine and ask that Crile, a senior surgeon, be censured.

Some scientists, following the ancients, have questioned whether surgery itself does not accelerate the cancerous process. This question, too, is a highly emotional one for surgeons.

Since surgery inevitably disrupts the tumor, the danger of cutting into the tumor and spreading cancer cells throughout the body is always present. "A single cancer cell left alive," according to a *Science* report on cancer research, "can spell a patient's doom" (Maugh and Marx, 1975).

Some authorities believe that even rubbing a tumor may spread cancer cells throughout the system. According to one textbook, *Clinical Oncology for Medical Students and Physicians* (published jointly by the University of Rochester School of Medicine and the American Cancer Society):

> Massage of a tumor is followed by massively increased numbers of circulating tumor cells in the bloodstream in animals. A few clinical studies suggest the same phenomena (Rubin, 1971).

This textbook goes on to warn of two additional dangers of surgery and/or biopsy (the removal of a specimen for analysis):

> Experimental data further suggest that surgical trauma decreases natural host resistance to the formation of metastases,

and

> Needle biopsy is occasionally used, [but] . . . a needle track may harbor nests of cells which may form the basis for a later recurrent spread. . . . Incisional biopsy of certain highly malignant tumors through an open operative field may be contraindicated because of risk of spread of the tumor throughout the operative field (ibid.).

Thus, surgical biopsy, a procedure used to detect cancer in its earliest stages and enable it to be cured, may contribute to the spread of cancer in some cases.

Other researchers have found, in experimental studies, that surgery per se has a deleterious effect on a patient's immune system and resistance to cancer. Drs. Gerald O. McDonald and Warren H. Cole, at the time of their studies at the University of Illinois, carried out an elaborate series of experiments to pinpoint the role of surgical stress in the spread of cancer. "Most surgeons," they told an American Medical Association meeting, "have encountered the patient whose cancer grows rapidly following operation, resulting in death within a few weeks" (McGrady, Sr., 1964:307).

In their animal experiments, the Illinois doctors subjected animals to various kinds of stress—operations, liver poisons, cold (of the type sometimes used as a "deep freeze" anesthetic), and chemical anesthetics. All of these, they found, decreased the animals' resistance to injected cancer cells. The chances of a tumor growing as a result of surgical operations increased anywhere from 50 to 450 percent. The liver poison, carbon tetrachloride, increased tumor take by 300 percent; ether, by 75 percent; and an anesthetic with deep-freeze properties, by 60 percent (ibid.).

The decreased resistance to cancer lasted two to three days after the stress—just the time when wayward cells in the human patient would be leaving the tumor site and attempting to establish themselves elsewhere in the body (ibid.).

Cole, now an honorary life member of the American Cancer Society, presented additional evidence that many cancer cells were left behind during surgery and possibly even stimulated to invade the body by the stress of the operation.

In half of the patients he studied, Cole found cancer cells already circulating in the bloodstream, before, during, and after surgery. But in an additional 17 percent, these circulating cells could be found *only during* surgery. It is possible that these cells were liberated by the surgery itself (ibid.).

Many other studies have shown that in 25 to 60 percent of patients, some cancer cells are left behind after an operation. Scientists have learned this by swabbing out the incised area after the operation and then examining the washings under a microscope. Such circulating cells *may* lead to further recurrences of cancer, although the subject is hotly debated among scientists (McGrady, Sr., 1964). At least one medical text has been devoted to the subject of doctor-caused cancer (Schmahl et al., 1977).

Such studies and statistics raise important questions about the extensive use of surgery in the treatment of cancer. But they leave out what may be the most important objection to the surgical treatment: the so-called human dimension.

Surgery hurts. Most of us are well aware of the excruciating pain that follows removal of a breast, a uterus, or a lung. Furthermore, the emotional pain may be worse than the physical. Much has been written about the psychological scars of mastectomy (Kushner, 1975). We might add the frightful prospect of laryngectomy, with the loss of one's natural voice; hysterectomy and oophorectomy, with the premature onset of menopause; the loss of limbs in such childhood diseases as osteogenic sarcoma; or the castration of thousands of men in the treatment of prostatic cancer. It is simply impossible to calculate the amount of human suffering caused by such surgery, as humanitarian and well-intentioned as it undoubtedly is in almost every case.

A team of psychiatrists, social workers, and psychologists studied the response of patients to their cures several years ago. They found that some "cured" patients had, quite simply, had their lives ruined by the successful therapy itself. For example, they cited the cases of

> —a previously dynamic corporation president confined to a wheelchair, with a nurse in attendance—ten years after successful cancer surgery.
> —a fifty-year-old woman "a prisoner in my bathroom" compulsively (and unnecessarily) irrigating a colostomy [an artificial opening for fecal wastes in the abdomen] for twelve hours every other day—six years after successful cancer surgery.
> —a thirty-five-year old mother with three children . . . a virtual recluse— five years after the loss of a breast in a successful battle against cancer.
> —a once-productive businessman, [who was prompted] to sell his business at a loss, become a non-functioning invalid, and settle down to await death— after successful cancer surgery eleven years earlier (Bard, 1973).

It must be emphasized that such patients figure among the *successes* of surgery and orthodox medicine—not its failures. Yet one of the psychologists who conducted this study was moved to remark:

> Such stories of "death expectancy" reveal untold suffering for people whose lives have been saved, and for their families. They suggest a disturbing thought—more and more lives are being saved, but *for what?* (ibid.:166)

It is little wonder, then, that "a great many patients fear cancer treatment as much as or more than death itself," according to Dr. Robert Chernin Cantor, who has counseled cancer patients for several decades.

And the greatest source of anxiety is surgery:

> Surgery is the most frightening of all treatment modalities. Consciously or unconsciously, everyone reacts to the recommendation of major surgery

57

with great alarm. . . . Surgery and mutilation are fused, bound together in the image of a helpless victim subjected to violent assault (Cantor, 1978).

For this reason alone—if for none other—the search for safer, more effective, and less traumatic methods of treating cancer is one of the imperatives of modern medicine.

« 4 »

Radiation Therapy

The second so-called proven method of treating cancer is radiation therapy. Enthusiasm for things nuclear declined in the last decade, especially in the wake of Three Mile Island and Chernobyl. And a sharp controversy continues to rage over the effectiveness of this set of techniques for the treatment of malignancies. Nevertheless, radiation continues in favor with much of the medical profession.

According to its defenders, radiotherapy, including X rays, cobalt rays, and newer techniques such as the proton beam accelerator, is both effective and safe.

"Radiotherapists are among the few cancer clinicians who speak in terms of 'cures,' " said the 1975 *Science* cancer report. They have claimed to be able to cure 55 to 65 percent of patients with locally inoperable cancer of the prostate. In fact, according to Frederick W. George 3d of the National Cancer Institute, by the mid-seventies, about 60 percent of *all* cancers were potentially curable with the current techniques of irradiation (Maugh and Marx, 1975).

Radiation was then being used on more than half of the cancer patients in the United States. Since only about a third of all cancers were being cured (five-year survival) at that time through the use of all methods, radiologists called for a stepped-up role for their technique.

'Radiation therapy, in use for seventy-five years, is more sophisti-

59

cated, accurate and effective, with fewer side effects,'' said the American Cancer Society (ACS, 1978). "Enormous improvements have been made,'' said Jane Brody of the *New York Times* in *You Can Fight Cancer and Win*, a book she coauthored with ACS vice president Art Holleb. "Cancer specialists are now using radiation more and more. . . . Radiation therapy is often effectively used as a primary treatment. . . . [It can] cure cancers by totally eradicating them . . . extend life . . . [and] make remaining life more pleasant" (Brody and Holleb, 1977).

"Although radiation therapy is not a new field," Morra and Potts wrote in the 1987 update of their book *Choices,* "research and improved technology especially in the past 15 years has made it a major treatment area for cancer. It is an area which is rapidly growing and changing" (Morra and Potts, 1987).

Memorial Sloan-Kettering, which concentrates on the most complex types of procedures, still averages 4.2 radiation treatments per patient and 6.6 X ray examinations. With a total of almost 195,000 procedures, this averages out to more than one X ray of some kind for every day that every patient is in the hospital (MSKCC, 1987).

Some of the many cancers now being treated by radiation, say Morra and Potts, are Hodgkin's disease and some lymphomas, cancer of the head and neck and of the uterine cervix, as well as early cancers of the bladder, prostate, and skin, certain brain and eye tumors, and some cancers of the bone (ibid.).

According to Brody's book, Senator Hubert Humphrey was a "famous beneficiary of modern radiation therapy." The reader will remember that the senator died of bladder cancer despite extensive surgery, radiation, and chemotherapy. The radiation treatment was the first line of defense, but failed to stop the relentless growth of his bladder tumor. Nevertheless, according to Brody and her American Cancer Society coauthor, he was a "beneficiary" because "he remained well for three years until the development of a new, more advanced cancer."

While many in the cancer field have called for more radiotherapists and for the utilization of existing methods "to their maximum capacity" (Maugh and Marx, 1975:102), radiation's critics dispute both the value and the safety of the procedure.

The kinds of cancer that can actually be cured by means of radiation are few. Eighty percent of patients in the early stages of Hodgkin's disease (cancer of the lymphatic system) have five or more years survival after radiation therapy. Radiation is also said to be very effective in cancers of the testicles, of the cervix, and of the prostate (Richards, 1972).

Dr. John Laszlo of the ACS in general represents a more sensible and humane tendency within the establishment. He acknowledges that "it is impossible to . . . give radiation treatments without injuring normal cells," calling high doses of radiation potentially "dangerous" and citing the case of lung cancer:

> For example, radiation therapy to a lung cancer may cause extensive inflammation followed by scarring of nearby normal lung, thus damaging lung function even if the tumor is completely eradicated. Naturally, the larger the dose of radiation or the larger the volume treated, the more danger there is of side effects (Laszlo, 1987).

In remarkably frank language for an ACS official, he continues:

> Depending on the site treated, large doses of radiation can cause nausea and vomiting, loss of appetite and reduction in bone marrow function. (Some of the same problems exist with chemotherapy. . .) (Laszlo, 1987).

Nevertheless, he believes that radiation is superior to other methods in a limited number of cases. For example, surgery for prostate cancer is not only risky but almost inevitably results in sexual impotence. "The importance of this used to be overlooked," he says. "Impotence was once considered (by the medical profession) to be a small price to pay for a potentially lifesaving procedure, but we have increasingly come to appreciate the emotional impact of impotence even in older age groups" (ibid.).

In the case of cancer of the vocal cords, a total laryngectomy involves loss of normal speech. Radiotherapy can make this unnecessary. Since both surgery and X rays are equally curative, "radiation is a very good treatment option and it is generally preferred" (ibid.).

Other scientists dispute claims for radiation therapy. According to the prominent French oncologist Dr. Lucien Israël, in early cases of some kinds of cancer

> radiotherapy sometimes gives brilliant results. Yet, apart from Hodgkin's disease and lymphosarcoma, there is much disagreement as to its effectiveness—indeed, there have been no conclusive trials. . . . Radiotherapists don't report their results . . . in such a way as to differentiate between the percentage of complete regressions and the percentage of objective partial regressions, and to indicate the distribution of length of those regressions (Israël, 1978).

In effect, Israël is saying that radiation therapy is an unproven—not a proven—method in many cases. Dr. Irwin D. J. Bross, formerly director of biostatistics at the famed Roswell Park Memorial Institute, went further:

> For the situations for which most radiotherapy is given, the chances of curing the patient by radiotherapy are probably about as good as the chances of curing him by laetrile. This is because the chances of curing any patient in advanced stages of cancer are very poor, regardless of the method employed (Bross, 1979).

Israël embraces the use of radiation therapy, but as a palliative. It is "absolutely irreplaceable" in bringing about an "attenuation of symptoms," such as relief of pain, in advanced lung, esophageal, pancreatic, breast, and colon cancer.

"It is obvious that the limitations of this method are similar to that of surgical resection," said the late Michael B. Shimkin, M.D., a prominent specialist formerly with the U.S. Public Health Service. "The cancer is curable only if it is destroyed entirely by being within the field of radiation at levels lethal to the cancer" (Shimkin, 1973).

"The majority of cancers," Prof. John Cairns has written, "cannot be cured by radiation because the dose of X rays required to kill all the cancer cells would also kill the patient" (Cairns, 1985).

Radiation is frequently used as an adjuvant—i.e., along with surgery or chemotherapy. Such use is becoming more common, critics charge, as more and more women opt for limited breast surgery augmented by radiation. Dr. Bernard Fisher of the University of Pittsburgh has disputed the value of this procedure. In a 1968 study of 3,000 women at over forty institutions, he found that those receiving postoperative radiation did no better than those receiving only surgery in the treatment of breast cancer (Fisher, 1968).

While this use of postoperative radiation is still subject to debate, it has become common practice in the United States. A 1989 study found that irradiation following lumpectomy significantly decreased the chance of recurrence in the affected breast, although it did not increase survival time (*New York Times*, March 30, 1989).

Israël noted that with adjuvant radiation

> we should observe a reduction in the rate of distant metastases. . . . [However], certain recent studies have thrown the medical community into confu-

sion by showing that metastases may be more frequent in cases that have received radiation. . . . (Israël, 1978).

Why, then, is radiation used so extensively—if it is of such limited and questionable value in most cases? Basically, says Bross, because doctors regard it as *harmless*. "It is an added precaution and doesn't cost anything" is the surgeon's attitude when he sends a patient to the radiation therapy department.* Many surgeons, adds the Roswell Park statistician, do not really believe in the value of the beam. "But if it's really harmless, it makes sense" (Bross, 1979).

Here we come to the nub of the controversy, for many critics charge that radiation is *not* harmless, but carries with it numerous dangers and drawbacks. In fact, they believe there is a massive, long-standing cover-up on the part of government officials and some scientists to hide the dangers of radiation. An integral part of that cover-up has been to minimize the dangers of radiation therapy while extolling its supposed virtues.

Charges of radiation's dangers have often been voiced, but most often these charges have been ignored. Initially this was because of the widespread enthusiasm for the new technique. In 1902, after one year of X-ray therapy at Memorial Hospital, the chairman of the board, John Parsons (the same Astor lawyer to whom Sims wrote his famous letter; see chapter 3), exclaimed ". . . the time is not far distant when a remedy for cancer may be found" (Considine, 1959).

Since radiation will often cause temporary remissions, some of the first reports were highly enthusiastic. William B. Coley, later to become famous for his Coley's toxins (see chapter 7), wrote at the same time of ten cases of abdominal cancer with

entire disappearance in one case of cancer of the cervix . . . marked improvement in three other uterine cases . . . more or less temporary improvement in most of the remainder. . . . In two cases of epithelioma of the head and face the tumors have entirely disappeared, one the size of a silver dollar on the forehead, one three-fourths of an inch in diameter on the face. . . . And one case of Hodgkin's disease, a practically hopeless condition, has shown the most remarkable improvement that has yet been reported. . . . The man has resumed his usual occupation (Considine, 1959).

*Of course, radiation treatment is not cost-free. It is "an expensive form of treatment because it involves a highly skilled team and extremely expensive facilities" (Laszlo, 1987).

Coley soon noted that in many cases there was "a recurrence within a year." Disappointment with radiation apparently increased his interest in even more innovative approaches.

Slowly it became apparent that the "quiet, dreamlike process, in which nothing of significance seems to happen" (Glemser, 1969), was fraught with danger. Radiation enthusiasts ignored these signals, and some of them as a result succumbed to the toxic effects of radiation.

Within a year or two after the discovery of X rays (1895), it was found that the rays could cause skin disease and systemic problems. By 1902, 171 cases of accidental X-ray burns had been reported in the medical literature, including those of radiation pioneers Henri Becquerel and Pierre Curie.

In 1902 a German doctor recorded the first case of human cancer caused by radiation: the tumor had appeared on the site of a chronic ulceration caused by X-ray exposure. Experimental studies performed in 1906 suggested that leukemia (cancer of the blood) could be caused by exposure to the radioactive element radium. By 1911, 94 cases of radiation-induced cancer had been reported, more than half of them (54) in doctors or technicians. By 1922, over 100 radiologists had died from X-ray-induced cancer, and many other research workers, laboratory assistants, and technicians had also succumbed (Hunter, 1978).

Many of these cases occurred because doctors refused to take warnings about radiation's dangers seriously. At Johns Hopkins, for instance, one of Halsted's students, Dr. F. H. Baetjer, became sick after administering X rays with few precautions. "Even when it began to be noised about by word of mouth and in the medical journals that patients and X-ray operators especially ought to be protected against possible burns," wrote a colleague, Dr. Bernheim, "Baetjer scoffed at it and then took only perfunctory precautions" (Bernheim, 1948).

Thus, although he "developed a huge private practice in X rays," Baetjer eventually developed cancer in his fingertips, which spread slowly and painfully to the rest of his body. After forty operations, he finally died of this X-ray-induced disease in 1933. This story was repeated dozens of times at most of the large medical centers in the country, and in many of the smaller clinics in which "X-ray fever" had taken hold. Both Marie Curie and her daughter Irène Joliot-Curie are believed to have died as a result of exposure to radioactive materials.

If the public needed convincing, proof of the danger of radiation came during the 1920s in a dramatic way. Soon after the discovery of X rays and radium, radioactivity was adapted for industrial use. One such use (employed until recently) was to luminize the dials of watches and instruments with a radium paint, which glowed in the dark.

There was tremendous demand for these instruments during World War I, and large factories were set up to process orders from the army. Working on a piecework basis, around the clock, the luminizers—mostly young women—developed a technique of expediting their work by sharpening the radium brush with their pursed lips.

Years later, veterans of this work began to succumb to one mysterious ailment after another. Out of approximately 800 women who had worked at a single New Jersey factory, 48 became seriously ill from radium poisoning, and 18 died of cancer of the jaw or related diseases.

Examples of industrial poisoning were not rare, of course, but what was unusual about this radium poisoning was the incredibly small amounts of the radioactive material needed to cause diseases, and the long latency period between exposure and clinical symptoms (Hunter, 1978). Yet radiation continued to be used in a careless way. Why was this so, if it was common knowledge that radiation was a two-edged sword, capable of great harm?

One possible motive was monetary. A medical practitioner, for example, admitted to the *New York Times* in 1914 that radium therapy appeared to do more harm than good:

> Something is created which kills many patients. I cannot tell, nobody can tell, for four or five years just what the results will be. I simply feel that I've shoved those patients over a little bit quicker (*New York Times*, January 27, 1914).

But "I can double my money in a year," he said frankly, "while charging 4¢ per milligram per hour" (ibid.).

The search for radium became a big—and frantic—business. Marie Curie's daughter Eve Curie notes in the famous biography of her mother that "radium had acquired a commercial personality. It had its market value and its press" (Curie, 1943). American businessmen, inspired by radium's selling price of $150,000 a gram, attempted to corner a monopoly on radium-bearing lands.

In 1913 James Douglas, chairman of the Phelps-Dodge copper-mining empire, founded a National Radium Institute in collaboration with the U.S. Bureau of Mines. Simultaneously Douglas made a $100,000 gift to Memorial Hospital, then struggling with serious financial problems. But, as Bob Considine, Memorial's official historian, notes, "Douglas's enormous gifts came with strings attached."

Douglas insisted first that his personal friend and physician, Dr. James

Ewing, be made chief pathologist (later medical director) of the hospital*; second, that the hospital treat only cancer patients; and third, that it routinely use radium in that treatment. Once this was arranged, Memorial Hospital became in effect the distribution center for a new and seemingly inexhaustible product: radium emanations. Ewing proceeded, according to Bob Considine, the Memorial historian, to push "radium beyond the capacity of that mighty weapon to produce results" (Considine, 1959).

A similar process went on at other major centers. Dr. Howard A. Kelly, one of the Big Four at Johns Hopkins Hospital, was Douglas's partner in the National Radium Institute. He constructed a private hospital adjoining his home in Baltimore. "One thing leading to another," wrote Dr. Bernheim, "he became owner of more radium than any other doctor in the nation." Under a convenient arrangement with Johns Hopkins, Kelly gave radium treatments to "all patients the Hopkins had—free as well as private" (Bernheim, 1948).

The press also had caught radium fever. "Radium Cure Free for All," cried *The New York Times* on page one in 1913, as it announced formation of the institute. "Not one cent's worth of radium will be for sale," proclaimed the head of the Bureau of Mines. "Every particle of the precious metal will be used in the cause of humanity" (*New York Times*, October 24, 1913; January 27, 1914).

"Our special object," said Kelly, is "reaching and relieving the poor and large middle class to whom all unexpected expenses are a sore burden in any emergency."

Douglas confided, however, that "all this story about humanity and philanthropy is foolish. I want it understood that I shall do what I like with the radium that belongs to me. . . . I shall use it any way I like" (Langton, 1940).**

Contrary to the newspaper stories, radium and X-ray therapy were hardly free. In fact, radiation helped to save Memorial from bankruptcy

---

*Ewing's monumental work, *Neoplastic Diseases*, was dedicated to the memory of James Douglas.

**Douglas's motives for his involvement with radium were complicated. To many of his contemporaries it appeared that he was out to corner a monopoly on radium-bearing lands for his own benefit. His National Radium Institute was eventually foiled by the opposition of other mineowners, including the Du Ponts. His belief in radium's value appears to have been genuine, however, since he used it on his daughter, dying of cancer, and even on his wife and himself, for trivial ailments. He died of aplastic anemia, probably caused by radium poisoning (*New York Times*, December 20, 1913; Considine, 1959; Langton, 1940.)

during the 1920s and 1930s. In 1924 the rules and regulations of Memorial stipulated that "an extra charge will be made for Radium Emanations used in the treatment of patients" (Memorial, 1924). In that same year, the Radium Department was the greatest single source of income for the hospital. It administered over 18,000 treatments and brought in about $70,000—a large sum for those days.

Millions of dollars were now invested in radium and X-ray machinery. By 1934 more than 25,000 X-ray therapy treatments were administered annually at Memorial Hospital. In 1937, after initial opposition from the surgeons, radiation therapy was recognized as a "proven" method of treatment by the American College of Surgeons (Bailey, 1971).*

By 1977 this had increased to 73,037 radiation therapy treatments and implants annually, and 102,700 X-ray examinations and special procedures at Memorial (MSKCC, 1977a). Eighty-nine professionals and technicians treated 160 patients a day with various forms of radioactivity (MSKCC *Center News*, July–August, 1977). In that same year, Memorial began a $4.5 million modernization program in the Department of Radiation Therapy, which aimed at replacing every piece of major equipment in the department by 1980.

The number of radiation treatments and implant procedures increased to 84,250 by 1983 and then began to decline. By 1987 the figure was down to 75,595. According to MSKCC, "the decrease in the number of radiation treatments and implant procedures beginning in 1984 is due to the increased complexity of procedures performed and greater time required for these procedures" (MSKCC, 1987). Despite this, it should be noted, such treatments still average over four per admitted patient (ibid.).

Radiation has always been lucrative—for hospitals, for equipment and film manufacturers, and for the radiologists themselves. Once millions of dollars are invested in capital equipment, there is a strong inducement to use that equipment, despite newer information suggesting its use should be curtailed.

In the late 1930s a more realistic attitude seemed to be forming toward the extensive use of radiation. In the 1934 *Annual Report* of Memorial Hospital, the doctors in the Breast Service wrote that because of excessive dam-

---

*Initial resistance to X-ray therapy was fierce, as it usually is to new methods of treatment. According to Dr. E. H. Grubbé of Chicago, the first man to treat cancer with X rays, the surgeons ridiculed and opposed his work. "They controlled medicine, and they regarded the X ray as a threat to surgery. At that time surgery was the only approved method of treating cancer. They meant to keep it the *only* approved method by ignoring or rejecting any new methods or ideas. This is why I was called a 'quack' and nearly ejected from hospitals where I had practiced for years" (Bailey, 1971).

age to the skin of their patients from "massive doses of high-voltage X rays," they had concluded that "this method of preoperative radiation was unsatisfactory" (Memorial, 1934).

Ewing continued to push the "continuous prolonged irradiation of the entire body" (ibid.) for practically every condition, but after his death even his most ardent supporters admitted that his view of radiation was excessively sanguine (Considine, 1959).

A realistic appraisal of radiation might have resulted if it hadn't been for the events of August 1945—the bombing of Hiroshima and Nagasaki, which ushered in the "atomic age." Suddenly radiation, which had been merely a medical subspecialty and an arcane branch of physics, moved to center stage in world history.

The question of radiation therapy's effectiveness and *especially its safety* became a burning political question. There were now powerful reasons, beyond the profitability of the procedures themselves, both to exaggerate its benefits and obscure its dangers. As the government pressed forward with its open-air testing program and its creation of a nuclear weapons arsenal, it ran into ever-increasing opposition in the United States and around the world (see, for example, Pauling, 1958).

Atomic medicine provided excellent public-relations copy for the purveyors of atomic bombs. Atomic energy "can be used for man's destruction or as a tool by which he can make himself a better world," said the chairman of the Atomic Energy Commission, Lewis Strauss. Strauss wore many hats: Wall Street investment banker, admiral of the U.S. Navy, trustee of Memorial Sloan-Kettering, the Rockefellers' personal financial adviser, and a "hawk" on matters atomic. The message clearly was that radiation per se was neutral but could be used for good or for ill. A "good" use was "the focusing of the powerful beams of deadly radiation on cancerous growths" *(New York Times,* April 8, 1954).

Key scientists, such as Cornelius P. "Dusty" Rhoads, director of Memorial Hospital, made public statements on the harmlessness of open-air atomic bomb testing during the 1956 Eisenhower–Stevenson campaign *(New York Times,* October 21, 1956). During this time, however, evidence was accumulating that radiation could have many deleterious effects on the body. High doses of radiation could cause acute radiation sickness. For example, an accident victim at the Los Alamos Scientific Laboratory (May 21, 1946) was accidentally exposed to about 2,000 roentgens of radiation.* According to Linus Pauling,

*A roentgen (named after the discoverer of X rays) is the unit used to measure the X rays or gamma rays to which a body is exposed.

During the first few hours he vomited several times. Then for several days his condition was good. On the fifth day the number of white cells in his blood fell rapidly, and on the sixth day his temperature and pulse rate rose. On the seventh day he had periods of mental confusion, then he gradually sank into a coma and died on the ninth day (Pauling, 1958:79).

This was a very large dose, but even seemingly minute doses, it was soon found, could cause various kinds of cancer and leukemia. It could also increase the probability of death and shorten a person's life span; cause chromosomal damage, affecting future generations; destroy the bone marrow and the vital immune system produced therein; and—in cancer patients—create burns, cell and tissue death (necrosis), and fibrosis of the internal organs (Israël, 1978:73; Pauling, 1958).

The Atomic Energy Commission was quite successful in hiding these troubling facts, not only from the general public, but from the medical community who actually administered the therapeutic beam. The AEC provided much of the information for the medical textbooks on radiation and its hazards. Thus, physicians generally received a biased education concerning the appropriate uses of radiotherapy (Bross, 1979).

The AEC's attitude toward low-level radiation was aptly summarized by Dr. Edward Teller, the "Father of the H-Bomb," and Dr. Albert Latter in *Life* magazine (February 10, 1958): "The only thing these statistics prove is that radiation in small doses need not necessarily be harmful—indeed may conceivably be helpful" (quoted in Pauling, 1958:119).

Even in 1979 *Science* magazine was forced to conclude:

> The radiation research community has lived almost entirely off the energy and defense establishments. . . . For anyone seeking objective scientific advice it is practically impossible to find someone knowledgeable who was not trained with AEC money *(Science,* April 13, 1979).

This may appear at first sight to be yet another honest debate over a scientific question—the danger of radiation versus the value of radiotherapy. But documents and investigations in recent years show that the pro-nuclear side of the argument consciously covered up what they knew to be real dangers of radiation and atomic fallout.

In the 1950s, President Eisenhower instructed the Atomic Energy Commission to "keep them [the public] confused" on questions of radiation. The commissioners sought to protect their bomb-testing programs from irate citizens. "People have got to learn to live with the facts of life," said one AEC commissioner, "and part of the facts of life is fallout." "It is certainly all right," said Strauss, "if you don't live next door to it." "Or *under* it," added another commissioner *(New York Times,* April 20, 1979).

Since that time the nuclear establishment has continued to promote industries and procedures which expose Americans to low levels of ionizing radiation. The rapid development of nuclear energy has added new pressure to declare low-level radiation safe. If it is *not* safe, then not only the nuclear arsenal but also the nuclear power plants are called into question, since such plants can emit radiation.

The nuclear waste problem erupted as a national scandal in 1988 and resulted in a shutdown of almost all U.S. weapons-production facilities by the end of that year. "The scope of the difficulties almost defies comprehension," the normally unflappable *New York Times* wrote (October 14, 1988).

For instance, it was revealed that for decades government officials had allowed radioactive wastes to leak into the environment, exposing thousands of workers and residents around the Fernald, Ohio, Feed Material Production Center. The amount of such pollution was truly staggering: thirteen *million* pounds from this one plant alone.

According to a Congressional panel investigating the disaster, there were three major forms of pollution: (1) plant runoff carried tons of deadly waste into drinking-water wells in the area west of Cincinnati and into the Great Miami River*; (2) storage pits, meant to store radioactive waste water, leaked into the water supply; and (3) the plant itself emitted radioactive particles into the air *(New York Times,* October 15, 1988).

The Fernald plant processed uranium for nuclear weapons and for military reactors. Its problems came to light after being shut down by a strike over wages and safety issues. There had been persistent questions about the health hazards posed by this and other plants. But it wasn't until late 1988 that the government admitted that it "knew full well that the normal operation of the Fernald plant would result in the emission of uranium and other substances" into the water and air (ibid.). Such emissions will remain dangerous for thousands of years.

But the Fernald situation was hardly unique. Similar scandals existed at other government nuclear facilities, such as the Savannah River plant near Aiken, South Carolina; the Rocky River Flats plant near Boulder, Colorado; and the Hanford Reservation in Washington State, where the plutonium for the Nagasaki bomb had been produced *(New York Times,* October 17, 1988).

It was also revealed that the Savannah River plant, operated by E. I.

---

*The Great Miami flows into the Ohio River. The Ohio empties into the Mississippi at Cairo, Illinois.

Du Pont de Nemours, had been the site of 30 reactor accidents between 1957 and 1985, according to another Congressional investigation. These accidents are considered "among the most severe ever documented at an American nuclear plant" *(New York Times,* October 3, 1988).

It is difficult to pinpoint the adverse health effects of this widely scattered pollution. But people living downwind of the Hanford plant claim that they have been subjected to higher-than-normal rates of cancer, miscarriage, and other health problems.

"We were all guinea pigs for the Government," said Betty Perkes, a 54-year-old mother of five who lives on a farm near Mesa, Washington. She believes that the loss of an infant and her family's many thyroid diseases were all caused by radioactive pollution from the plant.

"We know what caused all this," she said. "It was the Government. They never told us so we could protect ourselves" (ibid.).

Revelations about the federal Fernald, Ohio, facility certainly lend credence to such claims. For instance, the Energy Department admitted that when the plant was built in 1951, no provision was made for disposal of the solid waste generated by the production process. When the Atomic Energy Commission (AEC), predecessor of the Energy Department, proposed digging a pit in which to dump the waste, the plant's operator, NLO Inc., strongly objected that such a plan would contaminate local underground water sources. "The AEC disregarded NLO's warning and directed that the first waste pit be constructed," the government admitted in a court document *(New York Times,* October 15, 1988).

Additionally, in 1958, NLO told the Atomic Energy Commission that there was a crack in one of the tanks storing thousands of pounds of radium and other radioactive materials. The commission's solution was simple: they "let the leak continue until the level of radioactive waste in the tank dropped below the lowest crack" (ibid.). These tanks continue in use today, but are mercifully not filled above the level of the rupture.

It is hard to find words to describe such callous disregard of public health. At the very least, it calls into question the sincerity of the U.S. "war on cancer," when the same government simultaneously spreads millions of pounds of cancer-causing substances into the air, the soil, and the water. Between 1957 and 1975 there were 17 "comprehensive reviews" of tumors associated with diagnostic and therapeutic radiation (Schmahl, et al 1977). Nevertheless, U.S. scientists who have tried to expose the dangers and ineffectualness of diagnostic and therapeutic radiation have often suffered for their sins. Dr. Bross, who held important positions at both Roswell Park and Johns Hopkins and has published over 300 articles and communications, failed to get a renewal of his government grants when he spoke out on this topic. There was a congressional hearing on February 14, 1978, on this matter, and at that time he was asked to resubmit his proposal.

In 1979 Dr. Bross's grant application was approved by the National Cancer Institute, but only for $50,000 a year, far less than the $350,000 he claims is needed to answer the question, What are the long-term hazards of radiation therapy?

Bross pinpoints a thirty-year cover-up of radiation's hazards and, in particular, the role of doctors in promoting that danger:

> It is almost impossible to get "peer review" that will accept a study of iatrogenic [doctor-caused] disease. You just can't get people associated with the medical profession to accept a study that is frankly dealing with doctor-caused cancer. Everybody said I was crazy to do that, and they were right. But on the other hand if I called it something else and they turned me down anyway, then the public would not know why they turned me down. I figured it's better the public should know that the National Cancer Institute won't support this kind of research.
>
> For 30 years radiologists in this country have been engaged in massive malpractice—which is something that a doctor will not say about another doctor (Bross, 1979).

In conclusion, radiation therapy appears to be of limited value in the treatment of cancer although it is probably preferable to surgery in some cases, such as cancer of the larynx or prostate. There is little controversy over the number of patients currently being cured by radiotherapy—it is small. Many doctors believe that radiation is a relatively harmless procedure. They therefore recommend it to patients (especially advanced cases) as a palliative. It is also being used in earlier cases, such as in conjunction with limited mastectomy. Some researchers believe that this use of radiation is not only ineffective, but positively harmful for its recipients. It is part of a disastrous national policy that has always downplayed the hazards of radiation, while promoting its spread to every corner of the country.

« 5 »

Chemotherapy

Third among the so-called proven methods of treating cancer is toxic chemotherapy: the use of drugs to kill cancer cells. Few topics in medicine today are as controversial as the use of these agents.

In theory, a drug cure for cancer is highly appealing. Just as specific drugs cure many bacterial and parasitic infections, so should cancer chemotherapy ideally kill cancer cells without harming excessive quantities of normal tissue. In reality, however, orthodox chemotherapy has not yet developed an agent specific and safe enough to restrict its attack to cancer cells. Many chemotherapeutic agents work by blocking an essential metabolic step in the process of cellular division. Since cancer cells often divide more rapidly than normal cells, this lethal "antimetabolite" action should be directed preferentially against cancer cells. However, most normal tissues engage in cell division at varying rates. Thus chemotherapy poisons many normal tissues as well—especially the rapidly dividing cells of the bone marrow, intestinal wall, and the hair follicles.

The bone marrow is the foundation of the immune system, which seems to serve the dual function of preventing infections and combating the spread of cancer. The use of chemotherapy is often accompanied by destruction of this immune system. Chemotherapy often brings in its train a host of blood-deficiency diseases (such as leukopenia, thrombocytopenia, and aplastic anemia). These, in turn, can give rise to massive, uncontrollable infections.

Cancer patients on chemotherapy have been known to die of something as innocuous as the common cold.

Because of its effects on the immune system, chemotherapy stands in contradiction to another form of therapy: immunotherapy. This form of treatment is still considered experimental at most cancer centers. "Immunotherapy holds hope of enhancing the body's own disease-fighting systems to control cancer," says the American Cancer Society's 1988 edition of *Cancer Facts and Figures*. "This research area will take many years to find the proper role of these agents in cancer treatment" (ACS, 1988).

Since immunotherapy is generally used as a treatment of last resort, almost all patients receiving it have first received chemotherapy or are given drugs in combination with the immune-stimulating agents. Clinical results with immune modulators have generally been disappointing, and some doctors believe this is because the prior or concurrent use of immunity-destroying anticancer drugs wipes out whatever beneficial effects these newer agents may have.

Chemotherapy's effect on the gut can be equally disastrous. Cancer patients sometimes have difficulty in eating or absorbing their food. Cancer drugs may cause nausea, bleeding sores around the mouth, soreness of the gums and throat, and ulceration and bleeding of the gastrointestinal tract. Because most forms of chemotherapy particularly affect rapidly dividing cells most and because the mucous cells are quick dividers, this form of therapy has in some cases resulted in the sloughing of the entire internal mucosa of the gut. Death may result.

Some people withstand chemotherapy with few side effects. Many others become nauseated, vomit, lose their hair, or develop infections. Some have a wide range of toxic reactions.

There are approximately forty drugs in common use against cancer agents (see Table 1), which react with the genetic material of the cells (DNA). These drugs produce a cross-linking of the bases of the DNA chain, which blocks replication of nuclear DNA during mitosis, or cell division. The trade names of some of these drugs are BCNU, Cytoxan, and Platinol. Another category is derivations of nitrogen mustard, such as Leukeran, Mustargen, and Thio TEPA. Antimetabolites prevent cells from making nucleic acids and proteins essential to their survival. The drugs' molecules mimic necessary constituents in the cell. Methotrexate competes with folic acid and prevents this vitamin from being utilized. This leads to the death of the cell. It is thus literally an antivitamin. Other drugs in this category are 5-FU, Mithracin, and Thioguanine.

In addition, chemotherapists use antibiotics that have antitumor activ-

TABLE I

Some Anticancer Agents Commonly Used in the United States
(principal source: 1988 Physicians' Desk Reference)

Trade Name	Common Name	Marketing Company
ANTIBIOTIC DERIVATIVES		
1. Adriamycin	doxorubicin	Adria Labs
2. Blenoxane	bleomycin	Bristol-Myers
3. Cerubidine	daunorubicin	Wyeth, div. of Amer. Home Prods.
4. Cosmegen	dactinomycin	Merck Sharp & Dohme
ANTIESTROGEN		
5. Nolvadex	tamoxifen	ICI Pharma
ANTIMETABOLITES		
6. Efudex	fluorouracil, 5-FU	Hoffmann La Roche
7. Folex	methotrexate	Adria
8. FUDR	floxuridine	Hoffmann La Roche
9. Intron A	interferon alpha-2b	Schering Plough
10. Leukovorin	glutamic acid	Lederle, div. of Amer. Cyanamid
11. Methotrexate sodium injections	methotrexate	Cetus
Methotrexate tablets & parenteral	methotrexate	Lederle, div. of Amer. Cyanamid
Mexate and Mexate AQ	methotrexate	Bristol-Myers
12. Mithracin	plicamycin	Miles
13. Purinethol	mercaptopurine	Burroughs Wellcome
14. Roferon-A	interferon alpha-2b	Hoffmann La Roche
15. Thioguanine	6-thioguanine	Burroughs Wellcome
CYTOTOXIC AGENTS		
16. BiCNU	carmustine, BCNU	Bristol-Myers
17. CeeNU	lomustine, CCNU	Bristol-Myers
18. Cytosar-U	cytosine arabinoside	Upjohn
19. Cytoxan	cyclophosphamide	Bristol-Myers
20. Emcyt	estramustine	Pharmacia
21. Hydrea	hydroxyurea	Squibb

TABLE I *(continued)*

Trade Name	Common Name	Marketing Company
22. Matulane	procarbazine	Hoffman La Roche
23. Mutamycin	mitomycin	Bristol-Myers
24. Myleran	busulfan	Burroughs Wellcome
25. Neosar	cyclophosphamide	Adria
26. Platinol	cis-platin	Bristol-Myers
27. Vincasar	vincristine sulfate	Adria

HORMONES

28. Depo-Provera	medroxyprogersterone	Upjohn
29. Emcyt	estramustine phosphate sodium	Pharmacia
30. Estinyl	ethinyl estradiol	Schering Plough
31. Estrace	estradiol	Mead Johnson Laboratory
32. Megace	megestrol acetate	Bristol-Myers
33. Oreton	methyltestosterone	Schering Plough
34. Stilphostrol	diethylstilbestrol diphosphate	Miles Pharmaceutical
35. TACE	chlorotrianisene	Merrell Dow
36. Teslac	testolactone	Squibb

NITROGEN MUSTARD DERIVATIVES

37. Alkeran	melphalan	Burroughs Wellcome
38. Leukeran	chlorambucil	Burroughs Wellcome
31. Mustargen	mechlorethamine (nitrogen mustard)	Merck Sharp & Dohme
40. Thio TEPA	thiotepa	Lederle

STEROIDS and COMBINATIONS

41. Celestone	betamethasone sodium phosphate	Schering Plough

OTHER

42. DTIC-Dome	dacarbazine	Miles
43. Elspar	asparaginase	Merck Sharp & Dohme
44. Lysodren	mitotane	Bristol-Myers
45. Oncovin	vincristine sulfate	Lilly
46. Velban	vinblastine sulfate	Lilly
47. VePesid	etoposide	Bristol-Myers

ity, such as Adriamycin and Cosmagen, and plant alkaloids derived from the periwinkle plant, such as Oncovin and Velban.

All of these drugs have one characteristic in common: they are poisonous. They work because they're poisons. Methotrexate, for example, carries with it the following warning:

> METHOTREXATE MUST BE USED ONLY BY PHYSICIANS EXPERIENCED IN ANTIMETABOLITE CHEMOTHERAPY.
> BECAUSE OF THE POSSIBILITY OF FATAL OR SEVERE TOXIC REACTIONS, THE PATIENT SHOULD BE FULLY INFORMED BY THE PHYSICIAN OF THE RISKS INVOLVED AND SHOULD BE UNDER HIS CONSTANT SUPERVISION *(Physicians' Desk Reference,* 1988).

The package insert then goes on to describe the "high potential toxicity" of the product. This includes the abovementioned symptoms as well as malaise, undue fatigue, chills and fever, dizziness, and various problems of the skin, blood, alimentary system, urogenital system, and central nervous system. Finally, the doctor is warned that

> other reactions related or attributed to the use of methotrexate such as pneumonitis; metabolic changes, precipitating diabetes; osteoporotic effects, abnormal tissue, cell changes, and even sudden death have been reported (ibid).

Just how devastating these side effects can be is revealed in an anecdote told by Dr. John Laszlo, senior vice president for research at the American Cancer Society. Laszlo is considered an expert on the complications of cancer care. Not only do many patients suffer from extreme nausea and vomiting, he writes, but about one-quarter of the long-term patients become "conditioned" to experience these symptoms even in the absence of the actual drugs:

> We have seen patients drive into the hospital parking lot and promptly begin to vomit, or vomit when they smell the alcohol sponge used to clean off the arm prior to chemotherapy or even vomit when they see the nurse who administers the chemotherapy—even if that person is encountered out of uniform in a supermarket or elsewhere away from the hospital (Laszlo, 1987:52).

The author has even heard doctors jokingly refer to the drugs 5-FU as "Five Feet Under" and BCNU as "Be Seein' You."

In other forms of cancer, chemotherapy can offer palliation (partial or temporary remission of the disease) and, occasionally, prolongation of life. And, in fact, about 25 percent of all cancer patients are now receiving some form of anti-cancer drugs (ibid.).

Unfortunately, the types of cancer that respond to chemotherapy are generally among the least common forms of the disease. The most common forms of cancer—the big killers such as breast, colon, and lung malignancies—generally do not respond to primary treatment with drugs. Furthermore, according to Maugh and Marx, chemotherapy is not very effective against tumors that have grown large or spread. Its greatest successes are against small tumors that have only recently developed.

Chemotherapy has other drawbacks. There is an increased incidence of second, apparently unrelated malignancies in patients who have been "cured" by means of anticancer drugs. This is probably because the drugs themselves are carcinogenic. When radiation and chemotherapy were given together, the incidence of these second tumors was approximately twenty-five times the expected rate (ibid.:123).

Since both radiation and chemotherapy suppress the immune system, it is possible that new tumors are allowed to grow because the patient has been rendered unable to resist them. In either case, a person who is cured of cancer by these drastic means may find herself struggling with a new, drug-induced tumor a few years later.

Interest in cancer chemotherapy developed in part out of frustration with the limitations of surgery and radiation therapy. Even scientists sympathetic to these two methods admit that they "have been near the limits of their utility for many years" (Maugh and Marx, 1975).

The inspiration for cancer chemotherapy was the antibiotic revolution of the 1930s. Coupled to this was the "crash program" concept popularized during World War II.

"I am convinced that in the next decade, or maybe more, we will have a chemical as effective against cancer as sulfanilomides and penicillin are against bacterial infection," said Sloan-Kettering director C. P. "Dusty" Rhoads in 1953 (Denver Post, October 3, 1953).

"There is, for the first time, a scent of ultimate victory in the air," read an article on anticancer drugs in Reader's Digest in February 1957.*

*Reader's Digest is often a barometer of orthodox thinking on the cancer problem. Laurance S. Rockefeller, honorary chairman of the board of Memorial Sloan-Kettering, is a director of the magazine's parent company, and the Digest's founder DeWitt Wallace was, in turn, a major contributor to the New York cancer center. George V. Grune, chief executive officer of the magazine, is an overseer of MSKCC.

"We can look forward confidently to the control and ultimately the eradication of cancer," said the director of the National Cancer Institute in the 1950s. He promised Congress major new gains "in the next few years" (*Denver Post,* October 3, 1953).

In fact, announcing the imminent demise of cancer has become something of a subspecialty within the medical profession, especially around the month of April, when the American Cancer Society conducts its annual appeal drive.

"Nothing short of spectacular . . . a work of monumental importance" was how one New York chemotherapist described a new drug treatment for breast cancer (*New York Daily News,* February 17, 1976). Such promotion is not limited to chemotherapy but also affects the natural biological modifiers as well. The synthesis of interferon in 1980 unleashed a deluge of hype. "Like the genie in a fairy tale," the *Detroit Free Press* enthused "science came up with the key to the magic potion, a way to produce interferon in bulk" (cited in Nelkin, 1987).

Reader's Digest told its readers about the "wonder therapy," *Newsweek* about new "cancer weapons" and "the making of a miracle drug." *Time* spoke of "barely suppressed excitement among medical specialists" and a "gold mine for patients and for companies." *Saturday Evening Post* claimed that "punters in Wall Streets are already laying bets that interferon is a sure winner" (ibid.).

It wasn't until 1982 that reporters discovered the toxic side effects of interferon. That year four patients treated with the drug in France died. Suddenly there was widescale disillusionment: "From wonder drug to wall flower," as one reporter put it (ibid.).

Today interferon is approved for use in the treatment of two very rare forms of cancer, hairy-cell leukemia and juvenile laryngeal papillomatosis. It may also have limited use in a number of other rare conditions (*Merck Manual,* 1987). But it failed to live up to its promises. No sooner had its memory faded, however, than it was replaced by an even more virulent outbreak of "hype fever": interleukin-2, a protein produced by the T cells of the immune system.

"Cancer Breakthrough," screamed the cover story in *Fortune* that broke the story of the drug's development in the laboratory of Dr. Steven Rosenberg at NCI (November 1985).

"So powerful are the new weapons that many clinicians believe the odds in the struggle against cancer will soon be tipped in favor of the patient," wrote Gene Bylinsky in the five-page article.

A *Newsweek* cover and spots on all three networks followed. Rosenberg himself appeared on the "Today" show and called IL-2 "the first new kind of approach to cancer in perhaps 20–30 years" (quoted in *Science* 235, January 9, 1987).

Business Week was not far behind with a cover on "The New War on Cancer" (September 22, 1986). "Researchers are perfecting a potent weapon," the reader was told. "The body's own defenses." Not surprisingly, *Business Week* provided its readers with seven "biotech plays in the war on cancer" for those who wished to put their money where their hopes were.

(Many apparently did, for the stock of Cetus Corporation, the Emery-ville, California–based company that supplied the IL-2 to Rosenberg, soared from 16 to 33, "adding over $380 million to its market value before subsiding to 26" (*Financial World*, April 15, 1986).

"There's nothing [else] we have that's this exciting," said a NCI spokesperson. "This is not hype" (*Business Week*, December 23, 1985).

Soon after the initial announcement, however, doubts started to surface. On December 8, 1985, NCI announced that IL-2 had killed one of the patients in the experimental protocol at the Institute. Although his death had in fact occurred before the publicity, Rosenberg had failed to mention it on television or in the press (*New York Times*, December 9, 1985).

One year later, hype began to turn once again to disillusionment. Oddly enough, the cold water did not come from some unorthodox naysayers but from the very heart of the establishment itself. In an editorial in the *Journal of the American Medical Association,* Charles Moertel, the Mayo Clinic researcher famous for his negative tests of laetrile and vitamin C, charged that IL-2 was in fact highly toxic, inordinately expensive, and not particularly effective (*Science*, January 9, 1987).

"This specific treatment approach would not seem to merit further application in the compassionate management of patients with cancer," Moertel wrote. Commenting on the toxicity, he said "[T]reatment with IL-2 is an awesome experience." Patients require weeks of hospitalization in intensive care units if they are to survive the "devastating toxic reactions" (ibid.). The dollar cost, per patient is in the six figures. And the benefits are questionable.

The initial report had shown one complete remission out of 25, or 4 percent. A 1987 report claimed that widespread advanced cancers disappeared in 9 out of 152 patients—or nearly 6 percent—with partial responses in 20 others—about 13 percent. The majority of patients had no positive reaction to the treatment and four patients died from the therapy itself (*New York Times*, April 9, 1987).

The public has become cynical and disgruntled about such overstated claims, which usually succeed only in raising false hope in the minds of cancer victims and their families. "Cancer chemotherapists have a lingering poor reputation among large segments of the lay public," say the authors of the *Science* report, who are generally well-disposed toward the field. They attribute this in part to the "bitter disappointment" of chemotherapy's painfully slow progress (Maugh and Marx, 1975).

Many scientists have begun to question the basic premise of cancer chemotherapy, which is the use of toxic agents to kill every last cancer cell in the body. Dr. Victor Richards, for example, calls chemotherapy "at best an uncertain method of therapy" because it cannot harm or kill cancer cells "without producing comparable effects on normal cells." Chemotherapy succeeds because it is a systemic poison, and it fails for the same reason. Richards compares the use of such poisons to the difficulty of controlling

> an expanding colony of mice by shooting them with a smaller number of bullets than the number of mice. No matter how we calculate the firing system, one could see that inevitably, if even two mice capable of mating remained, doubling of the population would resume (Richards, 1972).

"With chemotherapy," he adds, "we have no sure shot. . . . It is clear that we can never eliminate the last cancer cell by using antimetabolites" (ibid.).

How successful are these drugs in combating cancer? This question is important: If they were highly effective, one might tolerate their admittedly harsh side effects to get the benefit of a cure.

It is generally agreed that in certain forms of cancer, chemotherapy is highly effective. Choriocarcinoma, a rare tumor that afflicts pregnant women, can be cured in 75–85 percent of cases with methotrexate and dactinomycin (*Merck Manual*, 1987).

Chemotherapy is now often given in various complex combinations, generally called "chemo cocktails." These are technically known by acronyms assembled from the generic or trade names of the drugs themselves. Thus many patients now receive CHOP (a combination of cyclophosphamide, doxorubicin, vincristine, and prednisone), FAM (fluorouracil, doxorubicin, and mitomycin), or MOPP (mechlorethamine, vincristine, procarbazine, and prednisone) instead of the single drugs favored in the past (NCI, 1987).

Another type of tumor that has yielded quite well to chemotherapy is Burkitt's lymphoma. Through the use of cyclophosphamide, methotrexate, and other drugs, doctors have been able to achieve about a 50 percent cure rate. However, this type of cancer is exceedingly rare in the United States.

It is found primarily in certain parts of Africa, where it is believed to be caused by a virus (Maugh and Marx, 1975:26).

Acute lymphoblastic leukemia, which most often attacks children, is in some ways the showpiece of the chemotherapists. Through the use of such drugs as daunorubicin, prednisone, vincristine, 6-MP, methotrexate, and BCNU, doctors at certain specialized cancer centers have been able to achieve 90 percent remission and 70 percent survival beyond five years. This is remarkably better than the grim prognosis for this disease only a few decades ago.

Other forms of cancer that have responded to chemotherapy include acute lymphocytic leukemia. Ewing's sarcoma, neuroblastoma, osteogenic sarcoma, ovarian cancer, and rhabdomyosarcoma. Testicular cancer has shown particularly good results in recent years (ACS, 1988).

Without diminishing the importance of advances in individual cases, it must be pointed out that almost all of these are uncommon forms of cancer.

In an excellent article in *Scientific American,* John Cairns, a professor of microbiology in the School of Public Health at Harvard University, evaluated the worth of various treatments currently employed against cancer.

His comments about chemotherapy are particularly telling. He acknowledges the successes of drugs in controlling such diseases as choriocarcinoma, testicular cancer, and Hodgkin's disease. But he points out that these are not only odd forms of the disease, but relatively rare. Choriocarcinoma finds its way onto every list of chemotherapy's triumphs, yet, Cairns points out, only about twenty or thirty lives a year are being saved through chemotherapy for this disease (Cairns, 1985).

For the common cancers "the results have been more often negative than positive," he writes. He also reminds us that

> many of the drugs used are known to be carcinogenic, and one of the long-term effects of chemotherapy is that somewhere between 5 and 10 percent of the surviving patients die of leukemia in the first 10 years after treatment (ibid.).

Nonetheless, despite the drawbacks, chemotherapy remains a growth industry. The Connecticut Cancer Registry, for instance, reports that one-quarter of all cancer patients receive some chemotherapy. The National Cancer Institute estimates that 200,000 patients receive cytotoxics nationwide each year. Yet "the number of patients who are being cured can hardly amount to more than a few percent of those who are treated. . . . For a

dangerous and technologically exacting form of treatment these are disturbing figures . . ." (ibid.).

"Whether any of the common cancers can be cured by chemotherapy
has yet to be established," Cairns adds (ibid.).

Cairns is himself a member of the establishment: polite, low-key, and
politic. Even so, he cannot help but point the finger at those responsible for
a failing strategy:

> Those who organize cancer centers and supervise the many clinical trials
> of chemotherapy look for ways to circumvent these relentless statistics. . . .
> It is surely an act of folly to pour hundreds of millions of dollars every year
> into giving a growing number of patients chemotherapy while doing virtually
> nothing to protect the population from cigarettes (ibid.).

Given the generally poor performance of chemotherapy, its often hor-
rendous side effects, and the limitations built into its very nature, why do
orthodox doctors continue to promote this form of treatment as the wave of
the future, and a proven method of treatment?

Among other factors are the economic forces that help shape the direction of cancer therapy, diagnosis, prevention, and management. Drugs
are central to the American economy, and it is perfectly logical from a
business point of view to seek a cure for cancer in the form of a patentable
and marketable drug.

The long-standing interest in such a cure, dating from before World
War II, has led to the creation of a "chemotherapy establishment" at all the
major medical centers. These individuals are tied to the pharmaceutical industry not only philosophically but often materially as well. Some of them
are consultants to drug companies, while others are directors or executives.
No law requires companies or consultants to reveal their relationships. Thus
it is possible that drug-company influence at cancer centers is greater than
appears from the public record. In addition, a number of drug-company
officials serve on NCI advisory committees.*

Grant money and gifts are available to those centers that work on

*Patricia E. Byfield, associate research scientist, Upjohn, served on NCI's Breast Can-
cer Task Force Committee; Hans J. Hansen, director, department of immunology, Hoffmann-
La Roche, on NCI's Developmental Therapeutics Committee; Bruce Johnson, analytical research department, Pfizer, on the Large Bowel and Pancreatic Cancer Review Committee; Irving Johnson, vice president for research, Lilly, on the Developmental Therapeutics Committee;
Gary L. Neil, head of cancer research, Upjohn, on the Developmental Therapeutics Committee;
and Arthur Weissbach, head, department of cell biology, Roche Institute on NCI's Cause and
Prevention Scientific Review Committee (NIH, 1979).

drugs in which the companies have a proprietary interest. Money is not generally available for substances or approaches in which drug companies have no such interest. Thus the invisible hand of the marketplace has chosen toxic chemotherapy for development and ignored other approaches that might be as promising from a medical, but not an economic, point of view (see chapter 17).

Chemotherapists are latecomers to the cancer scene. "[L]ack of regard for chemotherapists . . . has historically been exhibited by many surgeons and radiologists," according to the *Science* report on cancer (Maugh and Marx, 1975). Understandably, the chemotherapists have spoken in glowing terms about the effects of their agents while underplaying the drawbacks. A steady stream of positive reports has made chemotherapy fully acceptable to medical practitioners.

Finally, if cancer specialists were to admit publicly that chemotherapy is of limited usefulness and is often dangerous, the public might demand a radical change in direction—possibly toward unorthodox and nontoxic methods, and toward cancer prevention.

By constantly touting the promise of anticancer drugs, orthodox practitioners ward off this challenge to their expertise and scientists parry the threat radically new concepts represent to their long years of research. The use of chemotherapy is even advocated by those members of the establishment who realize how ineffective and dangerous it can be.

Richards, for example, admits that in the major forms of cancer (lung, bowel, stomach, pancreas, cervix, etc.), even *palliation* occurs only "for brief duration in about 5 to 10 percent of the cases." Yet he urges the use of drugs for such patients as well. His reason is revealing:

> Nevertheless, chemotherapy serves an extremely valuable role in keeping patients oriented toward proper medical therapy, and prevents the feeling of being abandoned by the physician in patients with late and hopeless cancers. Judicious employment and screening of potentially useful drugs may also prevent the spread of cancer quackery. . . . Properly based chemotherapy can serve a useful purpose in preventing improper orientation of the patient (Richards, 1972:215).

In Richard's view (and he is not alone), it is worthwhile to risk putting patients through possible nausea, vomiting, dizziness, hair loss, mouth sores, and even premature death simply in order to keep them "oriented toward proper medical therapy" and away from "cancer quackery."

Nor is the drug industry indifferent to developments in cancer research and therapy. "A cancer cure will be worth a fortune," a drug-company executive said in the 1950s (Applezweig, 1978). Although no infallible cure has yet been discovered for any form of cancer, by the 1970s chemotherapy had become a $200-million-a-year industry. A decade later this figure had nearly tripled (see below).

For many years the drug industry showed only lukewarm interest in investing its own money in the search for anticancer drugs. According to Alan Klass, a Canadian surgeon and former chairman of the Manitoba Cancer Institute,

> more effort is devoted in the [drug] industry towards research in the area of fast sellers, for the potentially unlimited market of coughs, colds, pain relief, depressions, tensions, than to grim cancer. Prospects of financial success are immeasurably greater in the less grim group (Klass, 1975).

"These [anticancer] drugs are costly to develop and sales are still limited," an industry analyst wrote some years ago (de Haen, 1975).

Other pharmaceutical spokesmen have worried that an effective cancer cure would upset the medical marketplace. "Nobody will be able to hold onto a cancer cure," a drug company executive predicted. "It would be too hot to handle" (Applezweig, 1978).

The president of Merck Sharp & Dohme told *Fortune:*

> I've always had a horror of Merck having an exclusive position in a cancer drug. It's just so emotional. I have a feeling that if we gave it away free, people would say we were charging too much (Robertson, 1976).

Despite these fears and reservations, since the 1950s all the major drug companies have maintained a presence in the cancer field. "All companies regard this work as a public service," Dr. C. Chester Stock of Sloan-Kettering Institute claimed in 1956. "For drug companies there won't be much money in anticancer drugs, but there will be a lot of prestige" *(Wall Street Journal,* February 8, 1956).

If only prestige were involved, however, as Stock claimed, the companies were working at it with unusual zeal. Between 1946 and 1953 Parke-Davis alone sent 1,500 different chemical compounds to Sloan-Kettering for testing, according to the president of that drug firm *(Wakefield* [Mass.] *Item,* September 17, 1953).

Many of the hundreds of thousands of compounds tested at Sloan-

Kettering or the National Cancer Institute were submitted by industry, usually by the largest pharmaceutical houses. A standardized legal agreement, drawn up by Frank Howard, a Standard Oil executive, was used to bring about a formal partnership between the company and Sloan-Kettering. The compounds were tested free of charge to the company. The agreement guaranteed a patent or a "perpetual non-exclusive, royalty-free license" for the company involved (Howard, 1962, contains a copy of the agreement). Howard was a firm advocate of patenting medical discoveries such as cancer drugs. Speaking at George Washington University in 1956, he said:

> To undertake a costly industrial research or development project without inquiring into the patent situation is like drilling an exploratory oil well without finding out who owns the property on which you drill (Howard, 1956).

"Dusty" Rhoads, who shared with Howard the original idea for a cancer-drug-testing institute, told a group of patent attorneys in 1940:

> In the near future patents may well control its [medicine's] entire development. . . . The patent lawyers can and do control the support of industrial science. I wish to establish clearly the need for, as well as the profits to be obtained from, intelligent study of the factors which influence the course of illness (Memorial, 1940).

In fact, almost every anticancer drug marketed since World War II has been patented by its manufacturer, although most of the research was done at government-supported institutions. The agreement between industry and Sloan-Kettering paid off in at least one case, that of methotrexate (or amethopterin), which was patented by Lederle Laboratories, a division of American Cyanamid, Inc., in 1951.* Under the standard form agreement, first used with Lederle, the company was given a patent, was allowed to keep drug research secret, and merely had to provide the substance for testing.

The agreement was so favorable to industry not only because of the business orientation of Memorial Sloan-Kettering's leaders but because of the difficulty of getting profit-oriented drug companies to invest in the "grim" field of cancer.

Sales figures for methotrexate in the 1970s were estimated at about $5 million a year. With the adoption of a high-dose methotrexate regimen for

*MSKCC overseer and former Sloan-Kettering chairman James Fisk, Ph.D., was a director of American Cyanamid, Inc. (see Appendix A).

a number of different cancers, however, these sales figures have probably increased considerably. Methotrexate cost around $9 for 500 milligrams in the mid-seventies (International Workshop, 1975); the high-dose regimen requires the use of hundreds of grams of this substance per patient.

In March 1989 the author conducted an informal phone survey of New York City pharmacies to determine the current price of methotrexate. Prices varied, of course, depending on both dosage and brand. Generics were considerably cheaper. But all showed a remarkable increase in the cost from that quoted above.

For example, a 2.5 milligram tablet (the usual oral dosage) is priced between $2.50 and $3.50. The price of a 500 milligram injection of methotrexate is now between $137 and $173: more than 15 times the $9 figure quoted in 1975.

Thirty milligrams twice a week is the usual dose. This works out to 24 tablets or about $72 a week for treatment. But the high-dose methotrexate regimen calls for "massive doses" of 350–5,000 milligrams per square meter of body area, followed by "leucovorin rescue" factor (Rubin, 1983). The human body area is generally in the 1–1.5 square meter range.

At this rate, a single treatment with the highest dose of methotrexate could cost in the range of $1,000–2,000 per treatment, and that's at discount rates. This does not include the cost of the rescue factor, which brings the patient back from the point of death, or the doctor's or hospital's charges for administering this life-threatening treatment. Clearly, the money adds up.

Drug companies have also been enticed into the field by government grants disbursed by NCI.

In 1955 the center of drug testing shifted from Sloan-Kettering Institute to NCI's Cancer Chemotherapy National Service Center in Bethesda, Maryland. Congress allocated $25 million to test 20,000 chemicals a year at "The Wall Street of Cancer Research," in the words of the center's director, Dr. Kenneth M. Endicott (*Newsweek*, January 20, 1958). Under this plan the government directly subsidized drug companies to do research that, if successful, would create new products for them. For example, Chas. Pfizer & Co. received $1.2 million in 1958, Upjohn & Co. $150,000, and Abbott Laboratories $208,000 (ibid.).

Most important in changing industry attitudes, however, have been market factors. The drug industry traditionally has been one of the most profitable businesses in the world. "For many years," says Dr. Klass, "the profits of the drug industry have been twice the average for all other American industries" (Klass, 1975:76). Most of these profits came from antibiotics, painkillers, or mood-altering drugs such as Valium.

As patents run out and as the industry faces increasingly costly government regulations and other problems, profitability also falls. From a pretax profit of 21 percent in 1973, the entire industry experienced a slump in the latter 1970s. "Drug profitability is not what it used to be," *Chemical & Engineering News* complained in 1976. "Profit margins have dropped to a 10-year low" (March 1, 1976). Besides these worries, "evidence of the slow-down in ethical pharmaceutical volume abounds," wrote Standard and Poor's *Industry Survey* (Standard and Poor's, 1979).

One of the main reasons for this drop was a lack of new markets to exploit. Patents had run out on many of the most profitable drugs of the 1960s and 1970s.

"What the drug industry needs is a major new product line," a Wall Street analyst told *Business Week*. Not surprisingly, one of the areas he pinpointed as a potentially lucrative area was cancer chemotherapy (*Business Week*, January 17, 1977).

Although new cancer drug research is usually shrouded in secrecy, it was known that such giant firms as Eli Lilly, Merck, and Hoffmann–La Roche had begun spending an increasing proportion of their research budgets on cancer (*Dun's Review*, December 1974; Robertson, 1976).*

General disappointment with cancer chemotherapy made the drug companies look in other directions for an effective (and patentable) cancer medicine. One candidate was interferon—or more accurately, the interferons. These are naturally occurring substances that appear to have anticancer and antiviral effects.

Interferon was discovered in the 1950s, and little interest was shown in developing its potential in the United States, mainly because of the difficulty of producing commercial amounts. Interferon is a natural substance formed by cells when they are attacked by viruses.

European studies showing anticancer results, plus an increased possibility of synthesizing an active anticancer drug, whetted the appetites of the drug companies. The American Cancer Society allocated $2 million to buy European interferon and test it in a "crash program" (ACS, 1978).

If interferon turned out to be an effective agent and a way had been found to market it (or a substance that could stimulate its production in the human body), it could have turned out to be a profitable breakthrough for the pharmaceutical industry. The potential profits to be derived from interferon production were huge, and the competition fierce.

Interferon, like radium seventy-five years ago, was fabulously expensive. One ounce of interferon in the late 1970s was worth $1.8 billion (*Omni*,

*The drug industry is said to be "notorious for secrecy" (*Dun's Review*, December 1974:55). Nevertheless, the chairman of Merck acknowledged that his company was working on a cancer vaccine (ibid.).

July 1979). In 1975 it was estimated that interferon treatment for cancer costs $500–5,000 per patient per day, depending on the dosage given (International Workshop, 1975:12). It was hoped at the time that new techniques would bring this cost down five to tenfold within a few years. But one industry spokesman said the price was likely to be *multiplied* by three (ibid.:85).

In 1979, 150 cancer patients were treated with interferon at ten U.S. cancer centers at an average cost of $50,000 per patient (*New York Post,* June 28, 1979). In the clinical trials conducted in Sweden at the Karolinska Institute, interferon was given three times a week for one and a half years. At 1975 prices, this cost between $117,000 and $1,170,000 per patient.

This represented a considerable potential market for the drug companies. Several patents were taken out on interferon purification processes. Nor surprisingly, there was intense competition for techniques, contacts, and markets.

The 1975 International Workshop on Interferon, chaired by Dr. Mathilde Krim, noted:

> A separate "workshop" session . . . dealt with the cost of production of human interferon. This session was attended by a number of representatives from the [drug] industry, obviously interested in the development of production facilities. However, there was considerable reluctance on the part of industry representatives to quote cost estimates in a public forum. (Interestingly enough, the same individuals were quite eager to discuss the problem in their competitor's absence.) (International Workshop, 1975:66)

When the American Cancer Society, Memorial Sloan-Kettering, National Cancer Institute, and the National Institute for Allergy and Infectious Diseases sponsored the Second International Workshop on Interferons at Rockefeller University, April 22–24, 1979, the list of contributors to the meeting read like a Who's Who of the drug field. It included Baxter-Travenol Laboratories, Bristol-Myers Co., Burroughs-Wellcome Co., Cutter Laboratories, Hoffmann-La Roche, Inc., Johnson & Johnson, Merck Sharp & Dohme, Miles Laboratories, Monsanto Co., Pfizer Inc., Schering-Plough Corp., Searle Laboratories, Smith Kline and French, U.S.V. Pharmaceuticals, and Warner-Lambert (Second International Workshop, 1979).*

*Industry speakers were well represented in most of the scientific sessions, which testifies to the seriousness with which it regarded this research. An Upjohn scientist spoke at the morning session (April 22) on "interferon inducers," a Burroughs-Wellcome researcher spoke that afternoon on "antiviral activities of interferons *in vivo,*" etc. In all, fifty-seven drug company representatives attended.

While a decade later interferon has been approved for sale by the FDA, it is only for a few very rare kinds of cancer.

Nor were the big companies neglecting the chemical approach to cancer, although it was, and is, plagued with disappointments. During this same period Bristol-Myers won approval for the commercial marketing of Platinol (cis-platin), a drug used in the treatment of bladder cancer (MSKCC, 1976). Bristol-Myers also won approval in March 1977 to market BiCNU. And ICI Americas received approval from the U.S. government to sell Nolvadex, a drug used in the treatment of advanced breast cancer (*New York Times,* July 23, 1978).

Cancer drugs represent a tantalizing possibility to the drug companies. In a few special instances it has paid off well. In the United States one of the best sellers has been adriamycin, an anticancer antibiotic noted for its extreme toxicity. It is owned outright by Adria Laboratories, a joint venture of Hercules, Inc., and the Montedison Group of Italy. The drug is said to produce regressions in such conditions as lymphoblastic leukemia, acute myeloblastic leukemia. Wilms' tumor, and various other kinds of carcinoma, including Hodgkin's disease (de Haen, 1975).

During its first year on the market (1974) adriamycin sold an impressive $10 million. And although the U.S. government routinely hides sales figures on drugs—"to avoid disclosing figures for individual companies"—it is believed that sales have increased considerably since then.*

Adriamycin illustrates how the public pays for these drugs to be developed and then pays again—this time at monopoly prices—to purchase these drugs from private companies. Montedison, the Italian conglomerate, attempted to find a U.S. licensee for its product in 1969. At that time, however, the U.S. drug industry still had little interest in investing in cancer drugs. The Italian firm finally made an arrangement with the National Cancer Institute under which the U.S. government and Sloan-Kettering Institute would test the drug in animals and humans. U.S. researchers did much of the work to develop the drug in this country and even obtained permission from the Food and Drug Administration to market it. Of course, U.S. taxpayer money paid for this expensive work. But the patent remained in the hands of its original owners, who have profited handsomely by this arrangement (Applezweig, 1978).

Even more profitable has been the Soviet drug Ftorafur. This compound has been patented by the Soviet Institute of Organic Synthesis, which has licensed the Japanese Taiho company to market the drug in Japan.

*Quote from a government report on pharmaceutical preparations (U.S. Department of Commerce, Bureau of the Census, 1977). "Data on new prescriptions are compiled privately for drug manufacturers by a company that copyrights its figures. Thus, they rarely work their way directly into public hands . . ." (*Wall Street Journal,* July 8, 1976).

Analysts were not sure of the exact composition of Ftorafur. It appeared to be an oral, relatively nontoxic form of the American drug 5-fluorouracil.*

In the 1970s Ftorafur was doing better than any American drug for cancer. Sales in 1976 were $100 million, or roughly ten times the best-selling drug in the United States.

The main reason for Ftorafur's success, however, was the unusual—some would say reckless—way in which the drug was marketed. "Some Japanese physicians," it is said, "now tend to identify 'precancerous' states, 'risk of cancer' or 'susceptibility to cancer' and treat the patient prophylactically [i.e., preventively] with anticancer drugs" (Applezweig, 1978).

This situation arises because Japanese physicians routinely sell drugs to their patients. Ftorafur reputedly came with a high retail markup, which naturally encouraged the physician to sell more drugs. If risk of cancer now makes one a candidate for an anticancer drug, then every Japanese (and American) could be considered a candidate for Ftorafur. Because of the radically different way in which drugs are marketed in the United States, however, it is unlikely that American companies could repeat the success of their Japanese counterparts (ibid.).

In fact, the best-selling cancer drug worldwide is Krestin, an immunostimulant produced by Kureha and marketed by Sankyo, both Japanese companies. With 1987 sales of $359.1 million, Krestin is in fact the nineteenth top-selling drug in the world (*Health Week,* March 6, 1987). Yet the drug is not available in the United States. Company officials indicated that Krestin was not being marketed in the United States in part because of the difficulty of obtaining FDA approval (Takaiwa, 1989).

The last decade has seen tremendous growth in the U.S. pharmaceutical industry, however. The Standard & Poor's Industry Survey calls the drug business "the brightest area of the health care universe" (December 15, 1988).

Profits for the industry as a whole were 24 percent in 1987 and close to 21 percent in 1988. It is "one of the nation's most profitable business enterprises . . . ," whose growth rate over the last ten years has been double that of the Standard & Poor's stock price index (ibid.).

The sales of chemotherapeutic agents have kept pace with this upward motion. They have more than doubled in four years. According to U.S. government figures, the market went from $270 million in 1983 to over $564 million in 1987 (U.S. Department of Commerce, 1983–1987).

But even this substantial growth rate understates the case. It does not

*The patent on 5-FU, as it is called, was held for seventeen years by Hoffmann-La Roche and the American Cancer Society (25 percent). Perhaps by coincidence, one of the founders of the ACS, Elmer Bobst, is a former president of Hoffmann-La Roche.

include "other pharmaceutical preparations affecting neoplasms, the endocrine system and metabolic diseases," which totaled over $109 million in 1987. Nor does it include the radioactive immunoassay market, which was over $50 million in 1982 and, by all expectations, should be about $100 million today. Detection and diagnostic kits add an additional $30 million (Teitelman, 1985). Thus *the actual figure for cancer drug sales is close to $750 million a year,* not to mention the huge amounts of painkillers, antibiotics, antiemetics, etc. that are used by cancer patients.

Bristol-Myers alone sold $153 million in chemotherapeutic drugs in 1984, making it the preeminent American manufacturer (ibid.). With top-selling drugs such as Platinol and VePesid, it controls close to 50 percent of the domestic anticancer market (Standard & Poor's, 1988). Some of the other major players in the market are Eli Lilly, with Oncovin; Adria Laboratories, with Adriamycin; and Hoffmann La Roche; with Matulane (ibid.).

Yet these figures only scratch the surface of what cancer could mean to the drug industry.

The developing market is divided into two components: the cytotoxic chemotherapy part and the biotech group. Traditional chemotherapy seems to have reached a plateau: its very toxicity generates a great deal of resistance, and except in the well-publicized dramatic cases, it has not proven highly successful. Most hopes therefore ride on biotechnology, on such exciting new products as tumor necrosis factor, monoclonal antibodies, and interleukin-2. In the mid-1980s, biotech investors even started to show up within the cancer establishment. For example, Frederick R. Adler, chairman of a number of biotech firms (Bio-Tech Gen Corp, Life Techs, and others), became a trustee of Memorial Sloan-Kettering Cancer Center.

The 1987 stock-market crash set in motion changes within biotechnology, however. Basically venture capital has dried up for the biotech section. The result has been a wholesale acquisition of the innovative core of those companies by the same large pharmaceutical giants they originally challenged for the cancer drug market. The result of this development on innovation remains to be seen ("Staying Alive in Biotech," *New York Times,* November 6, 1988).

The future, like the past, seems to lie with the largest companies. Bristol-Myers' Oncogen Division, which already controls almost half the U.S. market, is producing new drugs for cancer and AIDS. The vice president for cancer research at Bristol-Myers is Dr. Stephen Carter, formerly a top NCI official.

Of the new generation of drugs, only alpha interferon has been approved for marketing by the FDA, and that for a very rare form of cancer. But there has been a sharp increase in the number of cytotoxic drugs on the market. In the first edition of this book the number of commonly used anti-cancer drugs listed in Table I was twenty-two. The 1988 *Physicians' Desk Reference* lists seventy-one products.

To be sure, some of these are duplicates of older drugs that have lapsed into the public domain. In other cases, modifications of previously approved drugs have been marketed as new entities. Overall, without any conceptual breakthroughs, there has been an increase in the number of products. And the number of patients who receive chemotherapy has also increased greatly. It is now about 50 percent, although only about 5 percent could be said to significantly benefit from that treatment, according to an article in *Scientific American* (Cairns, 1985).

In Table I, are listed all these approved cytotoxic drugs, minus the duplications and also the hormones and steroids, which were usually not developed or sold specifically as anticancer agents.

In addition, there are several dozen drugs, not listed, that are currently awaiting trials at NCI. Many of these are being developed in conjunction with major drug companies (NCI, 1987).

A large number of drugs on the list come from a few companies— Bristol-Myers, Burroughs Wellcome, Adria and Hoffmann La Roche each, and Lederle and Merck.

It hardly seems coincidental that one of the most notable changes on the Memorial Sloan-Kettering board has been the ascendance of Bristol-Myers. The two vice chairmen of the Center are both now associated with that New York drug company. Richard L. Gelb, chairman of the board of Bristol-Myers, himself became chairman of the board of managers of Sloan-Kettering Institute and vice chairman of the overall board.

Meanwhile, James D. Robinson III, the American Express executive who is the other vice chairman of the Memorial Sloan-Kettering board, was made a director of Bristol-Myers.

Merck is represented on the MSKCC board by John K. McLaughlin, a director of the company and manager of MSKCC. The president of the Center, Paul Marks, M.D., is a director of Pfizer. (See Appendix A for fuller discussion).

At the national level, Gertrude Elion, Ph.D., the noted Burroughs Wellcome scientist and 1988 Nobel laureate, is a member of the select National Cancer Advisory Board until 1990 (*New York Times Magazine*, January 19, 1989).

By pointing this out, we don't mean to imply that these individuals are doing something illegal or immoral. On the other hand, it must be said that their drug company positions certainly predispose them to direct research in a manner consistent with the interests of the profit-making sector.

The drug industry is a kind of silent partner in the cancer research enterprise. It has managed to invest relatively little in the cancer problem, yet stands to reap tremendous benefits when and if a breakthrough is found.

Through its many interlocks with the research centers and the American Cancer Society, and through selective funding of specific research projects such as interferon, it maintains its presence in the field. The domination of investment bankers and industrialists over the cancer field is meant to guarantee that the ultimate cure for cancer will come marked "Patent Pending" and, they hope, "Made in U.S.A."

PART TWO

Unproven Methods

"It was from the inventions and temerity of quacks that physicians have derived some of their most active and useful medicines."

Benjamin Rush, M.D.

« 6 »

Unorthodox Therapies

The "proven" methods of treating cancer are in a state of crisis. Clearly, the cancer problem cannot be solved in any ultimate sense by sticking to today's "safe and sound" methods. Something radically new is needed—approaches that are fresh and daring.

Where will these radical new ideas come from? Many people believe they will come from the well-funded, orthodox research centers. It is only logical, they think, that those with the best credentials, finest equipment, and amplest research funds will make the big breakthroughs in cancer. No one can say with certainty that this will not happen.

Another possibility, however, is that the most fundamental breakthroughs will come from innovative clinicians or small research laboratories, which have the advantage of independence, so vital to a creative scientist. Many such laboratories exist around the world, and a number of them have put forward alternative views of the cancer problem—and alternative solutions. To the establishment, in general, such independent researchers are not innovators. Nor are they really scientists. They are advocates of unproven methods or, more bluntly, "quacks."

Quack is one of the ugliest words in the English language. The idea of exploiting a desperate, dying person's hope of a cure is so repulsive that

97

most people are instantly deterred from looking any further once this label is applied.*

If we are to find a cure for cancer, however, it is necessary to examine all alternatives. In the case of "quack" cures, it is necessary to ask, first of all, on what basis these methods are condemned.

Since the American Cancer Society has taken the lead in condemning such unorthodox procedures, its book *Unproven Methods of Cancer Management* can serve as a guide to orthodox thinking on quackery.

Unproven Methods (as well as the larger index and files that complement it) is part of a plan to investigate new methods in the treatment, diagnosis, and prevention of cancer. The American Cancer Society asserts that the book is meant only to be informative, and not to stigmatize any scientist. In fact, it resembles the list of "subversive" organizations once maintained by the House Un-American Activities Committee. Merely including a scientist's name on the list has the effect of damning that researcher's work and putting the tag of quackery on him and his efforts.

One scientist, added to the list in the late 1970s, noted that from 1973 to 1976 he received a basic research grant from the National Cancer Institute. But, he said, once his method was placed on the ACS's unproven list, "we could not get a renewal, by hook or crook—no matter how good the application itself was" (Gold, 1979).

The orthodox characterization of unproven methods is based on several serious charges. Each of these will be examined in some depth.

First, it is said that unorthodox practitioners and researchers are basically without the requisite knowledge of cancer to make any intelligent statements about the disease.

> The proponents of new or unproven methods of cancer management range from ignorant, uneducated, misguided persons, to highly educated scientists with advanced degrees who are out of their area of competence in supporting a particular form of treatment. A few hold Ph.D. or M.D. degrees. . . .
> They may have multiple unusual degrees such as N.D. (Doctor of Naturopathy), Ph.N. (Philosopher of Naturopathy), M.T. (Medical Technologist),

*The American Cancer Society changed the name of its Committee on Quackery to the Committee on Unproven Methods of Cancer Management in the 1950s (Young, 1967:398). But Richards (1972), himself affiliated with the Society, continued to use the designation *cancer quackery* and an ACS official in Rockland County, New York, called Michael Schachter, M.D., a "quack" for his use of laetrile and other unconventional therapies (*The Journal-News*, Rockland, New York, December 28, 1977). "Unproven method," for the American Cancer Society, appears to be simply a euphemism for quackery. In fact, the designation *quackery* burgeoned again in the 1980s, through the activities of the self-proclaimed "quackbusters" such as Stephen Barrett (Grossman, 1988).

DABB-A (Diplomate of American Board of Bio-Analysts), or Ms.D. (Doctor of Metaphysics); these degrees may have been received from correspondence schools (ACS, 1971b).

Table 2 lists seventy advocates of unorthodox therapies whose credentials are given in the ACS book on unproven methods.* It is immediately apparent that there is a discrepancy between what the ACS says about the advocates of these methods and the facts, as revealed in the Society's own chapters on the individuals involved.

According to information provided by the ACS itself, of these seventy, forty-one hold bona fide medical degrees from such universities as Harvard, Illinois, Northwestern, Yale, Dublin, Oxford, or Toronto. Two more are osteopaths who became medical doctors (M.D.'s) when the two healing professions merged in California in 1962. Only one individual holds a medical degree from what the ACS describes as a "class C institution which went out of existence."

Four of these medical doctors also hold doctorates (Ph.D's) in scientific disciplines from reputable institutions.

In addition, eleven other proponents of new methods received Ph.D.'s in such fields as chemistry, physiology, bacteriology, parasitology, or medical physics from universities such as Yale, Johns Hopkins, University of California-Berkeley, Columbia, and New York University.

Thus, over 77 percent of these "snake-oil salesmen," as they are sometimes called, are medical doctors or doctors of philosophy in scientific areas. In most cases, if they hold medical degrees, they have spent their working lives treating and/or researching cancer; the doctors of science have usually attempted to apply their knowledge of a particular area of research to the cancer problem.

Recall, however, that the ACS primer on unproven methods states that "a few" hold M.D. or Ph.D. degrees; a few in this case is 77 percent.

Of the other 23 percent, three individuals hold honorary doctorates of science (D.Sc.). There is also a dentist, a registered nurse, a chiropractor, a veterinarian, a bachelor of arts, and a naturopath. There are six laypersons for whom no degrees are indicated (see Table 2b).

An independent survey of 138 practitioners of unorthodox cancer therapies similarly found that 60 percent were medical doctors (Cassileth, 1984).

There are no M.T.'s, DABB-As, or Doctors of Metaphysics on the ACS list. In fact, in general it is difficult to distinguish most of these "quacks"

*In 1989, the ACS added the International Association of Cancer Victors and Friends, or IACVF, to its list (*CA* 39:1, January/February, 1989). No living advocate is mentioned in this article and consequently none is included in this table.

TABLE 2
Advocates of Unorthodox Cancer Therapies

(Information from American Cancer Society, *Unproven Methods of Cancer Management*)

Name	Sci. Degree(s)	From**	Professional Status
1. Jeanne Achterberg	Ph.D.	Texas Christian University	Assistant Professor, University of Texas Health Sciences Center, Dallas.
2. William P. Aiken	M.D.	Northwestern University	General practitioner; pulmonary specialist.
3. Eleanor Alexander-Jackson	Ph.D.	New York University	Bacteriologist, New York University; University Hospital, Michigan; New York State Dept. of Health; Cornell Medical College; College of Physicians and Surgeons, Columbia University.
4. Hariton Alivizatos	M.D.	[Athens Medical School]	Microbiologist; licensed in Greece
5. Manfred von Ardenne	Ph.D.	[not given]	"Connected with development of cathode ray and oscilloscope tubes and worked on the electron microscope." Work supported by E. German government.
6. H. H. Beard	Ph.D.	Yale University	Professor of chemistry and physical science, Tulane University.
7. Joseph Blaszczak	D.V.M.	University of Bologna	Veterinarian; vitamin therapy (B group).
8. Johanna Brandt	N.D., Ph.N.	First National University of Naturopathy	Advocated the "Grape Cure" for cancer.
9. Dean Burk	Ph.D.	University of California, Berkeley	Founder and head, Cell Chemistry, National Center Institute (ret.)

10. Lawrence Burton	Ph.D.	New York University	Cal Tech; NYU; St. Vincent's, NYC; IAT Clinic, Freeport.
11. Stanislaw Burzynski	M.D., Ph.D.	Medical Academy of Lublin	Assistant Professor, Baylor College of Medicine, Houston; Burzynski Research Institute.
12. Mildred Cates [Nelson]	R.N.	[not given]	Harry Hoxsey's nurse.
13. Robert R. Citron	M.D.	University of Illinois	General practitioner; member, American Medical Association.
†14. William B. Coley	M.D.	Harvard University	Chief of Bone Service, Memorial Hospital.
15. Ernesto Contreras	M.D.	Army Medical School, Mexico City	House Officer-Pathology, Children's Hospital, Boston; pathologist, Army Hospital.
16. William M. Crofton	M.D.	Dublin University	Fellow, Royal Society of Medicine; lecturer, University Hospital, Dublin.
17. Sergio M. DeCarvalho	M.D.	Lisbon University	Licensed to practice in California; laboratory medicine.
18. Philip L. Drosnes	[not given]	[not given]	"Convicted of practicing medicine without a license"; acquitted on appeal.
19. Isaac Newton Frost	M.D.	Memphis Hospital Medical College	General practititoner.
20. Max B. Gerson	M.D.	Freiberg, Breslau, Berlin Universities	Internal medicine, neurology, Gotham Hospital, N.Y.C.
21. Donald F. Gibson	M.D.	Yale University	General surgery and urology.
22. Thomas J. Glover	M.B. (M.D.)	University of Toronto	"Licensed to practice medicine in Ontario in 1913."
†23. Joseph Gold	M.D.	State University of New York–Upstate Medical College	Director, Syracuse Cancer Research Institute.

TABLE 2 *(continued)*

Name	Sci. Degree(s)	From**	Professional Status
24. Oskar C. Gruner	M.D.	Royal College of Physicians, London	Licensed to practice in Canada, 1936.
25. Henry G. Hadley	M.D.	Washington University, St. Louis	Certified by American Board of Internal Medicine; chest specialist.
26. Bruce Halstead	M.D.	College of Medical Evangelists	Marine biologist, Loma Linda University.
27. Wendell G. Hendricks	M.D. (D.O.)*	College of Osteopathic Physicians and Surgeons	"Accused of administering the Lincoln, Koch, and other agents. . . ."
28. John E. Hett	M.D.	University of Toronto	Developer of "Hett serum."
29. Harry M. Hoxsey	[none]		Developer of Hoxsey Method (herbs).
30. Andrew C. Ivy	M.D., Ph.D.	[University of Chicago, Rush Medical College]	Executive director, National Advisory Cancer Council; director, American Cancer Society.
31. Barbara J. Johnston	M.D.	New York University	Board-certified internist; head of oncology, St. Vincent's Hospital, N.Y.C.
32. Herman H. Kahlenberg	Ph.D.	University of Wisconsin	Assistant, Rockefeller Institute; laboratory owner.
33. William Donald Kelley	D.D.S.	Baylor University	Orthodontist.
34. William F. Koch	M.D., Ph.D.	[University of Michigan, Detroit College of Medicine]	Developer of Glyoxylide.
35. Byron Krebs	M.D. (D.O.)*	College of Osteopathic Physicians and Surgeons, Los Angeles	Full-time general practitioner.

36. Ernst T. Krebs, Sr.	M.D.	College of Physicians and Surgeons, San Francisco	Codeveloper of laetrile.
37. Ernst T. Krebs, Jr.	A.B.	University of Illinois, Urbana	"Biochemist"; co-developer of laetrile.
38. Michio Kushi	[D.Sc. (Hon.)]	[American Christian College, Tulsa]	East West Foundation.
39. Lillian Lazenby	[not given] [not given]	[not given] [not given]	"Convicted of practicing medicine without a license"; acquitted on appeal.
40. Rita LeRoi	M.D.	[not given]	Society for Cancer Research, Arlesheim, Switzerland.
41. Andrew J. Lewis	B.A.	John Carroll University	Owner, Lewis Laboratory for Cancer Research.
†42. Robert E. Lincoln	M.D.	Boston University	General practitioner.
43. Virginia Livingston	M.D.	New York University	General practitioner.
44. Jack G. Makari	M.D.	American University, Beirut	Research positions at Royal College of Physicians and Surgeons, England; WHO fellow, Harvard; fellow, Johns Hopkins; associate professor, University of Texas; immunologist, M. D. Anderson Hospital; director of research, Muhlenberg Hospital, New Jersey.
45. Harold W. Manner	Ph.D.	Northwestern University	Chair, Div. of Sci. & Math, Utica College of Syracuse University; Chair, Department of Biology, Loyola University, Chicago.
46. Mildred Miller	[not given]	[not given]	Administrator, Degenerative Disease Center, Las Vegas.

TABLE 2 (continued)

Name	Sci. Degree(s)	From**	Professional Status
†47. A. Ernest Mills	M.D.	Tufts University	Internist.
48. Norman Molomut	Ph.D.	Columbia University	Bacteriologist, Pasteur Institute, Michigan; College of Physicians and Surgeons, Columbia University; director of research, Waldemar Medical Research Foundation.
49. Paul A. Murray	M.D.	University of Pittsburgh	General practitioner.
50. Gaston Naessens	[not given]	[not given]	"Claims to have studied biology at University of Lille."
51. Perry L. Nichols	M.D.	University of the South	"A class C institution which went out of existence."
52. Paul Niehans	M.D.	University of Bern	Surgery: endocrinology.
53. James W. Ollerenshaw	B.Ch., B.M. (M.D.)	Oxford University	Fellow of Royal Society of Medicine; Associate of Industrial Medical Officers.
54. Robert C. Olney	M.D.	Eclectic Medical College, Cincinnati	Medical director, Providence Hospital, Lincoln, Nebr.
55. Morton Padnos	Ph.D.	New York University	Parasitologist, U.S. Army, New York Aquarium, Waldemar Medical Research Foundation.
56. James H. Rand, III	D.Sc. (Hon.)	University of Berlin	Development engineer, chemist, inventor; son of founder of Remington-Rand, Inc.
57. Wilhelm Reich	M.D.	University of Vienna	Associate of Sigmund Freud.

58. Emanuel Revici	University of Bucharest	M.D.	Director, Institute of Applied Biology, and Trafalgar Hospital, N.Y.C.
59. Jules Samuels	University of Gent	M.D.	ACS turned down offer to bring Samuels to U.S. to explain his "endocrinotherapy."
60. Michael J. Scott	Creighton University	M.D.	"Member of the College of Surgeons."
61. Franklin L. Shivley	Northwestern University	M.D.	Licensed to practice in Ohio.
62. O. Carl Simonton	University of Oregon Medical School	M.D.	Radiologist, Travis AFB; Cancer Counselling & Research Center, Fort Worth, Texas.
63. Leo L. Spears	Palmer School of Chiropractic	D.C.	Founder, 600-bed Spears Chiropractic Clinic.
64. Rudolph Steiner	[not given]	M.D.	Society for Cancer Research, Arlesheim, Switzerland.
65. Charles F. Swingle	Johns Hopkins University	Ph.D.	Plant physiologist in "government service."
66. Eli J. Tucker	Tulane University	M.D.	General practitioner; orthopedic surgery.
67. Henry K. Wachtel	University of Vienna	M.D.	Associate Professor of physiology, head of Cancer Research Dept., Fordham University.
68. Morvyth McQueen Williams	Yale University	M.D., Ph.D.	Certified in diagnostic roentgenology by American Board of Radiology.
69. Joseph W. Wilson	University of Pittsburgh Physicians and Surgeons	M.D.	General practitioner; general surgery.
70. George S. Zuccala	College of Microbiology, Chicago	B.S., D.Sc. (Hon.)	Serologist, City of New York, 1926–1944; laboratory owner.

†Name eventually removed from unproven methods list.
*California osteopaths became medical doctors (M.D.'s) in 1962.
**Information in brackets from sources other than ACS.

TABLE 2b
Statistical Analysis of Proponents of ACS Unproven Methods

Scientific Training	Proponent No. (total = 70)	Percentage of Total
M.D.	2, 4, 13, 14, 15, 16, 17, 19, 20, 21, 22, 23, 24, 25, 26, 28, 31, 36, 40, 42, 43, 44, 47, 49, 52, 53, 54, 57, 58, 59, 60, 61, 62, 64, 66, 67, 69 [total = 37]	52.9%
Ph.D.	1, 3, 5, 6, 9, 10, 32, 45, 48, 55, 65 [total = 11]	15.7%
M.D., Ph.D.	11, 30, 34, 68 [total = 4]	5.7%
Osteopaths (In Calif.>M.D., 1962)	27, 35 [total = 2]	2.8%
D.Sc. (Hon.)	37, 56, 70 [total = 3]	4.3%
Miscellaneous degrees (R.N., D.V.M., etc.)	7, 8, 12, 33, 41, 51, 63 [total = 7]	10.0%
Laypersons	18, 29, 38, 39, 46, 50 [total = 6]	8.6%
TOTAL		100.0%

from orthodox cancer doctors in matters of education, training, or scientific background.

A second common charge concerns the nature of the methods proposed by unorthodox practitioners. These are supposed to be highly bizarre and exotic, and therefore patently worthless and absurd.

In the 19th and 20th centuries, literally thousands of unproven cancer remedies were promoted or sold in this country. These ''remedies'' cover a wide range of materials, methodology and rationale.

Among the simpler ones are escharotic fluids used to treat external cancer; natural products, such as cobwebs saturated with arsenic powder liquid applied as a poultice, or clover blossom tea; and raw food diets, such as the ''grape cure'' . . . (ACS, 1971b).

Richards's book on cancer offers an alternative list of bizarre remedies:

UNORTHODOX THERAPIES

Tear extract? Ox bile? Llama placenta? Lemon juice enemas? Clam extract? Diamond carbon compound? These substances and many others have been or are currently being offered for the treatment of cancer (Richards, 1972:271).

This sort of commentary can have profound implications. In Justice Thurgood Marshall's 1979 decision concerning the legal status of laetrile, he cited the following in support of the government's argument:

> Since the turn of the century, resourceful entrepreneurs have advertised a wide variety of purportedly simple and painless cures for cancer, including liniments of turpentine, mustard oil, eggs, and ammonia; peat moss; arrangements of colored flood lamps; pastes made from glycerin and Limburger cheese; mineral tablets; and "Fountain of Youth" mixtures of spices, oil and suet (*New York Times,* June 19, 1979).

The fact is that none of these methods has been widely marketed for the treatment of cancer within living memory. Neither cobwebs, nor clover blossom tea, nor tear extract, ox bile, llama placenta, lemon juice enemas, nor *any* of the purported methods named in Marshall's decision are even mentioned in the ACS list.

The methods that Marshall mentions, if they once existed, did so at or before the turn of the century—not in the present period. They sound characteristic of an earlier age when patent medicines of dubious value dominated medical practice as a whole, not just the treatment of cancer.

But another point must be made. Many of the most effective orthodox medicines are derived from substances that, at first sight, do seem absurd and possibly even dangerous.

The well-known drug Premarin, used by millions of women to relieve the signs of menopause, is derived from *preg*nant *ma*res' *urine* (Epstein, 1978). Penicillin is derived from mold. The orthodox anticancer agent Mustargen is a form of poisonous mustard gas; another anticancer agent comes from the periwinkle plant. Digitalis, for the heart, comes from the common foxglove. The list goes on.

Imagine how possible it would be to attack these present-day conventional therapies, which are derived from mare's urine, mold, weeds, and poison gases. This is neither more nor less absurd than the lists given above. *Any* substance may offer a therapeutic effect: the only way to tell is to test the substance in the laboratory or with patients.

As the late Sloan-Kettering chemotherapist David Karnofsky once stated:

The relevant matter in examining any form of treatment is not the reputation of its proponent, the persuasiveness of his theory, the eminence of its lay supporters, the testimony of patients, or the existence of public controversy, but simply—does the treatment work? (Karnofsky, 1959).

The public, and much of the medical profession, is under the impression that unorthodox methods of cancer management are routinely subjected to fair and impartial analysis, before the "quack" label is pinned upon them.

This idea is embellished for the general reader in the chapter "Cancer Quackery" in Dr. Richards's book (the chapter was written by Denise Scott):

> Many agencies throughout the U.S. and indeed in many other countries carry on such investigations [of quackery] and report on their findings in a wide variety of scientific journals and other publications.
>
> These investigating agencies include the National Cancer Institute, the American Medical Association, the Federal Food and Drug Administration, the U.S. Public Health Service, and certain independent agencies. They have strict standards of investigation. These include examination of clinical evidence presented by the treatment proponent (such as the examination of biopsy slides and of X-ray pictures); analysis of the new drug; experiments in animals; tests for consistency (through treatment of a large number of patients); and reviews of the results of the autopsies of patients who have died after having received the new remedy or treatment (Richards, 1972:271).

This sort of investigation is so reasonable that, as the author states, "no honest and serious researcher can have any objection to scientific investigation of his method" along these lines. Unfortunately, such an investigation almost never takes place before a method is condemned as quackery.

Table 3 lists sixty-three unproven methods included in the ACS book in the 1970s and 1980s. In twenty-eight out of sixty-three cases (or 44.4 percent) *no investigation at all* was carried out by the American Cancer Society or any other agency before the method was condemned.

In seven cases, or 11.1 percent, it appears that the results of the investigation were not negative at all, but actually *positive*. This does not mean, of course, that these seven methods are cures for cancer. Rather, the scanty data points in a positive, rather than a negative, direction.

For example, one of the methods included on the ACS list is chaparral tea. This, it is said, is "an old Indian remedy made by steeping the leaves and stems of a desert shrub."

The American Cancer Society states:

TABLE 3
ACS Unproven Methods—Extent of Evaluation

Method	Nature of Investigation	ACS Findings*
1. Anticancergen Z-50	National Research Council	(−)
2. Antineoplastons	no investigation	(0)
3. Antineol	4 investigators, 15 patients	(−)
4. Bamfolin	no objective regression, but "subjective amelioration"—a French magazine	(+/−)
5. H. H. Beard Methods	test canceled midway by California Dept. of Public Health	(?)
6. Biomedical Detoxification	no investigation	(0)
7. Bonifacio Anticancer Serum	worthless—Commission of the National Institute for the Study and the Cure of Tumors, Milan	(−)
8. Cancer Lipid Concentrate	no investigation	(0)
9. Carcin or Neo-carcin	ineffectual—French Ministry of Public Health (undocumented by ACS)	(−)
10. Carzodelan	no investigation	(0)
11. CH-23	ineffective—Medical Association of Bavaria, quoted in *Journal of AMA*, Aug. 5, 1968	(−)
12. Chaparral Tea	some positive clinical data; effective in animal studies	(+)
13. Chase Dietary Method	no investigation	(0)
14. C.N.T.	no investigation	(0)
†15. Coley's Mixed Toxins	positive in double-blind study at NYU	(+)
16. Collodaurum, etc.	no investigation	(0)
17. Contreras Methods	no investigation	(0)
18. Crofton Immunization Method	no investigation	(0)

TABLE 3 *(continued)*

Method	Nature of Investigation	ACS Findings*
19. Dimethyl Sulfoxide (DMSO)	Natl. Acad. Science-Natl. Research Council	(?)
20. Ferguson Plant Products	positive effects in animals and possibly man	(+)
21. Fresh Cell Therapy	no investigations	(0)
22. Frost Method	no investigation	(0)
23. Gerson Method	data reviewed by AMA, NCI, and NY Medical Soc.	(−)
24. Gibson Methods	no investigation	(0)
25. Glover Serum	12 patients reviewed. Physician dissent.	(−)
26. Grape Diet	no investigation	(0)
27. "Greek Cancer Cure" (Alvizatos)	no investigation	(0)
28. H-11	mostly negative, but in some cases rate of growth appeared slow or inhibited	(+/−)
29. Hadley Vaccine	no investigation	(0)
30. Haematoxylon Dissolved in DMSO	hospital research committee, Harris County, Texas	(−)
31. Heat Therapy or Hyperthermia	no genuine investigation; now in use at most major cancer centers	(0)
32. Hemacytology Index (HCI)	conflicting reports: "must await further investigation"	(?)
33. Hendricks Natural Immunity Therapy	no investigation (license removed for violating Cancer Anti-quackery law by using banned methods, such as Koch, Lincoln, etc.)	(0)

34. Hett "Cancer Serum" and Gruner Blood Smear Test	no "independent clinical investigation"	(?)
35. Hoxsey Method	visiting committee of six doctors from British Columbia, for three days	(−)
†36. Hydrazine Sulfate	negative results at Sloan-Kettering [positive results by Gold, Gershanovich, et al. not cited]	(−)
37. Immuno-Augmentative Therapy (IAT)	no investigation	(0)
38. Iscador (Mistletoe)	no investigation	(0)
39. Issels Combination Therapy	five-day visit by English doctors	(−)
40. Kanfer Neuromuscular or Handwriting Test	"a means of separating high-risk groups from low-risk groups," worth "further investigation"	(+)
41. KC-555	positive in animals; tests terminated	(+)
42. Kelley Malignancy Index	no investigation	(0)
43. Koch Antitoxins	four medical commission reports	(−)
44. Krebiozen or Carcalon	NCI committee retrospective of 504 cases	(−)
45. Laetrile	retrospective on 44 patients; Mayo Clinic study	(−)
46. Lewis Methods	inconclusive—Cleveland Society of Pathologists	(?)
47. Livingston Vaccine	no investigation	(0)
48. Macrobiotic Diets	no investigation	(0)
49. Makari Intradermal Cancer Test	VA Hospital use, etc.	(+)
50. M.P. Virus	three patients tested: "does seem to affect malignant tissue" but dangerous	(+)

TABLE 3 *(continued)*

Method	Nature of Investigation	ACS Findings*
51. Mucorhicin	improvement in 2 out of 15 cases reviewed	(+/−)
52. Multiple Enzyme Therapy	no investigation	(o)
53. Naessens Serum, or Anablast	French Ministry of Public Health	(−)
54. Nichols Escharotic Method	Bureau of Investigation of AMA (1933); also 1943 study of 19 cases	(−)
55. Orgone Energy Devices	no investigation	(o)
56. Polonine	no investigation	(o)
57. Rand Coupled Fortified Antigen	"further investigative and re-search data" needed—Cleveland Academy of Medicine	(?)
58. Revici Cancer Control	33 cases evaluated in clinical trial	(−)
59. Samuels Causal Therapy	condemned after investigation by chairman of Amsterdam Health Council	(−)
60. Simonton Method	no investigation	(o)
61. Spears Hygienic System	no investigation	(o)
62. Staphylococcus Phage Lysates (Lincoln Method)	no objective evidence, but "marked symptomatic improvement" (since removed from list)	(+/−)
63. Ultraviolet Blood Irradiation	no investigation; resolution of Nebraska doctors against Koch methods	(o)

†Subsequently withdrawn from list
*Key: (−)   Ineffective according to data given in ACS book
(o)   Never investigated
(+)   Effective according to data given in ACS book
(+/−) Contradictory results found in investigations
(?)   Inconclusive results

After careful study of the literature and other information available to it, the American Cancer Society does not have evidence that treatment with chaparral tea results in objective benefit in the treatment of cancer in human beings (ACS, 1971b:55).

The story of chaparral tea began, it says, when an eighty-five-year-old man was brought to the University of Utah with a proven malignant melanoma (deadly form of skin cancer) of the right cheek. He refused surgery and instead treated himself with chaparral tea. "He returned eight months later," the ACS report continues, "with marked regression of the cancer."

Such regressions do occur spontaneously on occasion—but less than one in several thousand cases (Everson and Cole, 1966). University of Utah scientists then used the tea on other patients. "Four patients have responded to some extent to treatment with the tea, including two with melanomas, one with choriocarcinoma metastatic [spread] to the lungs and one with widespread lymphosarcoma." One of the other melanoma patients "experienced a 95 percent regression" whereupon the remaining growth was removed by surgical excision (ACS, 1971b).

Research then performed at the National Cancer Institute by Dean Burk, Ph.D., showed that in laboratory cultures "this is a very active agent against cancer," in the words of Dr. Charles R. Smart, associate professor of surgery at the University of Utah Medical Center (ibid.).

The tea was also being used by scientists at other medical centers, including the chairman of the biochemistry department at the University of Nevada. An Arizona scientist received an $81,000 contract "to investigate treatments which might be developed from desert plants," and doctors in Reno had begun to use chaparral tea on their cancer patients. And, in fact, many bona fide drugs originated as old Indian remedies (Vogel, 1970).

Dr. Smart does warn that in some cases the tea may have accelerated the growth of some tumors; otherwise, there is nothing negative about this treatment in the ACS summary. Yet based on the above information the Society placed chaparral tea on its unproven methods list.

A similar case is that of Ferguson Plant Products, otherwise known as the Jivaro Head-Shrinking Compound. This was given to an American explorer, Wilburn Ferguson, by an Indian chief in Ecuador.

In the early 1950s, the compound was analyzed by scientists at the Los Angeles County Hospital, who successfully isolated an active agent from the compound. It turned out to be a "highly potent antibiotic" (ACS, 1971b), which is significant, since antibiotics form one whole class of known anticancer agents.

The compound was then tried against known animal tumors and leukemias "with some degree of success," according to the hospital staff (ibid.:116). In 1952 a representative of the National Cancer Institute visited Ferguson in Ecuador and reviewed the scientific data that had been gathered there. He reported:

> Ferguson did not claim to me that he had a cure for cancer in humans, but did claim to have a cure for cancer in animals. He did say that he believed that his drug caused regression of human cancer and showed me evidence of this that was rather convincing. *All* of his treated patients still have cancer, some have died, but the ones which I saw, providing the previous observations were truthfully presented, had regressed considerably (ibid.).

The ACS report then adds that in the spring of 1953, the Merck Institute for Therapeutic Research, an offshot of the Merck Sharp & Dohme pharmaceutical company, "initiated studies with Ferguson anticancer material. A report on these studies has not been published."

Again, there is nothing negative in this account, which comes from the ACS article. Yet on the basis of the above facts the ACS added the Ferguson compound to its list, claiming that there was no evidence it "results in objective benefit in the treatment of cancer in human beings."

In some cases the ACS and its confreres have condemned a method only to silently remove it from the list years later.

Coley's toxins is such an instance (see chapter 7). Another was the case of Robert E. Lincoln, M.D. Lincoln's name was added to the ACS list in 1964, when the controversy over his work was still alive.

Lincoln was a graduate of Boston University School of Medicine, who had done postdoctoral work at Harvard, and then gone into general practice in the small town of Medford, outside Boston. For many years he was an unremarkable small-town doctor and a member in good standing of the American Medical Association and its state affiliate, the Massachusetts Medical Society.

In the 1940s, in the midst of an influenza epidemic, Lincoln made what he felt were some important discoveries concerning the bacterial origin of various diseases—discoveries he later extended to cancer. He also believed that he had discovered a possible cure for some forms of these diseases in bacteriophage—viruses that parasitically attack and destroy specific bacteria.

Lincoln began to treat patients with injections of these viruses and claimed to see some remarkable results, including remissions of cancer. In 1946, therefore, he submitted these clinical results to the *Journal of the American Medical Association*. His paper was rejected.

He then submitted the same paper to the *New England Journal of Medicine,* published in Boston. This time it was rejected for "lack of space" (Morris, 1977).

Undaunted, Lincoln wrote three letters in succession to an editor of the *New England Journal (NEJM)* asking for his assistance in preparing the article for publication. He received no reply to any of these letters. In March 1948 Lincoln asked the director of a large Boston hospital to visit him and study the clinical results he had assembled and the methods by which he had achieved them. The director wrote back that he "couldn't find the time."

The general practitioner next wrote to the Massachusetts Medical Society, asking for a chance to present his work to his colleagues at a meeting. The Society stalled, but in the meantime began sending out a form letter to inquirers stating that Lincoln's method was ineffective.

Lincoln was perturbed and wrote to the president of the AMA itself, asking him to send someone to Medford to investigate the situation. This medical leader, however, referred Lincoln back to the Massachusetts Medical Society.

This stalemate was dramatically broken when Lincoln happened to treat the son of Charles Tobey, a United States senator. Tobey, claiming that Lincoln had cured his son of cancer, excoriated the Massachusetts medical establishment from the floor of the Senate.

Stung by this criticism, the Massachusetts Medical Society finally dispatched a team of surgeons and radiologists to Medford, where they interviewed some patients on the back porch of Lincoln's house. They claimed to be unable to see any signs of actual, objective benefit, but did concede that there were some "cases of marked symptomatic improvement," which they attributed to "the tremendous force of faith and hope" (ACS, 1971b:197).

When Lincoln read this, he complained publicly of the "high degree of stupidity" shown by this report. The leaders of the Massachusetts Medical Society then demanded his resignation; when he refused to resign, he was expelled on April 8, 1952. One year later, Lincoln sued the Society for $250,000 for libel, but he died in the following year and the case never came to trial (Morris, 1977; ACS, 1971b).*

In 1975 the ACS quietly took Lincoln's name off the unproven methods list, a tacit admission of an error on its part. However, it is virtually impossible for cancer patients to receive his treatment.

But Lincoln is hardly alone in the treatment he received. Table 4 shows that 55.6 percent of the methods on the ACS list were either not investigated

---

*Much of the information on Lincoln comes from sources favorable to his approach, particularly Morris. The ACS account does not contradict these, but is scanty.

TABLE 4
Statistical Analysis of Investigations of ACS Unproven Methods

Kind of Investigation	Method Number (total = 63)*	Percentage†
I. No investigation made (0)	2, 6, 8, 10, 13, 14, 16, 17, 18, 21, 22, 24, 26, 27, 29, 31, 33, 37, 38, 42, 47, 48, 52, 55, 56, 60, 61, 63 [total = 28]	44.4%
II. Investigation made: method found to be useful (+)	12, 15, 20, 40, 41, 49, 50 [total = 7]	11.1%
III. Investigation made: contradictory data (+/−)	4, 28, 51, 62 [total = 4]	6.4%
IV. Investigation made: inconclusive results (?)	5, 19, 32, 34, 46, 57 [total = 6]	9.5%
V. Investigation made: method found to be ineffective (−)	1, 3, 7, 9, 11, 23, 25, 30, 35, 36, 39, 43, 44, 45, 53, 54, 58, 59 [total = 18]	28.6%
		100.0%

*See Table 3. †Rounded off.

at all before being condemned, or were actually found positive in the tests conducted. In another 6.4 percent the data was contradictory, while in 9.5 percent the investigators could not reach a definitive conclusion. *Thus, almost 72 percent of the methods on the unproven methods list have never been shown to be ineffective by any sort of rational scientific procedure.*

In the remaining 28 percent, some sort of investigation was carried out, and the method in question was judged ineffective by the investigators (if not by the proponent). But did these investigations conform to the fair and scientific standards outlined in the Richards book and in most other orthodox writings on quackery? Only very rarely, it turns out.

For many of these methods it is impossible to say whether the investigation was adequate, since the ACS critics rely on secondhand or thirdhand reports. Five investigations were carried out by foreign medical organizations, and for some the only source of information appears to be magazine articles. These may be valid investigations of fraudulent or worthless remedies, but it is hard to tell merely from the information the ACS provides.

For only about a dozen methods does the ACS offer documented evidence of failure. This in itself is significant, since it represents less than 20 percent of the total.

But were these methods subjected to adequate investigation before they were condemned? Again, the answer would have to be no.

Included in this "ineffective" category are such therapies as laetrile, hydrazine sulfate, Krebiozen, the Gerson method, the Hoxsey method, Glover's serum, Koch antitoxins, and Revici Cancer Control.

As the reader will see in the following pages, many of these methods have been tested and condemned in a one-sided manner. In *no* case, for example, was a clinical double-blind study carried out on any of these procedures before it was condemned. (A double-blind test is one in which neither the patient nor the physician knows the nature of the medication being given. It is generally considered the most objective form of testing.)

The National Cancer Institute long resisted performing such tests on Krebiozen, despite the fact that fifty-six U.S. Congressmen cosponsored a resolution calling for one (ACS, 1971b:2). For many years, of course, the establishment similarly refused to conduct a clinical trial of laetrile, on the grounds that this would be "a criminal abuse of hopes" (Dr. Daniel Martin in *Medical World News,* October 26, 1975. For the Mayo Clinic test, see chapter 8.).

Sometimes the investigation has been highly informal. Hoxsey's treatment, which on the surface may appear closer to true quackery than any in the ACS book, was never subjected to either animal studies or clinical trials of any sort. The only negative investigation cited in the book, in fact, was a three-day visit to his clinic by several Canadian physicians, who came away unimpressed.*

Glover's serum, which is a predecessor of the Livingston technique (see chapter 13), was subjected to some cursory animal studies and a review (but no clinical trial) of twelve patients before it was condemned.

It would be extremely surprising and unlikely if this list did *not* contain instances of mad delusion and outright fraud. After all, it purports to be an authoritative catalogue of quack remedies, and one would expect to find at least a few such treatments on it.

However, what is at issue here is whether or not these methods have been fairly and adequately tested before being condemned. Richards proposed excellent criteria for the testing of such methods: examination of clinical evidence, including biopsy slides and X-ray pictures; analysis of the drug or agent proposed for therapy; experiments in animals; testing in a large number of patients; and reviews of autopsies. In addition, one should add the trial of putative methods by means of double-blind studies.

* An excellent documentary about this controversy is *Hoxsey: When Healing Becomes a Crime* (1987), produced by Ken Ausubel and Catherine Salveson. See Appendix B. See also Ward, 1988c.

A careful examination of the ACS manual shows that these criteria are almost never met in the study of unorthodox therapies. Rather, the Society appears to have made an a priori judgment on the worthlessness of uncommon cancer therapies, and then stretched the facts to fit its preconceptions.

Not all these methods are valid, of course, and some are probably fraudulent. But, taken as a whole, the unproven methods are a repository of new ideas from which cancer scientists should be able to draw freely. The stigma of quackery attached to these methods by the American Cancer Society and others generally prevents them from doing so.

This opposition on the part of orthodoxy is antiscientific and ultimately self-serving. As the late Pat McGrady, Sr., for many years an American Cancer Society official, said:

> The Establishment has turned the terror of this ugly disease to its own ends in seeking more and more contributions from a frightened public and appropriations from a concerned Congress. Still, undismayed by the futility of funds dumped into the bottomless barrel of its "proven" methods, it remains adamant in refusing to investigate "unproven" methods. . . .
>
> Forgetful of the fact that of the few really useful treatments, all, or almost all, were initiated under the kind of abuse now heaped upon "unproven" remedies, the Establishment may be denying help for tomorrow's cancer patients as well as today's (McGrady, Sr., 1975).

(7)

Coley's Toxins

In the late nineteenth century a young New York City surgeon, fresh out of Harvard Medical School, stumbled across one of the most intriguing findings ever made in cancer research. His discovery was first tolerated, then ridiculed, and finally suppressed. Today, although given lip service by some doctors, its potential is still largely unexplored.

The doctor's name was William B. Coley, and his discovery is known as Coley's toxins, or "mixed bacterial vaccine."

Coley's first cancer patient was a nineteen-year-old named Bessie, sweetheart of the young John D. Rockefeller, Jr. She had a sarcoma of the bone. Coley amputated her arm, as was the standard procedure, and the prognosis seemed good. Yet a short while later Bessie died. The young doctor was devastated by his failure to effect a cure, despite the seemingly early detection of the growth (Nauts, 1976b).

Coley thus became aware of the limitations of surgery, a technique that was often dangerous, mutilating, and futile in the treatment of cancer. Nor could he accept the commonly held belief that cancer was incurable and unconquerable. This determined young man began a long and difficult search for a cure for cancer (ibid.).

Coley began by methodically searching the patient records at New York Hospital. Researching in the dusty archives, he went back fifteen years and examined the case records of all sarcoma patients treated at that hospital. He found over 100 such cases. Most of these predictably ended in failure and the death of the patient. To his amazement, however,

Coley discovered one patient who had been given up for lost by his doctors and yet had walked out of the hospital in apparently perfect health (Cancer Research Institute, 1976).

What had happened? On his deathbed, the patient had suffered two attacks of erysipelas, a severe and sometimes life-threatening infection of the skin caused by the bacteria *Streptococcus pyogenes.*

Today erysipelas is controlled by antibiotics, but at the turn of the century it was a fairly common infectious disease whose side effects included high temperatures and chills similar to those accompanying typhoid fever.

This one patient recovered from the erysipelas and, miraculously, his tumors also began to shrink and disappear. In a short while this man, on whom the doctors had operated four times to no avail, was discharged from the hospital. His doctors shook their heads as he left and called his case a spontaneous remission"—a cure with no apparent cause (Everson and Cole, 1966).

The man's records had lain in New York Hospital's record room until that day in 1888 when Coley dug them out and stared at them in amazement. Coley copied down the man's address and went to his house, but the man had moved. He found a neighbor who knew his forwarding address, and from there he went to yet another address. Up and down the stairs of New York's tenements Coley trekked in search of this miracle man. And, finally, he found him. It had been seven years since his discharge from New York Hospital yet despite that length of time, as Coley discovered, the man was still in complete remission of his cancer (Burdick, 1937).

Coley's next step was to try to create the same curative conditions that had occurred accidentally years before: he would deliberately infect a terminally ill cancer patient with erysipelas. One can imagine the consternation of Coley's surgical colleagues at this suggestion—after all, what was the sense in giving a patient with one fatal disease *another* nearly fatal disease to contend with?

After due preparations, however, a volunteer who had a sarcoma of the tonsil and neck was found, and was injected with a culture of strep. There was no reaction. Again and again, using different cultures, Coley injected his patient. Again nothing happened. What disappointment!—another dead-end lead. And there it might have ended, had not a friend brought Coley a particularly active, virulent culture of strep germs from the famous German microbe hunter, Robert Koch. When Coley administered this culture, in October, 1891, within 12 hours, the patient's temperature shot skyward and he contracted a severe case of erysipelas. And within a few days another "miracle" had occurred: the tumors on his tonsils and neck completely disappeared, and only a scar remained. The man, who could only swallow liquids and whisper when Coley started the treatment, made a complete recovery and ten years later was still free of cancer.

Coley inoculated nine more patients with live erysipelas microbes as part of a creative experiment with the microbial treatment of cancer that lasted over forty years. He studied a number of other cases of so-called spontaneous remission in cancer that had followed erysipelas infections. He discovered that over a dozen times before, doctors in Germany had deliberately infected patients with erysipelas in an attempt to cure their cancer. In 1893 he tabulated the results: of the seventeen cases of advanced carcinoma he studied, four were permanently cured, ten showed improvement that did not lead to a cure but added years to their lives, while three showed no improvement at all (Coley, 1893).

Coley realized, however, that using living cultures was dangerous and impractical. And so he started on a lengthy attempt to obtain potent and effective sterilized toxins from streptococcus. In 1893 he published his first paper on the new method, "A Preliminary Note on the Treatment of Inoperable Sarcoma by the Toxic Product of Erysipelas" (ibid.). Over the years Coley was to publish dozens of such papers, recording what he said was the success — and sometimes the failure — of his new treatment method. In sarcoma, cancer of the bone and connective tissue, Coley's claims were even more impressive: 41 percent complete cures. If these statistics were true, they were probably the best results ever achieved in cancer until that time. The results would even compare favorably with any mode of therapy used today.

Nevertheless, there were drawbacks to the erysipelas treatment. For one thing, it was an ordeal for the patient: high fever, malaise, and the danger of death from the infection itself. For another, live strep, an infectious agent, posed a potential health threat not just to the patients but to the workers and to others in the hospital. In fact, nearly 6 percent of the first group of patients died of streptococcal infection.

Another serious drawback was the uncertainty of erysipelas therapy. Often it was impossible to induce the disease or to cause a fever, even when the patient was placed in a so-called erysipelas bed—the unchanged bed of a recently deceased victim of the infection. Streptococcus was a temperamental microbe. Coley therefore greatly improved on his invention. Instead of using live bacteria, he mixed the toxins (normally formed during the metabolism of the microbe) from killed strep with those of a germ he had heard about in his studies, *Bacillus prodigiosus.* "Prodigiosus" in Latin means "wonderful," and the wonder of this germ was that it had the power of intensifying the activity of other microbes, such as strep. (Today it is called *Serratia marcescens.*)

The first patient treated with the mixture was a sixteen-year-old German immigrant boy who had a huge inoperable growth on his abdomen. The doctors at Memorial despaired of even treating him. As a last resort he was referred to Coley for treatment with the mixed bacterial vaccine. Coley began the treatment on January 24, 1893, injecting directly into the tumor, and continued injections for four months. Memorial Hospital records tell the story:

> These injections produced within eight hours a rise in temperature from 0.5 to 6 degrees, a pulse running from 100 to 106. The chill and tremblings were extreme. . . . [There were also] severe headaches. . . . The tumor gradually diminished in size, at times for a few days after injection it would be enlarged, but the final diminution was indisputable (cited in Nauts et al., 1953).

On May 13 the boy was discharged from Memorial—his tumor reputedly one-fifth the size it had been upon admission. Two weeks later the growth was no longer visible. Coley presented this patient a number of times to doctors at the New York Academy of Medicine and the New York Surgical Society. The patient lived on for another twenty-six years and died suddenly of a heart attack in 1919. At autopsy, the coronor is said to have found no evidence of cancer (Cancer Research Institute, 1976).

For those hearing of Coley's results for the first time, this will undoubtedly seem hard to believe. Yet, as Dr. Lloyd J. Old, a senior member of Sloan-Kettering Institute, and Dr. Edward Boyse, FRS, the American Cancer Society Research Professor there, wrote some years ago, "Those who have scrutinized Dr. Coley's records have little doubt that the bacterial products that came to be known as Coley's toxins were in some instances highly effective" (Old and Boyse, 1973).

Coley's voluminous results have been tabulated by his daughter, Helen Coley Nauts, executive director of the Cancer Research Institute, Inc., in New York City. In seventeen monographs and numerous papers, she and her medical colleagues have documented 894 cases treated with her father's vaccine.

Patients with inoperable tumors of various kinds had 45 percent five-year survival, while those with operable tumors had 50 percent. The best results were in giant cell bone tumors where 15 out of 19 (or 79 percent) of the inoperable patients and 33 out of 38 (or 87 percent) of the operable patients had five-year survival.

In breast cancer the results were equally impressive. Thirteen out of 20 of the inoperable (65 percent) and 13 out of 13 of the operable had five-year survival. Comparable results were seen in other types of cancer (for example, 67 percent in Hodgkin's disease, 67 percent in inoperable ovarian cancer, 60 percent in inoperable malignant melanoma) (Nauts, 1976a).

In addition, the toxin therapy brought other beneficial effects, including a marked decrease or cessation of pain, improved appetite and weight gain (up to 50 pounds), and a "remarkable regeneration of bone" in a number of cases (ibid.).

Since these results are generally much better than those achieved with any conventional therapy today, how is it that most nonprofessionals as well as many cancer scientists have never heard of this method?

From the start, many doctors were skeptical of Coley's unorthodox treatment, even when they saw what appeared to be proof before their very eyes. Today a cure for cancer is still a dream. A century ago it must have seemed like an impossibility, for most doctors believed that cancer was basically an incurable disease (Considine, 1959).

The claim that an unknown but ambitious young man was somehow curing cases they themselves were unable to cure may have irked some established cancer therapists. The fact that he, a surgeon, may have done so by nonsurgical means may have seemed disloyal.

Coley obtained the support of the powerful Huntington railroad family in his efforts. Not long afterward, however, Dr. James Ewing became medical director of Memorial Hospital, with the support of the even more powerful Douglas Phelps-Dodge interests. While Coley was not hostile to radiation, and in fact supervised the first tests of X-ray therapy at Memorial, Ewing was almost fanatical about the use of radium (see chapter 4).

The contrast between the two competing alternative methods could not have been greater. Radium was costly—a fabulous $150,000 a gram. Coley's toxins were remarkably inexpensive. The major cost was in paying the salary of a skilled technician to grow the germs properly. Since radium interests had invested millions of dollars in that metal, and since radium could be given in easily measurable and predictable doses, it had great appeal. Coley's toxins were more difficult to administer, and less certain in their results.

There were four basic reasons the toxins varied in their effects:

The preparations were made from living organisms that varied unpredictably in their strength (virulence). When they were made with care, under Coley's supervision, they appeared to be highly successful. But when Coley or a colleague did not supervise their production, the results tended to be rather less impressive. Parke-Davis, the pharmaceutical company, produced the toxins commercially for many years. Unlike Coley's collaborators, however, the company heated the formula for two and a half hours, thereby allegedly destroying much of its effectiveness. Yet despite its relative weakness, Parke-Davis formula #IX showed a 37 percent cure rate for inoperable patients.

Second, the toxins produced fevers, and not all physicians agreed on how to deal with temperatures ranging as high as 104° F. Many doctors felt that such fevers and discomforts should be combated with antipyretics, such as aspirin. Other doctors attempted to *use the fever itself* as a therapeutic tool—an idea said to date back to Hippocrates. These doctors appear to have achieved far better results.

Third, clinical results depended on the stage of cancer being treated— and this appears true of all treatment modalities. Those who received the toxins early in the course of their illness appeared to do much better than those who received the treatment when the disease had already spread. A high percentage of the patients in the operable group who received adequate toxin therapy remained free from recurrence five years or more (Nauts, 1976b).

Finally, the toxins worked best when they were given *before* other methods of therapy. These other methods, particularly radiation, suppressed and damaged the immune system. Coley's toxins appeared to work by jolting the immune system of the cancer patient into greater activity. One could therefore predict that attempts to give Coley's toxins to patients in a terminal condition who had already received surgery, radiation, and/or chemotherapy were unlikely to produce results that were as highly beneficial.

Such unpredictability, although based on controllable factors, was quite damaging to the reputation of Coley's toxins. Many doctors wrote to the New York surgeon and complained that they had received ineffective batches, especially those which had been prepared commercially.

Coley remained a member in good standing of the medical fraternity and was in fact highly honored. At the age of thirty-six he became the youngest Fellow of the American Surgical Association. In 1935 he was made an Honorary Fellow of the Royal College of Surgeons of England, a plaudit rarely given to an American (Burdick, 1937). At his retirement Coley was given a banquet at the Waldorf-Astoria. Even Ewing spoke in his honor. Coley was honored mostly for his work as a surgeon, however. His work with the toxins was rarely mentioned; it was treated as a kind of eccentricity.

After Coley's death on April 16, 1936, there was a real possibility that his innovative methods of treating cancer would be forgotten. This danger was not lessened when Coley's son, Bradley, succeeded him as head of

Memorial Hospital's Bone Service. In the 1936–39 hospital report, the younger Coley spoke of his father's "voluminous contributions" although oddly he omitted all mention of the toxins. With Coley gone, Ewing inserted a brief, backhanded compliment in the last edition of his encyclopedic *Neoplastic Diseases:*

> Coley's toxins have been used with other methods in certain cases of osteogenic sarcoma which recovered. I have been unable to form any definite estimate of the part played by this agent in the disease. But in some recoveries from endothelioma of bone, there is substantial evidence that the toxins played an essential part (Ewing, 1940:314).

Bradley Coley and a colleague did continue to give the toxins to patients in the Bone Tumor Department until they were forced to stop by Cornelius "Dusty" Rhoads, Sloan-Kettering's Director, in about 1955. The two doctors were "furious, as they were treating several patients at the time who were doing well," and had in fact "cured quite a few cases in the 40s and 50s" (Nauts, H.C., Personal communication, March 22, 1991). But Rhoads was a strident believer in chemotherapy and would brook no interference from competing methods.

In fact, Coley's work would most likely have been doomed to obscurity had it not been for members of his family: not just his son, who officially followed in his footsteps, but also his indomitable young daughter, Helen Coley Nauts. Without a scientific background, Mrs. Nauts believed that her father's work would vanish unless something were done to rescue it. On her own, she undertook the arduous task of verifying and publicizing Dr. Coley's work.

In 1945 she presented a paper at an American Association for the Advancement of Science (AAAS) meeting. She was encouraged to do so, despite the fact that she was a layperson, by Dr. Kanematsu Sugiura, Memorial's long-time chemist and a friend of her father (Nauts, 1976b). Mrs. Nauts's approach was to gather ironclad cases of cures or remissions definitely attributable to the toxins. She had hoped to gather 100, but after several years she had almost 1,000. These she published in 18 monographs and in papers delivered in China, England, France, Germany, Italy, Japan, Sweden, and Switzerland. These have been distributed to libraries and interested individuals around the world.

The response from the leadership of Memorial Sloan-Kettering was not encouraging. In the early 50s, Sloan-Kettering had produced a small amount of the toxins for research purposes. Parke-Davis had also continued to produce a small amount.

By 1953, however, all production of the toxins in the United States stopped. Nonetheless, through persistent pressure, Mrs. Nauts was able to get a clinical test performed at New York University–Bellevue Hospital, a double-blind study in which neither the patients nor the principal investigator knew who received the toxins and who a fever-inducing placebo.

This study was conducted by Barbara Johnston, M.D., and was supported by Mrs. Nauts's group. Dr. Johnston, who became head of medical oncology at St. Vincent's Hospital, New York, attempted to conduct a study that would eliminate the criticisms leveled at earlier studies. How she did this is part of the scientific record (Johnston, 1962). In addition to the double-blind test, a larger number of other patients were treated with Coley's toxins in relatively uncontrolled situations.

The results of both series of patients appear quite clear-cut. In the double-blind test, of the group treated with a placebo, only one patient out of 37 showed any sign of improvement: a questionable decrease in the size of the bladder tumor for a few weeks.

"Of the 34 patients treated with Coley's toxins," she wrote, "18 showed no improvement. Of the remaining 16, 7 noted decreased pain," while 9 showed such benefits as tumor necrosis, apparent inhibition of metastases, shrinkage of lymph nodes, and disappearance of tumors. The New York internist wrote:

> It is the impression of the authors that Coley's toxins has definite oncolytic [tumor-destroying] properties and is useful in the treatment of certain types of malignant disease (ibid.).

When the study was completed, however, the chairman of the Department of Medicine at NYU School of Medicine, Lewis Thomas, M.D., invited Dr. Johnston to leave the hospital. Thomas became the president (and is now the chancellor) of Memorial Sloan-Kettering Cancer Center (Johnston, 1976). "They let us finish [the test] so as to prove that it was wrong," Dr. Johnston has said. "But it didn't turn out that way" (ibid.).

To illustrate the doublethink that has surrounded the double-blind test—one of the few ever performed on an unproven method—one need only consider the manner in which the American Cancer Society interpreted this experiment when it included Coley's toxins in *Unproven Methods* in 1965.

"There was little objective basis offered for believing that bacterial toxin therapy had significantly altered the course of disease in any of the treated cancer patients," the ACS wrote (ACS, 1971b).

The Johnston articles contained striking confirmation of Coley's claims in both series of experiments. Perhaps most impressive are the photographs that accompany the article, which appear to show dramatic, objective remissions of tumors of the neck in a short period of time under treatment with bacterial toxins. But somehow this evidence was not enough to dissuade the ACS from issuing its negative judgment.

More recently Coley's toxins have been enjoying a kind of vogue in some research circles. Some scientists have tried to make Coley out to be a wise godfather of modern immunotherapy. The problem with such recognition is that *access* to Coley's toxins remains practically nonexistent.

Mrs. Nauts's contributions to this field cannot be overstated. For instance, she has corresponded with over 3,200 doctors in 67 countries about the treatment. Her overall strategy has been to attempt to bridge the gap between the cancer establishment and those who believe in Coley's toxins and other forms of immunotherapy.

To that end, a wealthy financier was made chairman of the board of her organization, a top Sloan-Kettering researcher is its medical director, and the ACS's Mary Lasker was appointed to the board of trustees.

In October 1975 the Cancer Research Institute, Mrs. Nauts's once controversial organization, was welcomed back into the fold at a Hotel Pierre banquet. Laurance S. Rockefeller gave the keynote address at the exclusive black-tie affair, and fifteen establishment scientists, including Drs. Old, Good, and Boyse of Sloan-Kettering Institute, received bronze medals and cash awards from the CRI (MSKCC, *Center News*, December 1975). The Cancer Research Institute became respectable.

Quietly in 1975, mainly through the effort of Mrs. Nauts and Dr. Old, the ACS removed Coley's toxins (as well as staphage lysate and hyperthermia) from its unproven methods list. But the desperate cancer patient, for whom Coley's method might offer hope, still finds it nearly impossible to get an injection of Coley's toxins in North America.

The Cancer Research Institute (CRI) has continued to progress along the path it took in the mid-seventies. In 1982 Mrs. Nauts stepped down as executive director of CRI and became director of science and medical communications. In 1983 the organization celebrated its thirtieth anniversary. CRI now has a budget of over $2 million and its own full-time director of public information (CRI, 1987).

As with Sloan-Kettering itself, CRI's board of directors has been dominated by leaders of Wall Street. These have included Chairman Oliver R. Grace, general partner of Sterling Grace Capital Management; investor Alan J. Hirschfield; Thomas S. Johnson, president of Chemical Bank; and William E. Mayer, managing director of the First Boston Corporation, who recently helped CRI raise $500,000 from "the Wall Street community" (ibid.). Lloyd Old remains the director of CRI's Scientific Advisory Council.

CRI gave out 78 two-year postdoctoral fellowships ($24–26,000 per year) in fiscal 1987. These went to scholars at thirty-nine institutions in thirteen states, as well as two foreign countries, working in many different areas of immunology. It is a laudable program. But judging from the titles of their projects, very little of this work was directed at understanding Coley's discoveries per se. Neither Coley's toxins nor mixed bacterial vaccine (MBV) are mentioned in a single such grant title, and even tumor necrosis factor (TNF) is only mentioned once, in the grant given to Richard A. Smith, Ph.D., of the State University of New York, Albany (CRI, 1987).

Coley's toxins were the subject of an illuminating historical overview by Patricia Spain Ward, official historian of the University of Illinois at Chicago (Ward, 1988a). This document, "History of BCG," was originally prepared under contract to the Unconventional Cancer Treatment Project of the Office of Technology Assessment (OTA), as were reports by Ms. Ward on the Gerson and Hoxsey therapies. The OTA staff at first refused to circulate these papers to its own advisory board; they were later disavowed by the staff as part of a bitter controversy (Ward 1988d).

Ward explains how the current work on tumor necrosis factor (TNF) ultimately derives from Coley, by way of M. J. Shear's 1943 discovery "that the biologically active substance in Coley's toxins is lipopolysaccharide (LPS, also called endotoxin) which occurs in the cell walls of gram-negative bacteria" (Ward, 1988a).

It was by injecting LPS into mice previously treated with *Bacillus Calmette-Guérin* (BCG), the tuberculosis vaccine, that Old and colleagues were able to cause the release into the serum of a substance that caused "hemorrhagic necrosis" of mouse tumors. It was this substance that was called tumor necrosis factor or TNF (Ward, 1988a).

A good description of the development of TNF is provided by Old in the *Scientific American* of May 1988. In it he speculates that TNF may activate some intracellular enzymes that liberate highly reactive molecules which may themselves kill cancer cells (Old, 1988-75).

In addition to the work on BCG, it appears that some unheralded trials have taken place with Coley's toxins. In 1982 Mrs. Nauts reported the results of the first randomized trials of mixed bacterial vaccine (or MBV, as Coley's toxins are now called), begun in 1976 at Memorial Sloan-Kettering. According to a talk that Mrs. Nauts gave at the International Colloquium on Bacteriology and Cancer in Cologne, Federal Republic of Germany, advanced non-Hodgkin's lymphoma patients receiving MBV had a 93 percent

remission rate as opposed to 29 percent for controls who received chemotherapy alone (Nauts, 1982).

As Ward notes, it has taken an extraordinarily long time for Coley's
basic discoveries to be acknowledged, much less used:

> It is now 100 years since William B. Coley first noted total regression
> of a recurrent sarcoma of the neck following erysipelas. . . . More than sixty
> years have passed since physicians reported that tuberculin . . . enhanc[es] the
> body's immune forces. . . . It is more than half a century since Sol Roy
> Rosenthal described the stimulation of the reticuloendothelial system by BCG.
> . . . The distance between these events and the recent beginning of clinical
> trials illustrates some important truths about the circuitous development of
> science and its susceptibility to extraneous social and political factors (Ward,
> 1988a).

In 1981, as a result of intense political pressure and scientific receptiv-
ity, the National Cancer Institute created the Biological Response Modifier
Program. But the exhaustive NCI *1990 Budget Estimate* reveals only passing
mention of TNF, and none of Coley's toxins (NCI, 1988).

The fact is, a century after Coley's initial success it still remains nearly
impossible for a patient to opt for this extraordinary therapy in any form.

« 8 »

The Laetrile
Controversy

Few controversies in cancer therapy have been as fierce or prolonged as that over the proposed anticancer agent laetrile.

According to the Food and Drug Administration, "Laetrile has been sold for treating cancer for around 25 years, yet there is still no sound, scientific evidence that it is either effective or safe. It is therefore classified as a 'new drug' " (FDA, 1975). In the words of an American Cancer Society official, Helene Brown, laetrile is "goddamned quackery" (Schultz and Lindeman, 1973).

According to its proponents, laetrile is neither new nor really a drug. And far from being quackery, when used correctly as part of an overall nutritional program, it is one of the most promising and effective treatments for cancer.

The widespread fear of cancer and the growing bitterness over orthodox medicine's failure to find a cure, despite billions of dollars spent, has fueled the laetrile controversy. According to Charles Moertel, M.D., of the Mayo Clinic, laetrile is "a dominant unresolved problem for American medicine today" (Moertel, 1978). Even after a negative double-blind study at the Mayo Clinic, laetrile continues to be used as part of a holistic cancer therapy at many unorthodox clinics. It is also the subject of continuing FDA raids on distributors (Schuster, 1989).

To understand why this is so, it is necessary to look more closely at the substance itself and the long history of its use.

Although the term *laetrile* is of relatively recent coinage,* the chemical most often sold as laetrile has been used as a folk remedy for cancer or related diseases for many centuries. The laetrile dispensed to cancer patients today is another name for amygdalin, a glycoside, or type of carbohydrate, that occurs frequently in living organisms, especially in plants and their derivatives. All glycosides have one thing in common: in reactions with water they can be split into a sugar (or sugars) and a noncarbohydrate substance(s). Usually an enzyme must be present to facilitate this cleavage.

There are different kinds of glycosides in nature. The kind we are concerned with releases cyanide (HCN) when broken down. It is therefore called a cyanogenic (or cyanogenetic) glycoside. Included in this category are plant chemicals such as prunasin, found most commonly in wild cherry bark; dhurrin, found in sorghum; lotusin, from the *Lotus arabicus* plant; and, of course, amygdalin.

Laetrile is found all over the globe, occurring naturally in about 1,200 different plants. One could compare it, in its ubiquity, to glucose. Like sugar, laetrile does not normally occur in a purified form but can be extracted quite readily from its sources.

We have all ingested amygdalin, or "taken laetrile," at one time or another—and some of us take it every day without knowing that we are engaging in medical controversy. Chick-peas and lentils, lima beans and mung bean sprouts, cashews and alfalfa, barley, brown rice, and millet—all these foods, and many more, contain laetrile. For commercial purposes laetrile is derived from the kernels of the apricot, the peach, and the bitter almond, after which amygdalin is named (Greek, *amygdale,* "almond").

*The definition of laetrile and its relationship to amygdalin can be confusing. Crystalline amygdalin was first isolated in 1830 from bitter almonds by two French chemists. The chemical formula of amygdalin is given in the Merck Index.

Laetrile, on the other hand, is a coined word, registered by Ernst T. Krebs, Sr., and Ernst T. Krebs, Jr., in 1953. It is a contraction of "*laevo*-rotatory mandeloni*trile* beta-diglucoside." This is a purified form of amygdalin, which turns polarized light in a left-handed (hence "laevo-") direction. For various reasons, the Krebses believed that only the "laevo-" form of this substance would be useful in cancer. Laetrile (with a capital L) usually refers to the Krebses' original product, whose purification process was patented by them.

In this book, laetrile (with a small l) refers to the commercial forms of amygdalin which are currently in use and around which the debate rages. Most of these are probably racemic (i.e., mixed left-turning and right-turning forms). Krebs, Jr., believes that these commercial products are less than one-third as effective as his original Laetrile (Krebs, Jr., 1979). This is more than a quibble, as many substances are biologically active only in their left- or right-turning forms (Hunter, 1987).

According to some experts, laetrile-rich foods, including fruit kernels, were eaten by our ancestors, including Peking man (Brothwell and Brothwell, 1969:130). Laetrile's use in medicine dates from the time of the great herbal of China, credited to the legendary culture hero Emperor Shen Nung (1st–2nd century A.D.), which is said to list kernel preparations useful against tumors. Ancient Egyptian, Greek, Roman, and Arabic physicians were all familiar with the biologic properties of "bitter almond water" *(aqua amygdalarum amarum)*. Celsus, Scribonius Largus, Galen, Pliny the Elder, Marcellus Empiricus, and Avicenna all used preparations containing laetrile to treat tumors. The same is true of the medieval pharmacopoeia (Halstead, 1977; Summa, 1972).

Such ancient use does not, of course, constitute proof that laetrile is effective. For those familiar with the course of medical history, however, it does remove it from the realm of simple quackery and make it a prime candidate for serious scientific testing. Other natural products have already demonstrated their usefulness in the treatment of cancer. Antibiotics such as bleomycin, dactinomycin, doxorubicin, mithramycin, and mitomycin C; plant alkaloids such as vincristine and vinblastine, and biologicals such as BCG and C. Parvum have all been accepted as orthodox treatments—but often after fierce resistance by the establishment. Ancient prescriptions are being rewritten in modern terms by cancer researchers. Remedies that were long thought of as pure quackery are now being found to have a rational basis.

Folk remedies from around the world have shown promise in cancer therapy. For example, the Penobscot Indians long used the mayapple *(Podophyllum peltatum)* as a folk remedy for cancer. This was even recorded in a medical book in 1849, but for over one hundred years it was scorned or ignored.

Most cancer researchers "shied away form such weird-sounding therapies, lest their scientific reputations suffer," according to Margaret B. Kreig in *Green Medicine,* a study of the search for plants that heal. A few researchers, like NCI's Jonathan Hartwell, decided to investigate mayapple and found that this quack cure actually retarded the growth of cancer. Now called VM-26, it has been found to be effective in the treatment of brain cancer in some cases, and is routinely used for certain warts, which are, after all, benign growths (Kreig, 1964; ACS, 1975).

The autumn crocus, which was advocated as a cancer cure by Dioscorides, the famous Greco-Roman physician and botanist, has been found to contain a chemical useful in the treatment of chronic granulocytic leukemia (Kreig, 1964).

Mistletoe *(Viscum album),* which was recommended by Pliny the Elder 2,000 years ago, was found to cause more than 50 percent tumor inhibition in mice in experiments at Roswell Park Memorial Institute, Buffalo New York (ibid.).

Garlic, ginseng, and other herbs have given some indication of anticancer activity (ibid; Brown University, 1976).

In fact, a group of NCI and Chinese scientists have shown that people who eat about three ounces a day of garlic, onions, scallions and leeks are only 40 percent as likely to get stomach cancer as those who eat few of these allium vegetables (Carper, 1989).

In 1975 the NCI announced that it was conducting tests on maytansine, a drug derived from an East African shrub. It, too, was used by natives to treat cancer (ACS, 1975).

Because of its natural origin, and the great antiquity of its use, laetrile would be a likely candidate for scientific investigation even if the current controversy had not developed.

Holistic Medicine

Howard Goldstein, M.D., an anti-laetrilist, has said: "There is no proven case of a person with bona fide cancer who has received no other treatment than laetrile being cured of his disease" (*Nyack* [N.Y.] *Journal-News*, December 21, 1977).

Even if this statement were true—and there are qualified physicians who would dispute it—it misses the point of the entire debate. Laetrile involves much more than the use of a single drug for the treatment of cancer. Laetrile and the movement that has grown up around it pose a major challenge to the current methods of treating cancer as they are practiced at most medical centers. This challenge has not only medical but also philosophic and socioeconomic implications.

Laetrilists are not just advocating a single substance but, like the advocates of other unorthodox therapies, are proposing a new kind of treatment for the patient's body and mind.

There is apparently an irreconcilable difference between laetrilists and orthodox doctors in how they understand cancer.

Since the time of John Hunter (1728–1793), orthodox physicians have tended to see cancer as a localized disease that, as Hunter said, "only produces local effects" (Shimkin, 1977). Such a disease should therefore be curable through localized means—for example, removing the growth through surgery.

Hunter's view led to an enormous increase in surgery and spurred the development of new operative techniques. Nevertheless, experiments in this century, and particularly in the past thirty years, have suggested that the body has natural immune mechanisms against cancer analogous to those that function in microbial infections. The logical corollary of this view is that cancer can be controlled by enhancing the body's normal immune functions, which orthodox methods tend to destroy.

Laetrilists are not alone in adopting this view, but they propose some novel methods of influencing the body's natural curative powers. First of these is with the cyanogenic glycosides, consumed either through the ingestion of laetrile-rich foods or introduced as medicine in a concentrated form. Laetrile per se is not an immune stimulant, but neither does it apparently harm the natural defense mechanisms. Since laetrilists regard this class of substances not as drugs but as vitamin B-17, they advocate its daily ingestion for the maintenance of a cancer-free state, as well as its use in concentrated form when cancer has already developed.

In addition, they utilize megadoses of recognized vitamins such as (emulsified) vitamin A and vitamin C, as well as other vitamins and minerals (e.g., selenium) believed to have anticancer properties.

Enzymes are usually added to this regimen, following the theory of Krebs, Jr. (1970) and Beard (1911) that the pancreatic enzymes—trypsin and chymotrypsin—are intrinsic anticancer factors. To free these enzymes to kill cancer cells, laetrilists advise their patients to eat only small amounts of animal protein. They also advise their patients to eat large amounts of fresh fruits and vegetables, in part to make up for the loss of animal protein and in part for the other enzymes and nutrients that these foods contain. Supplements are often given in the form of Wobe Mugos, which contain enzymes from pancreas, calf thymus, peas, lentils, and papaya (Wolf and Ransberger, 1972).

The laetrile diet of Ernesto Contreras also forbids such items as alcohol, coffee, soft drinks, white bread, ice cream, butter, canned and prepared foods, and it encourages the use of "health foods" such as whole grains, herb teas, and honey (see Table 5).

In addition, laetrilists sometimes employ other relatively nontoxic and unorthodox therapies, such as those mentioned in the following chapters of this book or included in the ACS handbook on unproven methods.

Finally, laetrile-using physicians generally attempt to treat the whole person—body, mind, and spirit—hence the designation *holistic medicine*. Although there is no single method of psychotherapy employed, there has been a great deal of interest in the work of Dr. O. Carl Simonton, who attempts to use biofeedback techniques to concentrate the patient's conscious and subconscious mind on the destruction of her tumor and the restitution of her health (Simonton and Matthews-Simonton, 1978).

TABLE 5
Laetrile Diet

	Laetrile Diet	Forbidden Food
Beverages	Chamomile tea, clear tea, mint tea, papaya tea, Sanka.	Alcohol, cocoa, coffee, milk, soft drinks.
Bread	Rye bread, soya bread, whole wheat or bran muffins, whole wheat bread.	All other. White bread.
Cereals	Buckwheat, cornmeal, cracked wheat, millet, oatmeal, sesame, finely ground grits, brown rice, barley.	All other. Refined and bleached flour. White rice.
Cheese	Cottage cheese only in limited quantities.	All other.
Dessert	Fresh fruits, stewed fruits, Jell-O.	All pastries, puddings, custards, junket, sauces, ice cream.
Eggs	Poached or boiled eggs, not fried; one a day.	Any other form.
Fat	Cold-pressed oils, preferably safflower or soya oil; soya-lecithin spread.	Butter, shortening, margarine, saturated oils and fats.
Fish	White-flesh fish only (very fresh).	All other fish and seafood.
Fruits	Fresh fruits only: apples, pears, apricots, bananas, cherries, currants, grapes, guava, mangos, melon, nectarines, papaya, peaches, plums, ripe oranges, quince, tangerines, avocados, ripe pineapple. Following dried fruits (unsulfured) can be stewed: apples, apricots, dates, figs, prunes, peaches, pears, plums, raisins.	Canned fruits.
Juices	Only fresh juices. May be selected from lists of fruits and vegetables permitted, including the following green leaves: chicory, endives, escarole, lettuce, Swiss chard, and watercress.	All canned juices and juices with artificial coloring and sweetening.

136

Meat	Lean, grilled, broiled, roasted, or baked beef, chicken, lamb, turkey, and veal. Internal organs: only heart and extra-fresh calf liver permitted.	No pork, fat, fried or smoked meat, sausages.
Milk	Yogurt, buttermilk, and nonfat milk allowed in limited quantities.	Other dairy products.
Nuts	All types of fresh raw nuts (except peanuts), almonds, 6 to 10 a day.	Roasted and salted nuts and peanuts.
Potatoes	Baked, boiled, and mashed. Potato salad seasoned with salad dressing substitute.	French fries, chips.
Salads	The following raw vegetables, shredded or finely chopped, separately or mixed: carrots, cauliflower, celery, chicory, green pepper, lettuce, radishes, Swiss chard, watercress, onions, ripe tomatoes, turnips, brussels sprouts, broccoli.	Any other.
Seasoning	Chives, garlic, onion, parsley, herbs, laurel, marjoram, sage, thyme, savory, cumin, oregano, salt substitutes or other potassium salt, and sea salt in small amounts.	Spices, pepper, paprika.
Soups	Vegetable soup; barley, brown rice, and millet can be added.	Canned and creamed soup, fat stock, consommé.
Sweets	Unpasteurized honey, unsulfured molasses, raw sugar, or dark-brown sugar. Carob.	Candy, chocolate, white sugar.
Vegetables	Raw or freshly cooked: artichokes, asparagus, carrots, cauliflower, celery, chives, corn, endives, green onions, spinach, green peas, green pepper, leeks, lentils, lima beans, potatoes, radishes, tomatoes, wax beans, yams, eggplant, squash. Any vegetables listed under salads.	All canned ones.

Any Variations in This Diet Should Be Done Only With Doctor's Permission.

(Information from Ernesto Contreras, M.D.)

All of this adds up to a new and radically different approach to cancer, one that many patients report to be a positive, healing experience, both mentally and physically. This is in sharp contrast to those methods currently employed in orthodox medicine that, whatever their medical value, are extremely trying on the patient's mind, body, and bank account. Opponents of the laetrile movement sometimes make the mistake of regarding the concept of holistic medicine as a clever ruse being used to fool a gullible public that simply doesn't want to take some very bitter medicine. Such an attitude is contradicted by the observations of two sociologists, neither of whom is connected to this movement, who view holistic medicine as a radical challenge to orthodoxy:

> In these revolutionary periods, nothing less than the very definition of the discipline is at stake. After a new paradigm emerges, all previous research in an area may be defined as irrelevant, if not false.
> Laetrile research is clearly an attempt at paradigm creation or revolutionary science (Markle and Petersen, 1977).

The fact that laetrile threatens to change current methods of treating a major disease accounts in part for the vehemence with which it has been opposed by the medical establishment.

Is Laetrile a Vitamin?

Laetrilists contend that purified amygdalin is not a drug, new or old, but a food factor—specifically, that it is vitamin B-17 (Burk, 1975). This concept has been attacked by Dr. David M. Greenberg in an article entitled "The Vitamin Fraud in Cancer Quackery" in which he proposes several properties that distinguish a bona fide vitamin:

(1) It is a nutritional component of organic composition required in small amounts for the complete health and well-being of the organism.
(2) Vitamins are not utilized primarily to supply energy or as a source of structural tissue components of the body.
(3) A vitamin functions to promote a physiologic process or processes vital to the continued existence of the organism.
(4) A vitamin cannot be synthesized by the cells of the organism and must be supplied *de novo*.
(5) In man and in other mammals, deficiency of a specific vitamin is the cause of certain rather well-defined diseases (David Greenberg, 1975).

Vitamin B-17 certainly conforms to requirements (2) and (4). Whether it conforms to the others hinges on a single, central issue: Does it help prevent cancer? If it does, it would certainly seem to be a vitamin—even by Greenberg's criteria.

Greenberg states that "no evidence has ever been adduced that laetriles are essential nutritional components"; "laetriles have never been shown to promote any physiological process"; and "no specific disease has been associated with a lack of laetrile in any animal." Yet no studies of the effect of laetrile on cancer are cited by this author, although such studies do exist.

There are three main arguments in favor of laetrile's vitamin status. None of these is ironclad, but each suggests that this theory deserves a serious reception.

First, cancer is a chronic, metabolic disease. As the well-known British chemist J. D. Bernal remarked:

> After the successes early in the century of the understanding and cure of such external deficiency diseases as scurvy (vitamin C) and beriberi (vitamin B), and internal deficiency diseases such as goitre (thyroxin) and diabetes (insulin), it began to be apparent that a very large number of chronic diseases were deficiency diseases, though in some cases the deficiency might be the effect of an earlier infection (Bernal, 1971:928).

Why should we rule out the possibility that cancer, or at least some forms of it, could be prevented or controlled by naturally occurring substances?

Second, there is epidemiological data suggesting that populations that have relatively large amounts of isolated laetrile in their diets are also relatively free of cancer. The Hunzakuts, who live in a kingdom near Pakistan, have often been reported to be virtually free of cancer. It is well established that apricots and apricot kernels form a staple in their diet to a degree unparalleled in the rest of the world (Leaf and Launois, 1975; Renée Taylor, 1960).*

Third, experiments performed to test laetrile's *preventive* value at Sloan-Kettering did show a prophylactic effect, according to Dr. Kanematsu Sugiura (see chapter 9).

The idea of laetrile as vitamin B-17 is therefore not simply a ruse or cancer quackery, but a scientific hypothesis deserving of serious attention.

---

*A great deal of nonsense has been written about this "paradise" principality, much of which seems intended to show that life is better under semifeudalism.

The Biochemistry of Laetrile

In the late 1940s, biochemist Ernst T. Krebs, Jr., purified a crude apricot-kernel preparation and proposed a biochemical rationale for its use in the treatment of cancer. On the basis of extensive work reported in the scientific literature, Krebs proposed a "cyanide theory" to explain laetrile's effect on cancer. Bruce W. Halstead, M.D., a toxicologist, summarized the long debate over laetrile's mode of action in 1977.

Two separate pathways have been suggested for laetrile's activity in the body. The first pathway is not controversial. The second—the one proposed by Krebs—has been sharply questioned by a number of critics (David Greenberg, 1975; J. P. Ross, 1975).

According to this second pathway, the glucuronide form of amygdalin is synthesized in the livers of people who ingest natural amygdalin. This glucuronide is then broken down at the tumor site to release cyanide, which selectively attacks the cancer cells but spares normal cells. Some scientists have in fact found glucuronide formation in the liver and, to a lesser extent, in the intestine and kidneys (Halstead, 1977).

In order for this glucuronide to be broken down, the enzyme beta-glucuronidase must be present. In some studies this enzyme has been found in cancerous tissues of the breast, uterus, stomach, mesentery, abdominal wall, and esophagus, in amounts about 100 to 3,600 times greater than is present in noncancerous tissues. When they went looking, Sloan-Kettering Institute researchers found that "in many cases beta-glycosidase and glucuronidase activities were higher in cancerous than homologous normal tissues. . . ." (Sloan-Kettering, 1974:60).

The breakdown of laetrile by beta-glucuronidase at the site of the tumor would cause general cyanide poisoning in normal cells were it not for the presence of another enzyme, rhodanese, which is capable of detoxifying cyanide.

Rhodanese was discovered by K. Lang in 1933, and a number of scientific reports have shown that normal cells contain a relatively high concentration of rhodanese and low levels of beta-glucuronidase (Halstead, 1977). Sloan-Kettering researchers found variable levels of rhodanese.

If the glucuronide is in fact formed in the liver, as Krebs postulated, and if this glucuronide then reaches the tumor site, where it is broken down by the high level of beta-glucuronidase, the resulting cyanide could conceivably poison cancer cells deficient in rhodanese, while sparing those normal cells that have high levels of this enzyme.

At the same time, benzaldehyde, a known painkiller, would also be released, accounting perhaps for the analgesic properties often associated with laetrile.

Some scientists believe that benzaldehyde itself may be an active anticancer chemical in laetrile. According to Andrew A. Benson of the Scripps Institution of Oceanography in La Jolla, California, the Japanese scientist Kenji Sakaguchi of the Kasei Institute of Biological Sciences in Michida, Japan, has found that benzaldehyde "is effective against human lung cancer" (*Science News,* February 3, 1979).

A number of other possible mechanisms of laetrile activity have also been proposed (Passwater, 1977; McCarty, 1975; Halstead, 1977). Krebs's original explanation is still widely respected among laetrilists and in some ways is the most appealing since it comes close to the long-sought "magic bullet" for cancer, which could kill cancer cells while leaving normal cells unharmed. Ironically, the basic principle behind laetrile's use resembles chemotherapy's rationale. In fact, when laetrile was originally proposed in the early 1950s, it was called chemotherapy. Halstead has summarized the current status of the controversy over laetrile's mode of action:

> Despite Krebs' critics and a number of unanswered questions about the "cyanide theory," it continues to remain the most biochemically rational explanation of some very complex chemical events revolving around the use of amygdalin (laetrile) in cancer metabolic therapy. This theory is now under critical review by a number of investigators and only time and further research will determine its ultimate reality (Halstead, 1977).*

The Question of Toxicity

A great deal has been made of the alleged toxicity of laetrile. In 1977–78 the FDA took the extraordinary step of posting large "Laetrile Warning" posters in 10,000 post offices and sending an FDA *Drug Bulletin* on the subject (November–December 1977) to hundreds of thousands of health workers. As a result, laetrile, once known as a remarkably nontoxic form of therapy, is today widely considered to be a dangerous and toxic drug.

*In November 1983 Dr. Halstead's Preventative Medical Clinic was raided. He spent two days in jail in November 1984. The following June he was convicted of seventeen felony counts of treating cancer patients with a Japanese anticancer "brew" called ADS. At the present time he is out on an appeal bond of $100,000 (Holcomb, 1988).

In the meantime, as a result of the "intensive prosecution against the use of metabolic cancer therapy," Halstead's clinic has "been forced to discontinue its clinical practice involving cancer patients of any type" (Fink, 1988).

The FDA *Bulletin* contained numerous misstatements about laetrile. For example, it stated that "this glycoside [amygdalin] contains cyanide." Of course, amygdalin does not contain cyanide, but can be hydrolyzed into benzaldehyde, hydrogen cyanide, and two sugars, given the presence of beta-D-glucosidase and beta-oxynitrilase (David Greenberg, 1975). This is more than a semantic difference. Unless the proper conditions are met, cyanide is as firmly bound in the amygdalin molecule as a brick in a solid brick wall. One might as well state that table salt is poisonous because it contains chlorine!

According to the poster, thirty-seven poisonings and seventeen deaths have been caused by "ingestion of laetrile ingredients (apricot and similar fruit pits)." Apricot pits are not ingredients of laetrile. If anything, laetrile is an ingredient of apricot pits (kernels), which also contain other substances, such as enzymes, not found in purified amygdalin. (The whole kernel contains only 2 to 4 percent laetrile.) The thirty-seven poisonings, culled from the entire world over many years, refer to circumstances quite different from those encountered by cancer patients ingesting laetrile as medicine.

In the United States, three deaths have been attributed by the government to laetrile ingestion. Two women died of apparent cyanide poisoning after swallowing vials of laetrile meant for injection purposes only (*Journal of the American Medical Association,* April 14, 1978).

The third case was that of Elizabeth Hankin, an eleven-month-old daughter of a laetrile-using cancer patient. According to the FDA, the child "accidentally ingested up to five tablets (500 mg./tab) of laetrile" and died. Laetrilists (including the parents) contend that the child may never have taken laetrile, and was off the critical list when doctors decided to administer a powerful anticyanide antidote. The child subsequently slipped into a coma and died (*The Choice,* December, 1977).

The FDA *Bulletin* contains other "warnings" that appear to be primarily designed to frighten cancer patients away from an alternative form of cancer therapy. For example: "Indeed, some deaths ascribed to cancer, particularly in debilitated patients, may have been either due to or accelerated by cyanide from the drug." A frightening prospect—but what is the evidence for this? The FDA hedges by saying, "Further studies should be undertaken to determine whether this is true or not."

It was estimated in 1978 that 50,000–100,000 cancer patients were taking over 1 million grams of laetrile a month (Moertel, 1978). Two or possibly three deaths were reported from accidental overdoses of this substance. Several cases of minimal toxicity were been reported. Based on these facts, laetrile does not seem to be a dangerous or toxic substance when taken correctly.

In 1978 anti-laetrile researchers killed dogs by infusing large amounts of cyanide into their stomachs through feeding tubes. The cyanide had been derived from laetrile prior to the "feeding." The amount necessary to kill the animals was figured out scientifically, and then the animals were given drugs to prevent them from regurgitating the mixture (Schmidt, 1978). This finding—that laetrile, when first broken down by enzymatic action or heat, can poison those who ingest it—made headlines around the world. But it is not really news. The potentially poisonous nature of a slurry of bitter-almond kernels has been known since the time of the pharaohs, when it was used to execute prisoners (Summa, 1972).

Since 1837 it has been known that under the proper chemical conditions amygdalin can be hydrolyzed to release hydrogen cyanide. This does not normally happen to a dangerous extent in the human gut, and certainly not when purified amygdalin (without enzymes) is administered by injections, which avoid the digestive tract. When administered properly by a physician, laetrile does not appear to be a significantly toxic substance. The record reveals no deaths or serious injuries of persons injected with laetrile.

This observation is borne out by Sloan-Kettering's five-year study of laetrile. In one case, laetrile was injected into mice in doses as high as 8 grams per kilogram of body weight per day, with no sign of acute or chronic toxicity. This is the equivalent of giving a human being a pound a day of this allegedly toxic substance! In another test, mice were given 2 grams per kilogram per day for thirty months. Sugiura reported that the treated mice in his experiments exhibited better health and well-being than the controls, which did not receive laetrile (Stock et al., 1978).

When advocates of orthodox chemotherapy accuse laetrile of being toxic, it is a case of the pot calling the kettle black. As was shown above, most standard chemotherapeutic agents are truly toxic in the extreme. Methotrexate alone can produce such blood diseases as anemia, leukopenia, and thrombocytopenia as well as liver atrophy, necrosis, cirrhosis, fatty changes, fetal death, congenital abnormalities, diarrhea, ulcerative stomatitis, and, occasionally, death from intestinal perforation (*Physicians' Desk Reference*, 1988).

In comparison to such agents, laetrile is indeed nontoxic, although one could certainly imagine situations in which it could be toxic or even fatal (the same is true of water or air). Paracelsus (1493–1541), sometimes called the father of chemotherapy, could very well have been commenting on this controversy when he wrote, "All substances are poisons; there is none which is not a poison. The right dose differentiates a poison from a remedy."

The Testing of Laetrile in Animals

Although spokespersons for orthodox medicine continue to deny that there have been any animal study data in favor of laetrile, this is contradicted by a number of studies, including—but not limited to—those at Sloan-Kettering.

For example, the SCIND Laboratories in California conducted several experiments in preparation for an Investigational New Drug (IND) application filed by the McNaughton Foundation in 1970. (The application was approved and then revoked a few days later, after it received unexpected publicity through Associated Press).

In their second study on carcinoma of rats (Walker 256), with amygdalin in dosages of 500 milligrams per kilogram injected intraperitoneally on days one, three, and six after tumor take, the following results were found:

DAYS SURVIVAL TIME

Controls: 19, 19, 19, 19, 20, 20, 22, 22, 22, 22, 24, 24, 24, 25, 25, 26, 26, 26, 26

Treated: 27, 28, 28, 28, 29, 29, 29, 30, 30, 30, 30, 30, 31, 32, 32, 32, 60, 60, 60, 60 (U.S. SENATE, 1977:419).

The mean survival time of the controls was thus 23 days, while of the amygdalin-treated group it was 38 days, or a 70 percent increase over the controls. Notice that the survival time of *every* amygdalin-treated animal was greater than that of *every* control animal.

As Dr. Carl Baker, then director of the National Cancer Institute, wrote in a letter to Congressman Edward Edwards, "The data provided by the McNaughton Foundation certainly indicates some activity in animal tumor systems" (McCarty, 1975). In Europe as well, a number of experiments were performed that appear to show anticancer activity in animal systems. For example, in a test by Dr. Paul Reitnauer, chief biochemist of the Manfred von Ardenne Institute, Dresden (East Germany), 20 of 40 H-strain mice were given bitter almonds in addition to their standard diet. Bitter almonds contain relatively high levels of laetrile.

Fifteen days after initiation of this regimen, all 40 mice were inoculated with 1 million Ehrlich ascites cells. The 20 control mice lived an average of 21.9 days following this injection. The 20 mice receiving the bitter almond supplement lived an average of 25.8 days, which was statistically significant (Reitnauer, 1973).

Dr. T. Metianu, director of research in pharmacology-toxicology of the Pasteur Institute, Paris, using an adenocarcinoma adapted for mice, showed that 10 mice treated subcutaneously with amygdalin two to three times per week for 20 to 25 days with 500 milligrams per kilogram lived an average of 58 days past the time of tumor take. A group of 10 control mice averaged 21 days survival time. A repetition of this experiment showed 47 days survival for the laetrile-treated mice and 27 for the controls. Less striking results were observed at higher dosages, and no effect was seen at 100 milligrams per kilogram in this system (cited in Burk, 1975).

Combination Therapy

Laetrile is rarely used alone in the treatment of cancer. Thus, laetrilists have always argued that research institutes such as Sloan-Kettering or NCI should use this "vitamin" in combination with other vitamins, minerals, and enzymes in order to achieve optimal results.

The first scientist to attempt such an experiment on a large scale in animals was Harold W. Manner, Ph.D. Dr. Manner, chairman of the biology department at Loyola University, Chicago, used a combination of emulsified vitamin A (A-mulsin, produced by the Mugos Company), the same company's Wobe Mugos enzymes, and laetrile.

The results were reportedly dramatic. As stated in Manner's book *The Death of Cancer:*

> After 6–8 days an ulceration appeared at the tumor site. Within the ulceration was a puslike fluid. An examination of this fluid revealed dead malignant cells. . . . The tumors gradually underwent complete regression in 75 of the experimental animals. This represented 89.3% of the total group. The remaining 9 animals showed partial regression. No attempts were made to determine increase in life span or changes in metastases (Manner et al. 1978a).

These startling results took place in mice which develop spontaneous mammary tumors, the female C3H/HeJ strain acquired from the Jackson Laboratories, Bar Harbor, Maine.

Manner's results were greeted with skepticism by most cancer researchers. Manner was criticized for first presenting his findings to a lay group—the National Health Federation—rather than to his scientific colleagues. Manner replied that it would take years before these results could be accepted and published, and that hundreds of thousands of people would die needlessly in that time.

In addition, Manner was criticized for not testing laetrile, enzymes, and vitamins separately. Specifically, his study did not determine if laetrile in and of itself had any effectiveness against cancer.

In a follow-up experiment involving a total of 550 C3H/HeJ mice, Manner attempted to clarify some of these problems. Enzymes alone, combinations of enzymes and laetrile, or of vitamin A and enzymes, produced between 52 and 54 percent total regressions of cancer. Laetrile alone had no appreciable effect, but a combination of enzymes, vitamin A, and laetrile was significantly more effective than just enzymes and/or vitamin A. The triple combination produced total regressions in 38 out of 50 cases, or 76 percent. Manner subsequently published these results (Manner, 1978b).

The establishment had much to say against Manner but, as the Chicago scientist often pointed out, orthodox cancer research doctors never availed themselves of the opportunity to refute his claims *by reproducing his tests.*

Manner subsequently took over the Cydel Hospital in Tijuana, Mexico, and renamed it the Manner Clinic. This 40-bed inpatient facility provided an eclectic mixture of treatments, including the "Manner cocktail" (9 g. laetrile, 10 cc DMSO, 25 g. vitamin C; see Fink 1988).

In May 1986 the metabolic cancer therapy of Harold W. Manner was included on the ACS's unproven methods list. According to the article in *CA,* the American Cancer Society's journal, there was no evidence that Manner's therapy "results in objective benefit in the treatment of cancer in human beings" (ACS, 1986).

Manner himself died suddenly of a heart attack in October 1988 at the age of 62. At this writing, however, his clinic remains in operation.

Clinical Studies

In modern times, laetrile was one of the first purified chemicals to be tried for cancer treatment in a hospital setting. The substance was used by the Russian physician Fedor J. Inosemtzeff in 1844; after several months "the patient was declared cured, and he left the hospital. He had received about one and a half ounces of pure amygdalin without showing any signs of toxicity" (Inosemtzeff, 1845).

Laetrile was employed in the treatment of cancer in the early 1950s by Ernst T. Krebs, Sr., a San Francisco physician, and a Los Angeles doctor, Arthur Harris. In a 1962 paper, Harris claimed that of the 82 cancer patients treated with laetrile between 1951 and 1953, 3 were alive and free of disease almost ten years later, 24 were alive with their cancers under control, and 55 had received only temporary, palliative results (H. H. Beard, 1962).

These and other early clinical reports were challenged in a retrospective study of 44 cancer patients treated with laetrile, reported in an article by the California Cancer Commission (CCC). The Commission claimed that laetrile was "completely ineffective" in humans, in laboratory animals, or *in vitro* (California Cancer Commission, 1953).

For many years this report stood as the definitive anti-laetrile study, but after twenty years it came under sharp attack. For example, all the doctors questioned by the CCC reported important subjective benefit from laetrile. In addition, the discussion of "toxic cellular changes" in cancer cells was omitted from the official 1953 report, even though the original laboratory studies had mentioned this occurrence. In addition, the patients had all received either very few injections or dosages considered to be minute by today's standards (Culbert, 1976:110).

Since that time, laetrile has been used by an extraordinary number of cancer victims. Although the aura of illegality that has surrounded laetrile in this country has undoubtedly discouraged scientific publication, there are a number of clinical papers that report positive results with regard to both safety and efficacy.

In 1962, for example, John A. Morrone, an attending surgeon at the Jersey City Medical Center, reported "a dramatic relief of pain" in ten cancer patients treated with laetrile, as well as other effects that "suggest regression of the malignant lesion" (Morrone, 1962).

At both the sixth and ninth International Cancer Congresses, sponsored by the International Union Against Cancer, Ettore Giudetti of the University of Turin and his colleagues reported positive effects of laetrile on cancer patients (Rossi et al., 1966).

One of the most prolific authors in the field has been a Philippine physician, Manuel D. Navarro. He has published almost twenty articles on his experiences with laetrile therapy since 1954 (bibliography in McNaughton, 1967). Navarro has called laetrile "the ideal drug for the treatment of cancer."

Hans A. Nieper, M.D., is a well-known West German oncologist who uses laetrile and synthetic analogs of laetrile in his medical practice. He is the author of several papers on laetrile, including one on the results of sixty cases treated with this substance (Nieper, 1970).

In 1977 John A. Richardson, M.D., published detailed case histories of cancer patients treated by him, selected from about 4,000 patients whom he claims to have treated with some success at his Albany, California, clinic. "Almost all of them have shown a positive response to their initial course of therapy before returning home" (Richardson and Griffin, 1977).

In addition, there have been numerous journalistic accounts of the Clinica del Mar of Ernesto Contreras, M.D., in Tijuana, Mexico, where cancer patients have been treated with laetrile since the early 1960s. (See Table 5, "Laetrile Diet," based on information from Dr. Contreras.) According to these accounts, Contreras claims that 35 percent of his patients (most of whom were terminally ill at the inception of treatment) experienced no response at all. Sixty-five percent received some benefit from laetrile, but almost half of these had recurrences of the disease after its temporary arrest; in the remaining cases, there were "more definite responses," ranging from slight improvement to the dramatic disappearance of all symptoms. Contreras estimates that perhaps 5 percent of the terminal patients he has seen have been actually "saved." These are modest claims, which belie the picture often painted of his Tijuana clinic as the haunt of crackpots and thieves. Nevertheless, Contreras has never published his results in a scientific form, despite numerous promises to do so (Schultz and Lindeman, 1973).

Today Contreras continues to provide therapy in Tijuana. He is said to have a staff of ten doctors, a pharmacy, a public relations office, restaurants offering the laetrile diet, and a motel and trailer park. His hospital has fifty beds. There is even "a nondenominational church adjacent to the clinic where Dr. Contreras preaches" (Fink, 1988:50).

The center emphasizes "immunotherapy, because this is most gentle" and "never harms the body" (ibid.).

The author knows of no scientific studies that Contreras has published to date, however, to back up his claims.

But there have been a number of other clinical studies attesting to laetrile's effectiveness, especially as a palliative. For years what was lacking was the kind of randomized, double-blind study that has become a standard part of new-drug testing in the United States. Responsibility for the lack of such double-blind tests rested mainly with the federal government and especially the FDA, which opposed such a test, even when it was proposed by established cancer scientists.

In 1978 the National Cancer Institute undertook a retrospective study of cancer victims treated with laetrile. This study came under criticism from the laetrile movement because it placed its main emphasis on tumor shrinkage as an index of anticancer effect, and omitted reduction in pain or other palliative aspects of laetrile's action. One pro-laetrile organization, the National Health Federation, therefore refused to cooperate in the government's study. The NCI sought patients who had received laetrile, and only laetrile, in the treatment of cancer. Twenty-two cases were finally found who met all of the NCI panel's criteria for judging drugs. These cases were then "blinded," i.e., reviewed in such a way that any pro- or anti-laetrile bias on the part of the reviewers was theoretically removed.

Of the 22 cases deemed evaluable by NCI, 2 showed complete responses, i.e., total elimination of their tumors; 4 showed partial responses, i.e., greater than 50 percent reduction in tumor size; 9 cases had "stabilized disease"; and "3 additional patients showed increased disease-free intervals." Thus 18 out of 22, or 82 percent, appear to have had a beneficial response to laetrile therapy (Ellison, 1978).

There is no way of knowing how typical these responses might be of laetrile patients in general, but such a response rate, if it were consistent for all patients, would compare quite favorably with orthodox methods of therapy.

Although NCI officials adduced other possible reasons for these results, Dr. Arthur Upton, the director of the National Cancer Institute, shortly afterward asked permission from the Food and Drug Administration to conduct clinical trials on patients at either NCI itself or at major cancer centers around the country (ibid.). More than a year later the FDA had still failed to grant approval for this test.

At the same time, according to one source, Hans Nieper, the German physician who uses unorthodox therapies, met at Sloan-Kettering with its vice presidents Lloyd J. Old, M.D., and C. Chester Stock, Ph.D., and with the honorary chairperson of the American Cancer Society, Mary Lasker. The meeting was held to arrange tests on new synthetic variants of laetrile, or mandelonitrile, which Nieper claims are far more effective than laetrile itself (Chowka, 1979).

The Legal Question

In part because of the federal government's intransigence on the question of testing, laetrilists took to the courts and the legislatures. Laetrile use was legalized in at least twenty states. In New York, pro-laetrile bills were passed by wide margins in the state legislature, only to be vetoed by an anti-laetrile governor.

Before the Supreme Court decision of June 1979, cancer patients were able to receive laetrile legally from their physicians under an affidavit system set up by federal district judge Luther Bohanon. The 1979 Supreme Court decision was widely interpreted in the press as a rebuff to Bohanon's opinions (*New York Times,* June 19, 1979). Yet according to Judge Bohanon's law clerk, Tim Kline, the main practical effect was to remand the case to the Circuit Court of Appeals for review (Kline, 1979).

Bohanon's original twenty-page opinion still contains valuable insights for everyone concerned with this controversy. Bohanon's ruling was not, as sometimes depicted, a call for unlimited freedom of choice without consumer protection. In the jurist's view the argument over laetrile was an un-resolved scientific dispute and needed to be treated as such:

> Unquestionably, the administrative record in this case reveals a substan-tial and well-developed controversy among medical professionals and other scientists as to the efficacy of laetrile.

> Advocates of laetrile's use in cancer treatment include many highly edu-cated and prominent doctors and scientists whose familiarity and practical ex-perience with the substance vastly exceeds that of their detractors. To deem such advocacy "quackery" distorts the serious issues posed by laetrile's prominence and requires disregarding considerable expertise mustered on the drug's behalf.

> While the record reveals an impressive consensus among the nation's large medical and cancer-fighting institutions as to laetrile's ineffectualness, a disconcerting dearth of actual experience with the substance by such detractors is revealed. . . .

> The current debate is fierce. The issue appears largely unresolved as to laetrile's true effectiveness, in large part because FDA has prevented adequate testing on humans. . . .

> It is only when the substance is openly used, and its results carefully observed and fully reported that this controversy will be resolved (Bohanon, 1977).

Conclusions

Laetrile's demise as a national phenomenon was as rapid as its ascent. After years of dickering, in July 1980 the National Cancer Institute finally agreed to test the substance in 178 patients with advanced cancer. The tests were conducted at four major U.S. medical centers—the Mayo Clinic in Rochester, Minnesota, the University of California at Los Angeles, the Uni-versity of Arizona Health Sciences Center in Tucson, and Memorial Sloan-Kettering in New York.

The results were presented at the late April 1981 meeting of the Amer-ican Society for Clinical Oncology (ASCO) by Charles Moertel, M.D., the man who was in charge of the Mayo Clinic portion of this trial. The results were intended to "close the book on laetrile" (Relman, 1982).

For various reasons, twenty-two patients were excluded from the re-sults announced at the meeting. This left 156 evaluable patients. According to Moertel, within a month of starting the laetrile therapy 50 percent showed evidence of cancer progression. Ninety percent progressed after three months. Fifty percent had died before five months and only 20 percent were alive by eight months. This was "consistent with that expected if patients had received no treatment," said Moertel, the same man responsible for the vitamin C double-blind tests.

Only one patient showed a reduction in tumor size. This man had a metastasized cancer of the stomach and was given laetrile at the Mayo Clinic as well as the University of Arizona. A tumor that had spread to his neck regressed for ten weeks but then progressed, despite the fact that he remained on laetrile therapy.

Nineteen percent did report improvement in how they felt at some time during the study, although the authors attributed this to the placebo effect (NCI, 1981).

Laetrile, Moertel concluded, is "ineffective as a treatment for cancer. We have tried very hard to conduct a scientifically honest trial," he added (*Science News,* May 9, 1981).

Laetrile advocates, who had been dubious about the test from the start, reacted bitterly.

While some laetrilists, such as Dr. Ernesto Contreras, had initially greeted the test with enthusiasm, others had been deeply skeptical of NCI from the start. The Committee for Freedom of Choice in Cancer Therapy and American Biologics, Inc. had offered to provide free laetrile to the investigators. When the offer was refused, they unsuccessfully tried to sue in California to have the trial stopped.

"Real laetrile is not the material being tested," a pro-choice publication, *Public Scrutiny,* said flatly (July 1980). In addition, they pointed out that 66 percent of the tested patients had already received chemotherapy, which can damage the body's natural immune mechanisms.

When the May 1981 results were released, the hard core of the movement was hardly surprised. "The whole thing, as far as we are concerned, is a put-up deal to discredit laetrile," said Robert Bradford, founder of the Committee for Freedom of Choice. Laetrilists, such as Michael Culbert, editor of the *Choice,* still believe that genuine laetrile was never tested (Culbert, 1988). It appeared, however, that for the general public, laetrile was a dead issue.

Yet according to Culbert, more laetrile is being used in the late eighties than it was a decade before. While that may be an exaggeration (70–100,000 used it in the late 1970s), it is certainly true that laetrile is now employed as an everyday part of eclectic "metabolic therapy" in a number of thriving clinics. These include the American Biologics-Mexico S.A. Medical Center, with which Bradford and Culbert are now affiliated, as well as over a dozen other centers (listed in John M. Fink's *Third Opinion*).

Because of the immense prestige of the Mayo Clinic and other centers, this large-scale test was a major public relations setback for unorthodox medicine. But in another sense it represented a step forward.

In the past, struggles over unorthodox drugs had been confined to the question of the efficacy of the method in question. When Krebiozen, for instance, was declared ineffective, the movement that had grown up in its support fell apart. But with laetrile, for the first time, a movement of patients was built in this country demanding the *right* to be treated with the medicine of their choice. And this idea did not go away after the Mayo study. It laid the basis for a more generalized patients' revolt, which continues to shake the foundations of orthodox medicine.

« 9 »

Laetrile at Sloan-Kettering: A Case Study

June 15, 1977, was a bright, balmy day on Manhattan's Upper East Side. Within Memorial Sloan-Kettering Cancer Center (MSKCC) that morning, almost one hundred reporters and observers and half a dozen film crews from the leading television stations had assembled to hear the long-awaited official verdict on laetrile from the world's most prestigious cancer research center.

On the dais of the new conference room sat men whose credentials in the scientific world, and even among the public, appeared impeccable: Robert Good, Ph.D., M.D., director and president of Sloan-Kettering Institute, whose face was familiar to many from the cover of *Time*. Lewis Thomas, M.D., president of the overall Center and author of popular books and articles on science. Dr. Daniel Martin, a leading cancer researcher at the Catholic Medical Center, Queens, as well as eight other Memorial Sloan-Kettering scientists.*

All of them agreed, apparently, in the words of the official press release prepared for the occasion, that "laetrile was found to possess neither preventive, nor tumor-regressant, nor anti-metastatic, nor curative anticancer

---

*C. Chester Stock, Ph.D., Kanematsu Sugiura, D.Sc., Isabel M. Mountain, Ph.D., Elizabeth Stockert, D.d'Univ., Franz A. Schmid, D.V.M., George S. Tarnowski, M.D., Dorris J. Hutchison, Ph.D., and Morris N. Teller, Ph.D.

activity," after almost five years of testing at the private research center (Zimmermann, 1977:127).

The officials of the center cleared their throats, reporters put down their danishes and coffee and picked up their pencils. Dr. Robert Good began to speak and, after general remarks condemning laetrile and its use, passed the microphone to one of his vice presidents, Dr. C. Chester Stock. Dr. Stock, at sixty-seven, was the director of chemotherapy research at Sloan-Kettering and head of its suburban Walker Laboratory. Originally an expert on insect control, he had switched to cancer research and for decades had supervised much of the animal testing of new drugs for Sloan-Kettering.

Stock attempted to explain some of the finer details of the testing, but as his voice droned on, the eyes of many turned toward another man to his left: a small, old Japanese scientist in a white lab coat, sitting upright and impassive, blinking at the lights through thick, rimless glasses.

When Stock finished and the conference was thrown open for questions, the first one was for this elderly gentleman, the eighty-six-year-old member emeritus of Sloan-Kettering, Dr. Kanematsu Sugiura. Most of those present were aware of reports circulating for years that Sugiura had claimed positive results with laetrile in his animal experiments. His presence on the dais this morning seemed, perhaps, to imply that he too now agreed with the negative verdict on laetrile.

"Dr. Sugiura," someone shouted out suddenly. "Do you stick by your belief that laetrile stops the spread of cancer?"

The television cameras swung in the old man's direction and began purring.

"I stick!" Sugiura shot back, in a voice startlingly loud and assertive. It was clear that rebellion still continued in the ranks of Sloan-Kettering on the emotional question of laetrile.

It is difficult to imagine a less likely rebel than Dr. Kanematsu Sugiura. Born in Japan in 1892, Sugiura had always been a grateful and loyal beneficiary of the establishment. He was brought to America by the railroad tycoon E. H. Harriman as a member of the first jiu-jitsu team ever to tour the United States. In 1905 he even performed at the White House for President Teddy Roosevelt. Sugiura proudly showed visitors pictures of himself as a handsome, athletic young man, standing barefoot in the snow in his *kendo* uniform (Sugiura, 1971).

After performing at many private homes and clubs, the entire team went home to Japan—all except young Sugiura, who chose to stay on as the house guest of Harriman's personal physician, Dr. William G. Lyle. Although Sugiura was terribly homesick, he knew that this was the only way he would be able to get an education: his father was a poor fencing master in Japan and could not afford to send him to school.

Sugiura's interest in science began early. After his day's study at Townsend Harris Hall high school in New York City, a school which specialized in training gifted young students, he would go to work at Roosevelt Hospital, where he would wash instruments, scrub containers, and help doctors with their experiments.

In 1909 E. H. Harriman died of cancer and left $1 million to establish a cancer research laboratory at Roosevelt Hospital. Dr. Lyle became its director, and in 1911 young Sugiura became assistant chemist at the newly founded Harriman Research Laboratory.

In the next year, Kanematsu Sugiura began his first experiments in the chemotherapy of cancer with colleagues at Harriman and at Cornell University Medical College. At the time, he was only twenty years old and hadn't even begun college. In those days, cancer chemotherapy was a highly unusual and unorthodox procedure, frowned upon by the surgeons who then held surgery to be the only acceptable method of treatment.

By 1917 Sugiura had received college degrees from the Polytechnic Institute of Brooklyn and from Columbia University, and was fully launched on his career as a cancer chemotherapist.* His lifetime in the field thus spanned the entire history of modern chemotherapy, and his work touched most of the chief areas of research and progress.

Sugiura's main influence was in developing the techniques of cancer research in rats and mice, and then in testing a wide variety of chemical and biological compounds in these rodents to see if they had an anticancer effect. In the pre-World War I days, Sugiura and his colleagues tested various inorganic compounds on cancerous animals. They were able to demonstrate that such chemicals did have a small, but real, anticancer effect in laboratory animals. These findings helped overcome skepticism about chemotherapy in medical circles and spurred interest in finding even more active chemicals.

In 1917, however, the Harriman family suddenly lost interest in cancer research and turned to politics. (E. H. Harriman's son William Averell later became governor of New York.) The Harriman Research Laboratory closed its doors, and the various staff members were forced to seek positions elsewhere (ibid.).

On November 1, 1917, Dr. Sugiura came to Memorial Hospital, then under the direction of Dr. James Ewing, to work as an assistant chemist.

---

*In 1925 he also received a doctorate in science from Kyoto Imperial University in Japan (*New York Times,* October 23, 1979).

(Before the founding of Sloan-Kettering Institute in 1945, both research and treatment were done at Memorial Hospital.) Recognizing Sugiura's talent, Ewing quickly sent him to the Crocker laboratory of Columbia University to learn the new techniques of tumor transplantation being developed there.

In the early days of 1917 the question of diet and cancer was receiving a great deal of attention, spurred by the wide-scale malnutrition caused by World War I. Reports had also begun to reach the industrially developed countries that the peoples in underdeveloped areas of Africa, India, and the East Indian Islands rarely developed cancer. Sugiura, who maintained a lifelong interest in nutrition, began to perform research in this field. He fed mice which had received transplantable tumors a diet composed solely of bananas—since bananas formed the basis of some tropical diets. The tumors grew very slowly. However, when Sugiura added protein and yeast, the tumors grew at a normal rate.

Another interesting experiment involved keeping the mice on a starvation diet. Mice fed one-third the normal amount of food showed much less tumor growth than animals fed normal rations. These studies were then extended to mice which had first had their tumors removed surgically. Sugiura found that if he then underfed the mice, few new tumors occurred either at the site of the operation or elsewhere (ibid.).

This early work on diet and cancer was greeted with little enthusiasm by the surgeons and radiologists of Memorial Hospital. There were a few halfhearted tries at applying this knowledge in the clinic, but by and large, doctors scoffed at the idea of "starving" an already weakened cancer patient. In fact, physicians who insisted that there could be a link between faulty dietary habits and the rising rate of cancer were looked upon as quacks (Sugiura, 1974).

A shy and retiring man, Sugiura never became embroiled in the controversies that raged over the link between diet and cancer. He remained aloof, and seemingly unaware of the larger issues involved. He was the laboratory scientist par excellence, content if he were left alone to do his work.

In the 1920s and 1930s, Sugiura studied the effects of such substances as coal tar–based dyes, hormones, and enzymes on cancer growth. He performed experiments showing that butter-yellow dye caused cancer in experimental animals. This led to the dye's removal from the food supply. Again, however, he shunned the limelight, and was never involved in the fierce controversy over this concept.

Despite the fact that he had lived in this country for many decades and had a daughter born in the United States, Sugiura was suddenly threatened with internment in a concentration camp with other Japanese after Pearl

Harbor. Intervention by Dr. C. P. Rhoads, Memorial's director, at the "highest levels of government" prevented this; Sugiura was "merely" placed under house arrest (*New York Times*, October 23, 1979).

Sugiura was therefore officially restricted to his apartment on the Grand Concourse in the Bronx for the duration of the war. He used to "wander" away, however, to do research at the New York Academy of Medicine or at the old, and by then largely abandoned, Memorial Hospital on 104th Street. Sixty-eighth Street, where the new hospital was located, was off limits to him (Sugiura, 1974).

After the war the entire scientific structure changed at the Memorial Center, as it was then known. Whereas previously the scientific as well as the clinical work had been done at Memorial Hospital, most of the laboratory research was transferred to Sloan-Kettering Institute after 1945. Sugiura was transferred as well and was made an associate member (later, a full member) of Sloan-Kettering.

C. Chester Stock was put in charge of a massive campaign to test thousands of compounds in an empirical search for a cancer cure. Sugiura now worked under him. Various drugs currently in use were discovered during this period, including methotrexate and the antibiotic mitomycin C.

In 1962 Sugiura officially retired and became member emeritus. In 1965 Dr. Stock helped gather Sugiura's more than 200 papers into a four-volume *Collected Works*. His introductory remarks summed up world scientific opinion about Sugiura:

> Few, if any, names in cancer research are as widely known as Kanematsu Sugiura's. . . . Possibly the high regard in which his work is held is best characterized by a comment made to me by a visiting investigator in cancer research from Russia. He said, "When Dr. Sugiura publishes, we know we don't have to repeat the study, for we would obtain the same results he has reported" (Sugiura, 1965).

A decade later, Sugiura was a fixture at the Walker Laboratory of Sloan-Kettering Institute in Rye, New York. He had an office on the second floor, which he shared with scientist Isabel Mountain. Every day he arrived at the low-lying suburban building at 8:00 A.M. Every day at 5:00 P.M. he left for his home in a nearby Westchester town, where he lived with his wife and daughter and her husband, Sloan-Kettering scientist Franz Schmid.

Sugiura had lived a long and full life, had been honored by his peers, and was well known and respected in both his adopted and his native lands. He had even received the Order of Sacred Treasure, third class, in 1960 from Emperor Hirohito of Japan for his contributions to medical research (*New York Times*, October 23, 1979).

By every indication, Sugiura would end his life as peacefully and quietly as he had lived it, content with his half-page niche in the National Cancer Institute-sponsored history of cancer research (Shimkin, 1977:404).

Instead, by 1973 Sugiura found himself unintentionally and uncomfortably the center of a furious controversy. Because he had merely done what he was told and recorded what he saw, he lived to see old friends desert and berate him, a close relative fail to support him, and former colleagues derisively question his sanity and competence.

What Sugiura did was to agree to test amygdalin (laetrile) in spontaneous animal tumors in the fall of 1972. In previous months, at the explicit request of the head of the President's Cancer Panel, Benno Schmidt, Sloan-Kettering had undertaken extensive tests of laetrile in transplantable tumor systems. The chemical failed to have any effects at all, thereby confirming all the statements and predictions made by orthodoxy about this "quack" remedy over a twenty-five-year period (*Science*, December 7, 1973).

But some scientists felt that transplantable tumors were not really similar to those that afflict the human cancer victim. What was needed was a more natural, spontaneous cancer that would simulate the clinical situation. Sloan-Kettering therefore obtained mice with spontaneous breast cancers from Dr. Daniel Martin of the Catholic Medical Center and gave them to its most experienced experimenter, Sugiura, for the testing of laetrile.

"Laetrile can't work on transplantable tumors," Dr. Sugiura said in 1974, in the course of a taped interview the author planned for the employee newspaper, MSKCC *Center News* (Sugiura, 1974).

"When I use it on a large spontaneous mammary tumor like this"—he made a circle with his thumb and forefinger about the size of a dime—"it has no effect. But a small tumor like *this*"—he made a tiny circle—"about one centimeter in diameter, laetrile stops the growth. Not permanently, but for a week, two weeks, three weeks. . . ."

"The most interesting part is metastases." (Metastases are secondary growths that migrate from the primary tumor and invade other areas of the body. Such secondary growths are often more lethal than the original tumor.) "When this mammary tumor grows to about two centimeters in diameter or more, about 80 percent develop lung metastases. But with treatment with amygdalin, it's cut down to about 20 percent" (ibid.).

"With all these positive results, why is there all this controversy?" Sugiura was asked during the interview.

"Many people still doubt my work, and so I show them all my work in this book—you see," and Sugiura took down from the shelf above him a volume, one in a long, uniform set of laboratory books, going back decades. "I keep records like this," he said, thumbing through the pages. "Here, amygdalin—"

The emeritus scientist pointed to pictures of small mice, each with an irregular circle on its breast—the outline of a tumor. The pictures were made with a rubber stamp Sugiura had used for over forty years. He used the stamped outline of a mouse and drew in not only the size of a tumor but its location on the body, in the belief that the location of the tumor might influence the curative ability of the drug in question.

In addition, Sugiura said, the laetrile-treated mice definitely seemed healthier and friskier than the saline-treated control mice. These results seemed remarkably similar to the reports of tumor growth inhibition and pain relief then filtering across the border from Tijuana, Mexico. Sugiura was therefore asked what he thought of these anecdotal reports.

"I think there must be some benefit. Dr. Old believes it," Sugiura added quickly. Dr. Lloyd J. Old was, with Stock, one of the two vice presidents of Sloan-Kettering Institute. "I think most people in this institution don't believe my work, although I show them results like this" (ibid.). Sugiura laughed sadly.

The senior researcher was asked if he had published any of these results.

"No, not yet." He hesitated, then said, "I'd like to, but it's up to the people downtown." (In Walker Laboratory parlance, "downtown" meant SKI headquarters in Manhattan.) "Dr. Old, Dr. Stock, if they want to publish it, they'll publish it." It would never have occurred to Sugiura to publish the results independently.

"Are you still doing work on amygdalin?" he was next asked.

"Oh yes, I'm now doing work on prevention. In the first experiments [i.e., the first six treatment experiments] the mice already had tumors, see? But in the latest experiment the mice have no tumors. At four months old, with no tumors, I started to inject amygdalin to see whether or not mammary cancer develops. These are strains of mice that are sure to get cancer in about 80 to 85 percent of the cases, during a lifetime of from two to two and a half years. Now it's eighteen months and we've gone through three-quarters of their life span, and I have found that the controls, receiving only saline injections, developed cancer in fifteen out of thirty cases. But the experimental animals, receiving laetrile, have developed only six tumors out of thirty mice, or about 20 percent.

"It would be interesting if it prevented it completely," Sugiura said, in a massive understatement. "One hundred percent prevention would be very interesting—then it would convince everybody. I never heard of anybody trying to repeat my experiment," he added. "Somebody should repeat my work," Sugiura said emphatically. "Not from this institution, somewhere else, a different institution."

Sugiura then drew a parallel between his own difficulties and those of William B. Coley, whom he had known at the old Memorial Hospital for twenty years.

"Nowadays, natural things are coming back more and more," Sugiura said. "Dr. Coley was working before 1900 with toxins prepared from bacteria. Doctors used to laugh at Coley as 'nonsense.' Now it's no longer nonsense. Bacterial toxins contain polysaccharides, which inhibit the growth of tumors in animals. Japanese scientists are finding that polysaccharides prepared from mushrooms can destroy tumors in mice.

"Amygdalin, too—people now are laughing at that, especially the director of the National Cancer Institute [Frank Rauscher] and the American Cancer Society. They even wrote a book, *Unproven Methods of Cancer Management*, with chapters on Coley's toxins, laetrile, and so forth."

"Why are they so much against it?" Sugiura was asked.

"I don't know. Maybe the medical profession doesn't like it because they are making too much money" (ibid.).

Although Sugiura's experiments were unpublished, they were no secret to the leaders of Memorial Sloan-Kettering Cancer Center. The elderly scientist had first achieved positive results with the apricot-kernel extract in the fall of 1972. In the summer of 1973 these results were leaked from Sloan-Kettering itself and used in a court case on behalf of Dr. John Richardson, then accused of violating the California antiquackery statutes (*Science*, December 7, 1973).

The positive results had been reported by Harry Nelson of the *Los Angeles Times* and Barbara Culliton of *Science* magazine. In the latter piece, Dr. Good had expressed an open-minded attitude toward the testing of all unorthodox methods, including laetrile.

Following the leak, the MSKCC Public Affairs Department had drawn up a cautious official statement for distribution:

> The Sugiura report is preliminary and part of a broad ongoing scientific inquiry. It would be premature at this time to draw specific conclusions on the basis of the Sugiura report (MSKCC, 1973).

Nevertheless, the attitude of MSKCC leaders toward laetrile and its advocates was definitely open and inquisitive. In November 1973 the Institute sent Lloyd Schloen, Ph.D., a young biochemist then working on laetrile under the direction of Dr. Lloyd Old, to the International Medical Society for Blood and Tumorous Disease Congress in Baden-Baden, West Germany, to report on the positive laetrile findings. Cancer researchers from more than fifteen countries were present (*Madison* [Wisc.] *Capital Times*, November 3, 1973).

About six hundred health professionals listened as Schloen detailed Sloan-Kettering's success with laetrile. Characteristic of the relaxed atmosphere then prevailing, Schloen was accompanied by Dean Burk and Raymond Brown, M.D., an aide to SKI vice president Old. Both men were considered advocates of unorthodox methods.

Schloen's statement to the congress, however, was a watered-down version of his original text. "Every hour on the hour [Schloen] was getting telephone calls from Sloan-Kettering to keep taking this out and that out," Burk recalled. "There wasn't too much left when he got through" (Burk, 1977).

Despite this, enthusiasm for laetrile seemed to mount throughout 1973 and 1974. A Laetrile Task Force was created at SKI, and prominent members of the unorthodox community were welcomed on the thirteenth floor of the Howard Building—SKI headquarters. The minutes of one "meeting on amygdalin" (July 10, 1973) shows the following individuals in attendance: Dr. Old; Dr. Brown, New York Cancer Research Institute Fellow; Dr. Burk; Dr. Ernesto Contreras, the prominent Mexican laetrilist; Dr. Contreras's son; Dr. Raymond Ewell, a retired University of Buffalo professor interested in unorthodox approaches; Dr. Good; Dr. Vincent F. Lisanti of the Council for Tobacco Research; Mr. Andrew McNaughton, sponsor of the laetrile movement; Mrs. Helen Coley Nauts; Dr. Morton K. Schwartz, a MSKCC biochemist; and Dr. C. Chester Stock. Dr. Old, the new vice president, chaired the meeting and was believed to be the driving spirit behind this unprecedented reconciliation effort (Sloan-Kettering Institute, 1973).

Yet many at Sloan-Kettering were disturbed at Old's apparent drift toward unorthodoxy. "Had Good chosen Andrew Ivy, promoter of the discredited cancer drug Krebiozen, as his deputy, the reaction of some members [of SKI] could not have been more categorically negative," said a former MSKCC official (Hixson, 1976a).

Simultaneously, advocates of other unorthodox approaches, such as Virginia Livingston, Eleanor Alexander-Jackson, Joseph Gold, and Hans Nieper, were also invited to Sloan-Kettering. The "Vatican of cancer research" also sent an observer to the convention of the International Association of Cancer Victims and Friends, a pro-laetrile organization (Schloen, 1973).

This détente with the unorthodox was a highly unstable affair from the beginning. It had no wide base of support at Sloan-Kettering, for relatively few scientists and staff members were invited to these meetings on the thirteenth floor of the Howard Building. Of those invited, some were disinterested or downright hostile, including those most closely tied to the current methods of treating cancer, such as the chemotherapists.

The main support for the new policy seems to have come from a few top administrators, especially Robert Good and his deputy, Lloyd Old. Not surprisingly, within about a year, the new policy had collapsed. The would-be innovators were back in the fold, condemning methods they once had greeted enthusiastically.

In retrospect, this change appears to have been the result of powerful economic and political forces that tended to discourage serious investigation of unorthodox approaches. At the time, however, a single incident triggered a retrenchment on the part of Sloan-Kettering's more innovative leadership.

In April 1974 the world was shocked by a scientific scandal at Sloan-Kettering Institute. Known as the "Summerlin painted-mouse affair," this bizarre story of cheating in high places raised serious questions about the conduct of cancer research in general and about Sloan-Kettering's behavior in particular.

William Summerlin was a thirty-five-year-old dermatologist with a promising future. A protégé of the recently appointed president Dr. Good, Summerlin had been brought in as a full member and made head of a clinical department at adjacent Memorial Hospital (Hixson, 1976a).

Most researchers spent decades working their way up the ladder until they became full members (the equivalent of professor). Dr. Sugiura, for example, had been at MSKCC forty years before attaining this honor. Summerlin's instant success stirred resentment at the Institute.

Dr. Summerlin's éclat was due to a novel application of a technique known as tissue culturing. Using this technique, the young doctor claimed to be able to take skin, or other tissues, from one person and make them "stick" to another person. He backed up his claims with dramatic animal work: white mice which showed dark blotches of black skin, from unrelated other mice, on their backs.

Generally, skin from one animal will not make a permanent graft to another animal. After a temporary attachment it becomes inflamed, ulcerates, and falls off. This is because the immune system of the receiver recognizes the new skin as foreign and rejects it. (The main exceptions to this rule are identical twins in humans and inbred strains in mice.)

By tissue culturing—first soaking pieces of skin in a special bath—Summerlin claimed to be able to make these transplants take perfectly.

The implications of this work were revolutionary. Organ transplants can be often difficult and precarious, since the recipient's immune system will often reject the new organ as foreign in short order. To prevent this, the patient is given drugs to suppress the immune system. But these drugs have many drawbacks, one of which is heightening a patient's susceptibility to cancer. If Summerlin's technique were valid, organ transplants might have become relatively common and easy. Cancer patients, for example, whose disease had not spread beyond a single organ, could receive a suitable replacement—provided that replacement had first been soaked for a while in Summerlin's magic fluid. Burn victims would also be major beneficiaries of the new technique.

The Summerlin technique also had major theoretical importance. Cancer, after all, is a kind of foreign tissue in the body. If Summerlin had figured out what made the body accept a new piece of skin as its own, perhaps others could figure out why the body of a cancer patient accepts his tumor. Clearly, then, Summerlin had a big idea.

For Summerlin himself these ideas and claims had already taken him farther than most thirty-five-year-olds ever dream of getting: to a top post at a world-famous private research center.

Other scientists were watching Summerlin's ideas with great interest. Surgeons, for example, would benefit enormously by these new techniques. In fact, the entire medical world was buzzing with news of the imminent breakthrough at Sloan-Kettering.

But, above all, Dr. Good was at Summerlin's side, directing him, encouraging him, coauthoring his papers. Good had been brought in by the MSKCC trustees to make such breakthroughs and firmly reestablish SKI as *the* leading cancer research center, a position in jeopardy because of the government's recent largesse to other institutions. What better way to prove his worth than with this startling finding? It was no secret, either, that Good was hoping for a Nobel Prize in medicine. He had made several important discoveries in the field of immunology, but none of them seemed to warrant the prize. Sponsorship of Summerlin's work would have been a crowning achievement for the Minnesota pediatrician.

In 1973–74, at the same time that Lloyd Old was advocating the testing of unproven therapies, Good was trumpeting Summerlin's work. About this work *Time* magazine wrote, in a cover story on the director, "No one appreciates [its] potential more than Good, . . ." who predicted that, as part of immunology, "it will enable us to understand the basic processes of life" (March 19, 1973).

In the middle of 1973, however, scientists began to write to Summerlin and Good that they could not reproduce the young dermatologist's techniques or results. Yet no one made these doubts public. Dr. Peter Medawar, a member of the SKI Board of Scientific Consultants, and a Nobel Prize winner, later explained why *he* had not said anything to contradict Summerlin, despite strong doubts at the time:

> I simply lacked the moral courage to say at the time that I thought we were the victims of a hoax or a confidence trick. It is easy in theory to say these things, but in practice very şenior scientists do not like trampling on their juniors in public (*New York Review of Books,* April 15, 1976).

Medawar certainly deserves credit for his honesty in admitting this. Nevertheless, it is quite revealing of the way frauds and cover-ups can be perpetrated in high places.

Good now put pressure on Summerlin to reproduce his famous results. This Summerlin could not do—perhaps because they were faked from the start, or perhaps because they were simply a one-time fluke that he didn't know how to repeat.

The showdown came on the morning of March 26, 1974. In the elevator of the Howard Building, on his way to Good's office, Summerlin quickly painted black splotches on two white mice with a felt-tip pen. The touch-up job escaped Good's notice. But an astute animal handler noticed the unusual patches while he was taking the mice back to their cages. Using a little alcohol, he removed the ink markings and immediately notified several young doctors working with Summerlin (Hixson, 1976a).

These doctors then went to Good and told him of the fakery. Good in turn informed Lewis Thomas, president of the Center. The recently appointed public-affairs director, T. Gerald Delaney, was also brought in on the secret.

Suddenly Summerlin's spectacular breakthrough had become a major problem for the new administration. Instead of confronting the issue head-on, however, the administration sat on the story for weeks.

"No written word about the trouble circulated within or outside the institution," wrote Joseph Hixson in his 1976 book on the scandal, *The Patchwork Mouse.* Delaney was simply given a short statement to read to the press "in case there was a leak."

As long as there was no leak, however, the administration said nothing, and there is no indication they ever intended to say anything to the public unless they were forced to do so. Finally, almost three weeks later, somebody tipped off the *New York Post*'s science reporter, Barbara Yunker, who broke the story (ibid.).

A peer review committee was appointed by Good, made up of five long-time members of the Institute: Drs. Stock, Burchenal, Clarkson, Sonenberg, and Boyse. This committee issued a lengthy report, which gave a detailed history of the facts of the case seen from the administration's point of view.

The committee concluded, basically, that Summerlin was entirely to blame for the incident: "In several instances Dr. Summerlin did indeed grossly mislead his colleagues" (ibid.). They attributed Summerlin's fraud to such things as his personal "disarray," the "desultory conduct of his everyday affairs," and other aberrations. After lengthy consultations with lawyers, Summerlin was declared to be mentally unbalanced. He was dismissed but given $40,000 severance pay (one year's salary) and told to see a psychiatrist (ibid.).

Summerlin is currently a practicing dermatologist in the South. Like former President Richard Nixon, he had "suffered enough" and never faced any charges from the medical society or the state. The peer review committee also exonerated Good of any guilt, although his name was on the fraudulent papers and shortly before Summerlin's downfall he had presented the young dermatologist's work at a scientific soirée thrown by the American Cancer Society's Mary Lasker (ibid.:106).

The only criticism of Good was for "prematurely" promoting the young researcher to full membership and for "undue publicity surrounding Dr. Summerlin's claims, unsupported as they were by adequate authenticated data." This criticism focused on individuals but sidestepped the significance of such fraud for the war on cancer, which was just then attempting to get into stride.

Prominent scientists noted at the time, however, that "the episode reflected dangerous trends in current efforts to gain scientific acclaim and funds for research, as well as the possible misdirection of research at Sloan-Kettering itself" (*New York Times*, April 17, 1974). It followed by only a year the Zinder Report, which had discovered evidence of financial irregularities in the government's virus program (see chapter 1).

Science magazine pointed out that "Sloan-Kettering, these days, is not a happy place. It is rich and getting richer, but not happy. . . . It appears that a high-pressure environment that drives individuals to exaggeration and fosters hostility is not ideal for the kind of achievements in research that Good, like everyone else, would like to see" (May 10, 1974).

Summerlin himself later alleged there was a "pressure-cooker atmosphere" at SKI. He blamed his problems on the "frenetic situation" at the Institute and especially on the "extreme pressure put on me by the Institute director to publicize information . . ." (Hixson, 1976a:101).

The Summerlin affair was a major embarrassment for Sloan-Kettering, and especially for its new director. It put a damper on the enthusiasm for new research and reestablished the position of the conservatives who had viewed Dr. Old's ascent to vice-presidency with trepidation. Laetrile testing thus got caught up in the Summerlin backlash. Good, who had said "we will test anything," became susceptible to pressure from outside and within to bring this open-minded policy to an end.

The evidence for such pressure is not merely anecdotal. In the course of researching a story on the unorthodox German Janker Clinic, Pat McGrady, Jr., son of the former ACS official, happened upon a revealing letter in the files on unproven methods at the American Cancer Society's headquarters. Before he could be stopped, he had copied the text and later reprinted it in a leading magazine. Written in January 1974 by ACS executive vice president Arthur Holleb (a former Memorial Hospital breast surgeon) to Good, it appears to be an attempt to bring Sloan-Kettering under ACS's umbrella, at least on the question of the unproven methods:

> I wish I knew how one could better control the unfortunate and premature publicity which links my distinguished alma mater to the promotional side of these unproven methods. We have both agreed that the public will be best served if tests are properly conducted in a prestigious institution, but the exploitation of the good name of the Sloan-Kettering Institute is becoming embarrassing. Perhaps your staff would be willing to consult with us and review our files before commitments are made (cited in McGrady, Jr., 1976).

There is no open threat here. Nevertheless, it could not have failed to escape Good's notice that ACS contributed almost $1 million a year to Sloan-Kettering at a time when MSKCC itself was suffering from what officials called a "disquieting deficit of $5 million" due to "expansion of research programs for which funding was simply not available" (MSKCC *Center News,* January, 1975).

On January 10, 1974, Dr. Good declared that "at this moment there is no evidence that laetrile has any effect on cancer." Most of Sugiura's highly positive results were already in the files, however. Shortly afterward, Dr. Holleb of the American Cancer Society told reporters at the ACS Science Writers' Seminar that "subsequent tests could not confirm the initial results" of Sugiura. The story was carried nationwide with such headlines as "Cancer 'Drug' Called Worthless" (*New York Daily News,* March 25, 1974).

Other establishment leaders also stepped up the attack on laetrile, completely ignoring the positive SKI data. "Every study to date has not found any evidence of efficacy" with laetrile, Dr. Alexander M. Schmidt, then commissioner of the FDA, told reporters on March 25, 1974. "If there was one shred of evidence from animal or cell systems I would issue an IND," that is, permission to test the substance in humans (Burk, 1974b).

A week later, Frank Rauscher, Ph.D., then director of the National Cancer Institute, said on the *60 Minutes* television show, "I would certainly not turn off laetrile if it had an iota of activity that we could pinpoint. Unfortunately, there's no evidence at all" (ibid.).

Dr. Jesse L. Steinfeld, former Surgeon General and an anti-laetrilist since the early 1950s, said, "There is no basis for the use of laetrile in man based on data derived from experiments in animals" (ibid.).

And Dr. Charles Moertel of the Mayo Clinic said, "Extensive animal tumor studies conducted independently at two outstanding cancer research centers—New York Memorial Sloan-Kettering and the Southern Research Institute—have shown this drug to be totally without evidence of anticancer activity" (ibid.).

How could Sloan-Kettering's leaders allow other prominent members of the establishment to so distort its own research findings? And how did these leaders get the idea that laetrile had, in fact, been proven ineffective? Was it the result of Dr. Good's January 10 statement, cited above?

No clear answers have emerged to these puzzling questions. One possibility, however, is that these statements coincided with MSKCC's difficulties with the Summerlin affair. Perhaps the New York leaders were unable to defend themselves at this critical juncture, and therefore the misleading or uninformed statements slipped by unchallenged.

In an apparent effort to set the record straight, however, a meeting was held at the Food and Drug Administration headquarters in Beltsville, Maryland, on July 2, 1974. According to the minutes of that meeting (obtained under the Freedom of Information Act by Representative John Kelsey of the Michigan House of Representatives), Sloan-Kettering leaders still maintained their belief in laetrile's effectiveness, as shown by Sugiura's studies (FDA, 1974).

The top leaders of MSKCC were present—Good, Old, Stock, and Lewis Thomas. In addition, a dozen other establishment leaders from the FDA and NCI were in attendance.

Dr. Good emphasized that "studies on amygdalin are a *small* part of Sloan-Kettering's program" (emphasis in original), no doubt to correct the opposite impression circulating among the doyens of orthodoxy. Lloyd Old then presented the case for laetrile. He recounted his search for clinicians who had actually used the substance. According to the minutes:

> Dr. Old has written to several world users of laetrile, including Drs. Contreras and Niepes [Nieper] and others. He found two groups: (1) Those who used it and found it of value [e.g., Contreras] and (2) Those who had *not* used it and did not believe in it (ibid.).

Old confirmed Sloan-Kettering's belief that laetrile had no effect on transplantable tumors but presented data, complete with accompanying charts, from Sugiura's studies to show that laetrile "inhibited metastases to the lung."

He even implied that laetrile might be useful against other chronic diseases:

> It was mentioned that amygdalin may be useful in sickle-cell anemia because of thiocyanate levels. The Sloan-Kettering group believe their results show that amygdalin used in animals with tumors show: a decrease in lung metastases; slower tumor growth; and pain relief. The Sloan-Kettering group are thinking of a study in man on pain relief (ibid.).*

After this buildup for amygdalin at the FDA meeting, it is rather curious to read:

> Sloan-Kettering is not enthusiastic about studying amygdalin but would like to study CN [cyanide] releasing drugs (ibid.).

Such drugs could be patented and marketed in conventional channels and would have the additional advantage of unequivocally coming under the jurisdiction of the FDA, a point that would hardly need emphasizing in that company. Laetrilists had in fact postulated exactly such a scenario, in which laetrile's name and chemical structure would be modified by Sloan-Kettering in order to make it more acceptable to market forces (Griffin, 1975:464).

At the conclusion of the FDA meeting, everything seemed encourag-

---

*The idea of laetrile as possibly useful in sickle-cell anemia was first proposed by Robert Houston in 1973, based on a hypothesis of Ernst T. Krebs, Jr. (Houston, 1974).

ing. The final proposals indicated that the meeting and the presentation had been a success for SKI's leaders:

> A discussion ensued on where we should go from here. Agreements: (a) Sloan-Kettering Institute and NCI will consider clinical trials aimed at treatment of cancer and for the relief of pain and will request consultation with ACS; (b) There are no regulatory policy problems preventing the study of amygdalin in man; (c) A standard scientific approach to studying amygdalin is recommended, meaning the drug should be worked up by standard approaches; (d) FDA will publicly endorse good research on amygdalin as in the public interest (FDA, 1974).

None of these proposals was carried through at the time. It was to be four years before a new director of NCI called for clinical trials aimed at treatment of cancer and for the relief of pain. The FDA never came out for good research on amygdalin; on the contrary, it maintained its stand that laetrile had been adequately tested and found without an iota of value. Nor did the FDA declare publicly that there were no regulatory policy problems preventing the study of amygdalin in man. On the contrary, it maintained that such studies would be unethical.

How were these excellent proposals sabotaged, and by whom? There is a gap in our information here: we just do not know.

During the remainder of 1974 and 1975, in fact, the controversy only heightened. Sugiura continued to get positive results, this time adding the AKR system to his growing list of experiments. In these mice, doomed to die of leukemia, he saw a decided shrinkage of the swollen internal organs, the spleen, thymus, and the lymph nodes. This is normally taken as a sign of anticancer effects by cancer researchers (Kassel et al., 1977).

In preliminary tests, other SKI researchers had also gotten highly positive results with laetrile. Dr. Lloyd Scholen, the same man whom SKI had sent as its spokesperson to Baden-Baden, had reproduced Sugiura's results in Swiss albino mice. All the mice receiving the highest dose of amygdalin were healthy at the time of "sacrifice" (death); all those receiving lower doses, or only a saline injection, were sick. In addition, in one small experiment combining laetrile and an enzyme (after the manner of Hans Nieper, whom Scholen had visited in Germany), the young researcher got 100 percent cures. Dr. Elizabeth Stockert, another SKI researcher, got 25 percent cures in the same way (Second Opinion, 1977).

Stockert, however, entered the lists *against* Sugiura in March 1975 when she failed to confirm his experiments with the CD_8F_1 mice. Sugiura felt that she was unable to do so because she had failed to follow the protocols of his experiments. In particular, Sugiura always used a microscope to examine the mice's lungs and considered microscopic evaluation the sine qua non of all such research. Stockert chose not to use a microscope at all and relied instead on gross visual observations (ibid.).

Another problem—at least early in the year—was the inability of another SKI researcher to duplicate Sugiura's work. This researcher was Walker veterinarian Franz Schmid, Sugiura's son-in-law, who also worked under C. Chester Stock. In his first test, Schmid also did not use the microscope and was not able to confirm Sugiura's results. In this experiment, however, the treated mice lived somewhat longer than the controls.

In Schmid's second experiment, he used a dose that was one-fiftieth of Sugiura's. This dosage had been suggested by Dr. Stock, who felt that it was more analogous to the amounts being received by humans in the laetrile clinics. Again, there was no positive effect on metastases, according to Schmid's "eyeball" observations, but the laetrile-treated mice lived 50 percent longer. Nevertheless, the experiment was interpreted as a failure for laetrile, and no one outside the Institute knew that the treated mice had lived longer until a reporter extracted the information from Dr. Stock more than a year later. Nor was it generally known that Schmid had used a fractional dose (ibid.).

Far more serious a challenge to laetrile was presented by the appearance of Dr. Daniel S. Martin of the Catholic Medical Center, Queens, New York. Martin had supplied the mice for the early Sugiura experiments and had taken part in the first collaborative experiment, which ended inconclusively.

In 1974 Martin had performed his own experiment with laetrile, which he claimed had disproven Sugiura's contention. A study of this 1974 experiment showed that he changed a number of elements in Sugiura's original protocol (ibid.). Despite these changes, Martin publicly proclaimed he had evidence that Sugiura was wrong.

Late in 1974 Sugiura traveled to Queens to take part in another collaborative test with Martin. Martin declared the experiment further proof that laetrile did not work. On the other hand, Sugiura pointed out that, *even by visual examination,* there were twice as many metastases in the animals which did not receive laetrile as in those that did.

The issue might have been settled by recourse to a microscope—the most common way of determining whether or not secondary growths are present. But Martin did not believe in using the microscope to make such determinations. He relied on a relatively less common test called a "bioassay."* By this bioassay test, Martin claimed there was no difference between the treated and the control animals.

One could hardly imagine a greater contrast than that which existed between these two scientists, Sugiura and Martin. Sugiura, who died on October 22, 1979, at the age of eighty-seven, was modest and deferential, a retiring scholar content to perform his humdrum tasks day in and day out for over sixty years. Martin, chairman of the Committee on Unorthodox Therapies of the American Society of Clinical Oncology, was outspoken and assertive. While Sugiura talked in hushed tones to his friends and colleagues, Martin blared his opposition to the world at scientific meetings, on the Op-Ed page of the *New York Times,* and in public debates.

"I flatfootedly and categorically tell you," Martin once said, "that laetrile is without activity against spontaneous tumors in mice—period" (*Medical World News,* October 26, 1975). "Laetrile has been found absolutely devoid of activity, period. It's just that simple" (MSKCC, 1977c). When *Science* magazine asked him if the Sloan-Kettering tests weren't addressed to scientists, he replied, "Oh, nonsense. Of course this was done to help people like [Benno] Schmidt and congressmen answer the laetrilists" (*Science,* December 23, 1977). Benno Schmidt is an investment banker who served as vice-chairman of Memorial Sloan-Kettering Cancer Center and head of the President's Cancer Panel.

Despite Martin's outspoken opposition, by 1975 Lloyd Old and others were back at work trying to push quietly forward with a clinical trial of laetrile. Two Mexican oncologists, Dr. Mario Soto de Leon and a colleague, went to SKI and arranged for the Institute to collaborate in a clinical trial of laetrile on Mexican government workers with cancer.

Old wrote Soto on January 24, 1975:

> It was indeed a pleasure to have you and Dr. Sanen visit our Institute and share with us your clinical experience with amygdalin in cancer patients. I was pleased to hear from Dr. Sanen that our proposed collaborative controlled trials have the approval of your hospital. We are looking forward to a fruitful exchange of information (Committee for Freedom of Choice, 1975).

No such trials took place. Again, it is not clear who or what aborted this plan. However, the schism within orthodoxy was clearly growing. On

---

*In the bioassay, as was used by Martin, "all the lungs of each animal are shredded (by scissors) and injected subcutaneously into two male CD_8F_1 mice. . . . If a tumor subsequently arises at an injection site, it indicates that cancer cells (at least 10^5 cells) were present in the lungs" (Second Opinion, 1977).

March 4, 1975, another meeting was called, this one at the National Cancer Institute's headquarters in Bethesda, Maryland, "to decide on what further course of action should be undertaken with this controversial compound" (Stephen Carter, 1975).

Thirty-two top cancer establishment figures were present, including the director of the National Cancer Institute and eighteen of his assistants, six top leaders of MSKCC—this time including a surgeon and a chemotherapist—and officials of the FDA, the ACS, and the Mayo Clinic. Finally, there was Dr. Martin.

Once again, and for the last time as it turned out, Sloan-Kettering's leaders defended Sugiura's work. Lloyd Old summarized Sloan-Kettering's results:

(1) No tumor regression was observed.
(2) There is a variable slowing of primary tumor growth.
(3) There is a decrease in the incidence of pulmonary toxicity [i.e., metastases] from roughly 80% to 20%.
(4) There is no evidence of toxicity (Stephen Carter, 1975).

This time, however, unlike at the FDA meeting in the previous year, the opposition had found its voice. "Dr. Daniel Martin, of the Catholic Medical Center in Queens, New York then briefly summarized his results in the CD_8F_1 mouse system. . . . He has performed two experiments with Mexican amygdalin. . . . Both experiments were completely negative" (ibid.).

Sloan-Kettering officials contradicted this claim, calling Martin's results "limited data" and saying that only one of his experiments duplicated Sugiura's methods.

Dr. Old responded by citing the human, clinical data provided him by Soto and his colleague on their visit. "With one exclusion, there was a 46.6 percent objective response rate, with an objective response rate defined as a [greater than] 40 percent tumor shrinkage" (ibid.).

The Sloan-Kettering spokesman said that Soto was "going to undertake a trial of amygdalin in his hospital and would like to have help in the protocol design, if possible, and would welcome observation. Dr. Old felt that this was an opportunity to have a clinical trial of this compound undertaken, which might give us some believable data" (ibid.).

A "prolonged discussion" ensued in which two sharply divided sides emerged. One side, representing the views of SKI's top leadership, held that "the nontoxic nature of amygdalin made it a superb candidate for a double-blind evaluation" (and it should be noted that it was taken for granted in all these discussions that laetrile *is* nontoxic). It said that "the preclinical data are not that critical since the drug is being extensively used" (ibid.).

The anti-laetrile side countered that ". . . the preclinical data, only, clearly do not support a clinical trial being undertaken . . . there are no convincing clinical data to date [and] undertaken, a clinical trial in the U.S. would be fraught with many consequences on many levels." Unfortunately, the notes do not tell what those consequences would be.

After three hours of debate, the final consensus decision was to send a group of American cancer specialists to Mexico to help set up Dr. Soto's clinical trial there "and observe the results of any trial undertaken." Three doctors volunteered to participate in this study: Dr. Stephen Carter of NCI, Dr.Charles Moertel of the Mayo Clinic, and Dr. Irwin Krakoff, then of SKI (ibid.).

A trial in Mexico offered many advantages and was an excellent way out of the dilemma. Principally, a Mexican trial would not have to be approved by the U.S. FDA, but if the test were supervised by three prestigious American doctors, positive results would certainly clear the way for a U.S. trial.

Again, however, this compromise plan was aborted. Sloan-Kettering wrote to Soto and Sanen and informed the Mexican doctors that the proposed collaborative trial was off.

This was followed by a dramatic turnabout on the part of the top MSKCC leadership. On April 2, 1975, Lewis Thomas told reporters at the ACS Science Writers' Seminar that two years of testing laetrile had demonstrated:

> No protective effects against cancer.
> Failure to provide any prolongation of life.
> An inability to reduce the size of a tumor.
> Failure to inhibit the growth of a tumor (*San Diego Evening Tribune*, April 2, 1975).

The story was circulated nationwide by the American Cancer Society's public information department.

One month later the *New York Times* carried a front-page story, "Coast Ring Smuggles Banned Cancer Drugs" (May 26, 1975). It told how an assistant U.S. attorney was preparing grand jury indictments against the top leaders of the laetrile movement, including some of those (such as Krebs, Jr., McNaughton, and Contreras) who had been respectfully received at Sloan-Kettering not long before. Now they were accused of masterminding "an international smuggling operation" comparable, said the government official, to the Mexican brown heroin traffic.

Justification for the prosecution, said the *Times,* came from no less an authority than Memorial Sloan-Kettering and its respected president:

> Dr. Lewis Thomas, president of Sloan-Kettering [sic], reported April 2nd while in San Diego, that the institute's study showed that laetrile had absolutely no value either in combatting cancer, prolonging life or inhibiting tumor growth (ibid.).

In July, Sloan-Kettering leaders amplified their beliefs in another front-page story in the *Times.* Sugiura's extensive results were now called "spurious" and the result of "the vagaries of experimental variation" and "unfamiliarity with the animals used." The CD_8F_1 system was, indeed, a relatively new system. But Sugiura had used the Swiss albino mouse system, in which he also saw positive results, since World War II.

Not only did Sugiura disagree with this new judgment on his work, but he now claimed, in August, that the most recent results, with the AKR leukemia system, confirmed his earlier findings. "No compound affects AKR about the same as amygdalin," he said in a private conversation. "There's something there" (Sugiura, 1975).

Sugiura himself said nothing in public, however, to refute or challenge the remarks of his superiors. He maintained his attitude that it was "up to downtown" what they would do with his results. His job was only to conduct research, not get involved in controversy. He emphasized that in sixty years no one had ever found cause to contradict his work.

In early August, Dr. Stock was interviewed by *Medical World News,* and he amplified the Institute's new position. "We have found amygdalin negative in all the animal systems we have tested," he said (*Medical World News,* August 11, 1975).*

Because this and the previous statements seemed completely out of line with the reality of laetrile testing at SKI, a number of the Center's employees privately decided to take action to counter the misstatements. (The author was one of these employees.) After failing to obtain a retraction through the normal channels, copies of Sugiura's laboratory notes—photocopies obtained from Sugiura himself—were sent to a number of writers.

By September, these notes and other documents had been reprinted by

---

*Stock claims to have been misquoted by MWN's David Leff. "I'll never live down the misquote I should have corrected," he wrote in 1977, after his statement had become a matter of public controversy (Stock, 1977).

the Committee for Freedom of Choice in Cancer Therapy, Inc., a pro-laetrile group centered in California, under the title *Anatomy of a Cover-Up*
(Committee for Freedom of Choice, 1975).

David Leff of *Medical World News,* who also had received a set of
notes, was granted an interview with Sugiura; he was the first reporter who
questioned the elderly Japanese scientist at length on his laetrile experiments. Sugiura repeated his belief in the validity of his results (*Medical
World News,* October 6, 1975).

Before the leak, Memorial Sloan-Kettering officials had hoped to close
the book on laetrile, and especially laetrile testing in humans. "Clinical
trials?" Benno Schmidt, vice-chairman of MSKCC, had said in August.
"No way! There's no way, I believe, that they can convince the people at
Sloan-Kettering there's any basis for going further (*Medical World News,*
August 11, 1975.)

The leak may have convinced the administration to perform further
tests, since a new trial was now called for. "He [Sugiura] will have another
chance to check [his] belief, in a collaborative experiment with Dr. Schmid.
. . . This time the two men are working together, with Dr. Schmid random-
izing 15 controls and 16 experimental mice, Dr. Sugiura (who pioneered in
tumor-transplantation techniques) doing the injecting, and both evaluating
the grossly visible metastases. Results of this newest laetrile test are expected by late this year, depending on when the last animal dies" (*Medical
World News,* October 6, 1975).

This experiment differed from Schmid's previous ones in that the dosages given were the same as in Sugiura's experiments; the microscope was
utilized; and Sugiura did the actual injecting of the mice, on the theory that
results may be affected by the way in which the compound is given.

The results were a confirmation of Sugiura's work. According to
Schmid's observations, there were 80 percent metastases in the control animals and 44 percent in the treated. Sugiura found 100 percent metastases in
the controls and 38 percent in the treated. The Pathology Department of
Memorial Hospital found 80 percent in the controls and 31 percent in the
treated"—they show that the positive results were very unlikely to have
been due to chance (Stock et al., 1978).

"A dramatic reversal of Dr. Schmid's previous tests" was what reporter Mort Young of the *San Francisco Examiner* called this experiment in
a front-page story (November 12, 1975). Sugiura's enthusiasm dampened,
however, when Schmid refused all comment on the test, wouldn't talk to
reporters to confirm his findings, or even to people in the MSKCC Public
Affairs Department.

Sugiura was confused and disappointed by this; this situation was made even more difficult by the close family relationship between him and Schmid. "The cooperative experiment came out my way," Sugiura said some months later. "Schmid's data confirmed my original contention. I try my best. I report what I see" (Sugiura, 1976a).

Instead of interpreting these results as a confirmation of Sugiura, the administration scheduled yet another test, this one a "blind" experiment at Dr. Martin's Catholic Medical Center in Queens. Sugiura would not know which mice were receiving the laetrile and which were receiving only the saline solution. Only Dr. Martin would know which was which, and he would keep this secret from Dr. Sugiura.

In late November 1975 the plans for the blind test were made public. Apparently, though, Sugiura was told nothing about it, although he was the principal party concerned. "Maybe I'm supposed to do it," he said in mid-February 1976, "maybe somebody else. Nobody has told me anything" (ibid.). By May 1976 the plans for the blind test were finalized by Stock and Martin. The experiments were to be performed in Dr. Martin's laboratory, under his supervision. Sugiura would travel to Martin's facilities in Queens several times a week to observe the mice.

This first blind test ended in bitter controversy. Sugiura had traveled from Rye to Queens each week, as planned, and had weighed the mice, measured their tumors, and observed their lungs, whenever possible, for secondary tumors.

In addition, bioassays were performed on the lungs of the sacrificed animals (those killed just before their natural demise, to prevent decomposition of their bodies before measurements could be taken).

In July 1976 Sugiura said privately that he was generally happy with the way the experiment was progressing. There were seventy mice, divided into fourteen cages, five to a cage. Four weeks into the test, Sugiura surmised that the first seven cages housed control animals (receiving saline injections) while the second group of seven cages housed the laetrile-treated animals (Sugiura, 1976b).

"There are seven new tumors in the first group of thirty-five," he said, "and only one new tumor in the second group. About 50 percent of the small tumors in the second group stopped growing, but far fewer in the first group. Nine animals are still alive in the 'control' group," he added, "and fifteen are alive in the 'treated' group. There is also a difference in the number of metastases" (ibid.).

"Couldn't Dr. Martin have mixed some of the laetrile-treated mice in among the controls?" he was asked.

Sugiura answered that in his opinion there would be too much chance of a mix-up in this way, it would be too difficult for the technicians to function without confusing the treated with the untreated and ruining the experiment. They would probably have to be arranged with each cage housing either treated or controls and the simplest way would be to form two distinct large groups (ibid.).

Sugiura added that he had seen Dr. Martin only once since the start of the experiment. He had wanted to speak to him because an unusual number of animals were dying suddenly, apparently from faulty injection procedures.

"I cannot criticize him," Sugiura said. "He's the expert, I can't ask to see his mice or feel them. But a funny thing: a couple of times I performed a bioassay procedure, and only three or four days later, when I came back, a tumor had already developed—much less time than normally. Very strange!" (ibid.).

Sugiura wrote in his interim progress report to Stock and Old that the first thirty-five animals were the treated animals and the second thirty-five animals were the controls. Was he right?

On September 9 Sugiura was jubilant. "Last Friday, Dr. Stock told me that I picked the controls and the experimental *correctly*. The first seven cages are the control group and the second seven cages are the laetrile-treated group. I don't have to rewrite my progress report" (Sugiura, 1976c).

According to his tally, there were 70 percent metastases in the controls and 30 percent in the experimental, a significant difference in favor of laetrile (ibid.).

Soon after Sugiura filed this progress report, the SKI administration declared the experiment invalid as a blind test. "We've lost the blindness aspect of it," Dr. Stock told reporters (Moss, 1976). He told *Science* the experiment "went badly because of clumsy injection procedures" (*Science*, September 10, 1976).

Consequently, another blind experiment was scheduled, this one to take place at SKI itself.

At around this time, Second Opinion began publishing a bimonthly newsletter of the same name at the Center. Second Opinion was composed primarily of employees and former employees of MSKCC, who had begun meeting in the fall of 1975 to discuss problems at the Center, including what they perceived as a cover-up of the laetrile results.

The group had sent a number of letters to MSKCC administrators, asking them to release full details of the laetrile experiments and to publish Sugiura's results. To protect the anonymity of the MSKCC employees, only those Second Opinion members who had no affiliation with the Center signed these letters. The employees felt that they would be fired if they publicly voiced criticism of the administration.

The first issue of the newsletter *Second Opinion* (November 1976) contained the following characterization of the blind test:

> Although the test was "blind" Dr. Sugiura surmised which mice were being treated with laetrile and which were receiving the inert saline solution. . . . As soon as Dr. Sugiura correctly surmised which group was which, his SKI superior, Dr. Stock, declared the entire test invalid!

According to the official Sloan-Kettering report on laetrile, however, this account is wrong, because Dr. Martin, who controlled the experiment, says that the animals never were grouped into two distinct sets of thirty-five. Rather, he says, the cages were randomly alternated between control and treated animals.

A four-month investigation by Richard Smith of *The Sciences,* a publication of the New York Academy of Sciences, was unable to unearth any proof that Sugiura had in fact guessed correctly or that the cages had later had their designations altered (Smith, 1978).

The second blind test was no less controversial. From the start, in private conversation, Sugiura had objected to the way in which the mice were to be arranged in their cages. He expressed fear that since the treated and untreated animals were to be put in the same cages, the technicians might inadvertently give laetrile injections to the control animals and saline injections to the treated animals. This would completely destroy the validity of the experiment. Since the animals were distinguished only by punch marks in their ears, and such holes can be torn in the course of an experiment, he felt that such a possibility was not at all farfetched (Sugiura, 1976c).

This is precisely how the administration decided to perform the test, however. "They must be smarter than me," Sugiura said ironically (ibid.). Although on this occasion Sugiura was vocal about his dissatisfaction with the setup, Stock later claimed he knew nothing about the senior scientist's reservations. "Sugiura never expressed to me dissatisfaction with the experiment," Stock later wrote. "I heard of it after the results were in, and not in confirmation of his own experiments" (Stock, 1977).

The second blind test also did not come out in Sugiura's favor, according to the SKI administration. A memo from the director of public affairs on January 26, 1977, stated:

> Stock insists the results from the experiment do not confirm the earlier positive findings of Sugiura. He further states that he has not found encour-

agement in the data to take laetrile to clinical trial. . . . In general the results do not confirm Sugiura's earlier findings (Delaney, 1977a).

Sugiura was not only disappointed by these results but upset by what he saw as discrepancies in the data. "There's something funny here," he said. "The small tumors stopped growing 40 percent of the time in the saline control group and only 27 percent of the time in the treated group. We people in chemotherapy use saline solution because it does *not* affect tumor growth. Now this happens. They must not forget to mention that there was more stoppage in the controls than in the treated. I won't give in to this" (Sugiura, 1977a).

One possible explanation for the discrepancy, he suggested, was that the technician had inadvertently given some of the control mice amygdalin, thereby causing temporary tumor stoppages, one of the three antitumor effects Sugiura had seen in his previous laetrile experiments. Another possibility was that the control mice, which are coprophagous (feces-eating), had ingested some of the amygdalin-laden wastes of their treated cagemates (ibid.).

In MSKCC public affairs the professional staff was instructed to tell reporters who were carefully following the story that the second blind test had proven in general that the "results do not confirm Sugiura's earlier findings" without telling them that Sugiura himself thought the experiment flawed and invalid (Delaney, 1977a).

At a Monday morning public-affairs staff meeting, the author informed the director of public affairs that he could not give out that statement, since it failed to mention the inexplicable tumor stoppages in the control animals and since it did not mention Sugiura's own reservations about the outcome of the test.

T. Gerald Delaney, director of public affairs, replied that the author could put that in a memo to Dr. Stock, but that he would probably be fired for doing so. All the other staff members present then agreed to be cosigners to this memo. As the author prepared to write it, Delaney modified his stand and agreed to talk to Stock about these omissions.

On February 1, therefore, Delaney issued an amended statement for the press. It included a new sentence: "Dr. Stock also points out that Dr. Sugiura continues to believe in the validity of his earlier findings" (Delaney, 1977b). Sugiura told reporter Mort Young point-blank, "The tests were not done to my satisfaction."

Five years of testing had ended in controversy and confusion—not a pleasing outcome for the leaders of the world's most prestigious private cancer center. Nevertheless, about twenty positive experiments with laetrile

179

had been performed by three researchers: Sugiura, Schloen, and Schmid. Quite a few negative experiments had also been performed. In April 1977 Second Opinion issued an appraisal of the paths open to the Memorial Sloan-Kettering administration:

> If, on the one hand, they publish the truth about laetrile they will have to say something like this: we have been unable to reach any definitive con-clusion on this substance. Dr. Sugiura, one of the most experienced research-ers, has done many studies showing positive effects. Other researchers have claimed negative results. We think this issue can only be settled through a study on willing human volunteers with cancer, and we would like to conduct such a study here at Memorial.
>
> That would be honest, but it would also be disastrous from a fund-raising point of view, since it would bring down the wrath of the American Cancer Society, and the National Cancer Institute, from whom MSKCC receives most of its research funds, not to mention the Food and Drug Administration. . . .
>
> The other choice is to publish a totally one-sided report. . . . This is the most likely prospect at the moment, but it too will bring down wrath and exposure—from tens of thousands of individuals around the country.

Sloan-Kettering took the latter course. In mid-June 1977 the aforemen-tioned press conference was called and the public affairs office sent out a news release summarizing the ninety-page set of papers on the laetrile test-ing (reprinted in Zimmermann, 1977).

Despite Sugiura's "I stick!" the comments of all the other administra-tors were totally negative.

"We have no evidence that laetrile possesses *any* biological activity with respect to cancer, one way or the other," said Thomas (MSKCC, 1977c).

"We have found no reproducible evidence that amygdalin, or laetrile, is active," said Good (ibid.).

"Laetrile has been found absolutely devoid of activity, period. It's just that simple. It's all there in black and white if you take the trouble to read the paper," said Daniel Martin (ibid.). Meanwhile, MSKCC public affairs functionaries had been instructed by Delaney to stash copies of the paper itself behind a curtain in an adjoining room and give them out to reporters only if they explicitly asked for them. Only a handful did.

Laetrile's "failure" was carried on nationwide television that evening. Release of the report to the lay press, almost a year before its actual publi-cation in the *Journal of Surgical Oncology,* coincided with the debate then raging on laetrile legalization in New York State. The measure subsequently passed the legislature but was vetoed by Governor Hugh Carey.

It also came less than a month before Senator Edward Kennedy's hearings before the Subcommittee on Health and Scientific Research, "Banning of the Drug Laetrile from Interstate Commerce by FDA."

The Kennedy hearings were an unprecedented showdown between the pro-laetrile and the anti-laetrile forces after twenty-five years of skirmishes. It would have been embarrassing in the extreme if the pro-laetrile side had been able to present unpublished—apparently suppressed—documents from Sloan-Kettering showing that laetrile was indeed effective in some circumstances. This did not happen; Thomas came armed with a strongly worded anti-laetrile statement when he appeared before Senator Kennedy on July 12, 1977.

Thomas told the senators:

> There is not a particle of scientific evidence to suggest that laetrile possesses any anticancer properties at all. I am not aware of any scientific papers, published in any of the world's accredited journals of medical science, presenting data in support of the substance, although there are several papers, one of these recently made public by Sloan-Kettering Institute, reporting the complete absence of anticancer properties in a variety of experimental animals (U.S. Senate, 1977).

In his prepared statement Thomas did not cite the many studies conducted worldwide showing laetrile's anticancer effects, nor did he mention Sugiura's work. Under questioning by Senator Richard Schweiker (R.-Pa.), Thomas admitted that "it did seem in Dr. Sugiura's experiment [laetrile] would inhibit the number of metastatic lesions in the lung." He claimed, however, that the number of mice involved in these tests was small and that this observation was made only on "two or three occasions" (ibid.:19–21).

In the summer of 1977 a group of MSKCC employees, including members of Second Opinion, met to discuss the latest developments in the controversy. It was decided at this meeting to write a counterreport to the official laetrile papers. In studying the Sloan-Kettering papers, the Second Opinion investigators decided that there were numerous errors in the SKI version. To err is human, of course. But one characteristic of these errors was that, big or small, they always seemed to be made to the detriment of laetrile and of Dr. Sugiura.

One such error concerned the effect of various drugs on Dr. Martin's CD_8F_1 mouse. The SKI paper stated that the alleged failure of laetrile to stop the growth of cancer in these animals was highly significant, since other, conventional anticancer drugs were active against the tumors:

Of those eight agents declared clinically active against human breast cancer by the National Cancer Institute, all eight agents also are active against this murine breast cancer. . . . Thus, the negative laetrile findings in this animal tumor model appear particularly significant (cited in Second Opinion, 1977).

Apparently laetrile had failed where chemotherapy succeeded—an important charge, since the relative value of orthodox chemotherapy was also clearly at issue in the laetrile controversy. This point was emphasized a number of times at the June 15 press conference.

Research into scientific literature by the Second Opinion group during the summer of 1977 revealed that when chemotherapy was used in the same way as laetrile had been tested, it too was ineffective against the primary breast tumors. Proof of this came from Dr. Martin's own papers, written between 1970 and 1975, which concluded:

Cure has thus far been impossible to achieve by chemotherapy alone on large primary tumors. Hence, this most difficult methodology has been largely shelved. . . . (Martin et al., 1975).

Of the nineteen drugs and two immune-stimulating agents that had been "studied at length in the treatment of this tumor," all "proved to be quite resistant to influence by chemotherapy alone" and "ineffective in this spontaneous tumor system" (ibid.).

But this discarded method of testing drugs had been taken down from the shelf to test laetrile. When laetrile failed where other drugs had also failed, this was interpreted as "particularly significant."

The Second Opinion investigators also took issue with the manner in which SKI judged anticancer effects. According to the Second Opinion report:

In AKR leukemia, a recent publication by Robert Kassel [in a book edited by Robert A. Good] makes clear that while prolongation of life is the most certain sign of anticancer effects, it is very rare. Scientists therefore take a shrinkage of internal organs greater than 20 percent to be a sign of anticancer activity. While Sugiura saw such effects, and commented on them in memos, this is never mentioned in the text of the report.

Much was made at the SKI press conference about Martin's inability to reproduce Sugiura's results with lung metastases. Although it was admitted that Martin used a different method from Sugiura, the presentation maintained that Martin's method—bioassay—was superior to Sugiura's method—visual gross observation plus microscopic slides.

Second Opinion found that Martin's method had not been adopted by many researchers. According to references in *Citation Index*, a standard bibliographic tool, no group other than his own had published papers on experiments employing his bioassay method. Between January 1976 and February 1977 there were eight articles dealing with the question of metastases in rodents in the journal *Cancer Research*. All but one of these used the macrovisual and/or microscopic techniques favored by Sugiura. The one that didn't was by Martin and his group (Second Opinion, 1977:8–10).

These are technicalities, but it was on technicalities such as these that laetrile had been condemned as totally ineffective.

On November 18, 1977, Second Opinion called a press conference at the New York Hilton and released its forty-eight-page report. The author, who was part of the Second Opinion group from its inception, decided to make his criticisms public and associate himself with the report. He was fired on the next working day for failing "to properly discharge his most basic job responsibilities," according to an official MSKCC statement (MSKCC, 1977d).

Two days later, Second Opinion received a letter from Sugiura, who had been sent a copy of the report. The elderly scientist wrote:

> I read your paper in the Monograph [the report] with great interest. Your critical review of my positive results and negative results of three investigators at Sloan-Kettering Institute is very well done and accurate. Please accept my sincere congratulations (Sugiura, 1977b).

Others at Sloan-Kettering had a less positive evaluation of the report. At first the administration dismissed the charges as minor inconsistencies which an "irresponsible and malicious" group had "blown all out of proportion to their scientific significance" (MSKCC, 1977e).

The medical establishment realized it would have to take the charges more seriously when an article on the controversy appeared in *The Sciences* echoing the Second Opinion criticisms.

The president of the New York Academy of Sciences, which publishes *The Sciences*, stated that the "misinterpretation by Dr. Martin was not excusable" (*New York Times*, December 13, 1977). Concerning Martin's claim that other drugs could cure breast cancer in the CD_8F_1 mouse, Stock told the *New York Times*:

We accepted the statement from Dr. Martin as submitted. I did not check the original publications to be certain of the appropriateness of the statement. It should not have been used in the context of this report, and therefore it has been deleted (ibid.).

The final version of the SKI paper, as published in 1978 in the *Journal of Surgical Oncology,* contains an addendum by Daniel S. Martin, C. Chester Stock, and Robert A. Good.

While clearly meant to refute unnamed critics who questioned the erroneous statements, the addendum threw fuel on the fire by stating that "the finding that laetrile is devoid of anticancer activity is particularly pertinent" and "laetrile's lack of anticancer activity in the CD_8F_1 animal tumor model is particularly significant" (Stock et al., 1978).

However, until his death Sugiura continued to hold to his original belief:

> I still think my experimental results on the effect of amygdalin (with high doses) on spontaneous mammary tumors (adenocarcinomas) are correct—stoppage of growth of small tumors temporar[il]y; prevent the development of lung metastases 80 percent against 20 percent in control group (saline); delayed the development of spontaneous mammary cancers for three to four months (Sugiura; 1979).

In sticking by his own results, Sugiura is not unique in science. Experienced researchers, confident in their own abilities, often will hold out against a crowd of vociferous opponents—and often they will be vindicated in the end.

Nobel Prize–winner Sir Peter Medawar, who serves on Sloan-Kettering's Board of Scientific Consultants, has related a similar instance in his own career:

> Several people tried to repeat our work and failed. There were, however, always good reasons why they did so; either they had introduced into our techniques little "improvements" of their own, or they were too clumsy or something. These failures did not disturb us in the very least: we knew we were right—and we were—so we did our best to tell those who were struggling with our techniques how best to carry them out (*New York Review of Books,* April 15, 1976).

But Sloan-Kettering did not want to hear any more about Sugiura's laetrile experiments, nor did it want the public to hear. In 1979 reporters seeking to interview the elderly researcher were told by him: "I am not allowed to talk about laetrile" (Pressman, 1979). A few months later he was dead.

Thus ended the most extensive study ever carried out on an unorthodox method of treating cancer.

« 10 »

Hydrazine Sulfate: Unorthodox Chemotherapy

Since the end of World War II, the battle between the orthodox and unorthodox camps in cancer has often centered on the controversial question of chemotherapy.

To the orthodox scientists, pure chemicals are the most desirable forms of therapy, since each batch of these drugs is identical to the preceding one, and dosages can be set as precisely as the rads of a cobalt beam. To the unorthodox, however, such chemical treatments are anathema since, it is claimed, the human body has not evolved to handle substances so completely foreign to its normal metabolism as methotrexate or 5-FU.

This is the general outline of the debate. Nevertheless, there are certain exceptions to this rule. Some drugs, highly unnatural by anybody's standard, are scorned by the establishment and embraced by many advocates of unorthodox therapy. One example is the simple, off-the-shelf chemical hydrazine sulfate.

Unlike most anticancer agents, which have been discovered by trial and error, hydrazine sulfate's use was the end result of a series of logical deductions—a rational quest for a specific type of therapy.

In 1968 Joseph Gold, M.D., of Syracuse, New York, published a scientific paper in which he proposed a new departure for cancer chemotherapy (Gold, 1968). Chemotherapy was still a relatively new field, but it had become apparent, even by this time, that the principle upon which it was based—toxicity—limited the ability of these agents to kill cancer cells without also damaging the healthy cells of the body.

Perhaps it was not necessary to kill cancer cells directly with poisons, Gold suggested. Possibly the same or even better results could be achieved if scientists were able to block the cancer cells from inflicting damage on the patient's body.

Gold had studied the work of the great biochemist Otto Warburg, winner of the 1931 Nobel Prize in physiology and medicine for his discovery of a respiratory enzyme. One of Warburg's most controversial theories concerned the nature of cancer cell metabolism—the way in which such cells obtained their energy. Warburg's work formed the theoretical underpinning of Gold's innovation (Warburg, 1930).

Normally human cells obtain their energy through respiration—taking in oxygen and giving off carbon dioxide and water. This is a complex—but highly efficient—way of generating energy. There is, however, another, far more primitive and wasteful way of generating energy: fermentation. This type of energy production is common to some simple forms of life, such as the bacteria which cause milk to sour or the yeast which makes bread rise.

There are also times when our human cells employ fermentation. One is when the muscles or brain require a quick burst of energy. Another, said Warburg—and this is the essence of his controversial theory—is in cancer. According to Warburg, all cancer cells live by fermenting sugar in what are essentially airless (anaerobic) reactions. Find a way of stopping this fermentation, and you might have a way of stopping cancer.

Warburg's theory was eclipsed in the 1950s, but in the following decade, before Gold began his work, Dr. Dean Burk and others at the National Cancer Institute had attempted to iron out some of the problems and restore the credibility of this aspect of Warburg's contribution. Burk himself won a scientific prize for his demonstration that, in at least some cases, Warburg's proposal that cancer ferments had been correct (Burk, 1965).

Warburg's theory has remained controversial over the years. "Unfortunately," wrote Pat McGrady, Sr., "Warburg was only partly right; some tumor cells, to a great or small degree, can adapt to a respiration mode of life, and some normal cells have fermenting mechanisms." A drug that blocked fermentation, oxalic acid, was tried as a cancer treatment but was toxic and gave only mixed results (McGrady, Sr., 1964).

"The relation between the Warburg effect and transformation [of normal cells to cancerous ones] is still unclear," the *Science* cancer report noted in 1975. "Warburg's theory does not account for the aberrant properties of tumor cells" (Maugh and Marx, 1975).

Gold took Warburg and Burk's studies as his starting point, but then attempted to pursue this concept further than anyone had yet done in the practical application of these ideas to cancer. He reasoned as follows: A prime cause of death in cancer is the weight loss and debilitation often seen in the disease. This is known medically as cachexia. If cancer cachexia could be interrupted, the disease itself might be brought under control, much as diabetes is controlled by a daily injection of insulin.

But what causes cachexia—a frightful condition that often reduces the dying patient to skin and bones while his tumor grows with apparent vigor? Orthodox science had no answer. Gold's research indicated that cachexia is the result of cancer's ability to recycle its wastes, but at the energy expense of the body. It thus imposes a severe energy drain on the body, eventually resulting in emaciation.

Specifically, Gold pointed out, cancer uses glucose (sugar) as its fuel but only incompletely metabolizes, or combusts, it. The waste product of this incomplete combustion is lactic acid. This lactic acid then spills into the blood and is taken up by the liver and kidneys (normal, noncancerous tissues). But the body must now expend a great deal of energy from these normal tissues merely to reconvert this lactic acid back into glucose.

Ironically, the body then returns an ever-increasing amount of this new glucose back to the tumor for fuel, and the process is repeated over and over again, to the great benefit of the cancer and the great detriment of the normal tissues of the body. "The net result is a loss of energy from normal body energy 'pools,' " says Gold. "As the cancer grows, its production of lactic acid grows, imposing on the body a condition in which the normal body energy 'pools' become more and more depleted" (Syracuse, 1979).

Eventually the body reaches a point where it can no longer keep up with these constant energy losses. The result is rapid weight loss and debilitation—in other words, cachexia.

Gold reasoned that

> cachexia is but the end result of an insidious process—unrecognizable at first, but slowly taking its toll of the body's reserves until a "point of no return" is reached. Cachexia begins with the very first cancer tissue. What we need is a way to stop the vicious cycle and thereby put a halt to the leading cause of death in cancer: cachexia (Gold, 1968).

Armed with his theory, Gold now went in search of a drug that could interrupt this "sick relationship" that had developed between the liver and the cancer. He toyed with various drugs, diets, and compounds, including the amino acid tryptophane. In the early 1970s, however, he found a scientific paper stating that hydrazine sulfate could block a key enzyme in the liver that allowed lactic acid to be converted into glucose.

Before beginning clinical trials, Gold put hydrazine sulfate through a battery of animal tests. In four different transplantable tumor systems, hydrazine sulfate performed well. It also appeared as if the chemical was working according to Gold's innovative theory. For one thing, the drug did *not* damage cancer cells in the test tube, yet it did destroy them in the animal's body. This suggested that the drug worked by some indirect mechanism. Second, examination of the animals' tumors suggested that the cells were, in fact, not directly poisoned, as in conventional forms of chemotherapy (Gold, 1971a, 1973).

Gold also found that hydrazine could be used to enhance the effectiveness of most of the major cell-poisoning drugs in tumor-bearing animals (Gold, 1971b, 1975a).

The toxicity studies also seemed promising. A very high dose could certainly kill the animals. But at the optimal dosage, anticancer effects were accompanied by a minimum of side effects (Gold, 1975a).

Shortly after Gold's first animal studies were published, he gave a talk about his new concept at the New York Academy of Sciences. After the talk, a doctor came up to the Syracuse physician and said, "Dr. Gold, I have a patient who will certainly die in three or four days. I would like to try hydrazine sulfate on her." Gold and the doctor exchanged information on probable dosages and routes of administering the compound. Shortly afterward, according to Gold, the woman experienced a remarkable change in her condition. Within a few weeks she was up and about, greatly improved. A number of other patients also appeared to experience dramatic remissions (Wayne Martin, 1977).

By August 1973 there were about twenty or thirty patients taking hydrazine sulfate in different parts of the country. By the middle of September, there were about two or three hundred. And by October there were over one thousand.

When hydrazine sulfate at the optimal dose had been shown to be relatively nontoxic and effective in animal studies, the Food and Drug Administration cautiously began to give out a few Investigational New Drug (IND) permits to a handful of doctors. For example, they granted an IND to the Medical College of Virginia to study the substance. Another permit went to the California drug company Calbiochem, Inc. But the number of INDs granted was very few, and many individuals began to obtain the drug on their own and treat themselves. The American Cancer Society and the National Cancer Institute officially maintained silence, but Gold began to experience difficulties in his requests for funds from NCI.

However, not everyone at NCI was negative. Dr. Burk, then the head of cell chemistry at the government's cancer center, was understandably enthusiastic over Gold's work. Since the death of Warburg in 1971, one author had written, "Burk could well be called the world's greatest biochemist, and he has borne the torch of Warburg's life work since then" (ibid.). Gold's finding seemed to vindicate Warburg and Burk's work on cancer cell metabolism.

Burk declared hydrazine sulfate to be "the most remarkable anticancer agent I have come across in my forty-five years of experience in cancer." He predicted that the FDA would make hydrazine freely available to cancer patients, but added, "It would make little difference with hydrazine sulfate if the FDA wanted to balk, because this material is so cheap—and it is cheap because it is made by the trainload for industrial purposes" (Burk, 1974a).

In mid-August 1973, Burk met with top officials of Sloan-Kettering Institute in New York to tell them about hydrazine's successes. Burk thus presented his case:

> Let me tell you this perfectly true story. There is nothing mystical or poetic about it—and I could give you many [such stories]. A woman with Hodgkin's disease who had been flat on her back for seven weeks, who had no appetite and who had lost all her weight—a "paper-thin" patient—took hydrazine sulfate. One week later she was shopping in the grocery store with her own bag; five days later she was spending most of the day in her garden. I don't give you that as any miraculous story—it is simply the plain truth (Burk, 1974).

According to Burk, some of the leaders of Sloan-Kettering were highly enthusiastic about the early reports on hydrazine sulfate. Some of them were immunologists who considered themselves the heirs of Dr. Coley. But hydrazine sulfate was no immune-stimulating natural agent, like Coley's toxins; it was a drug, pure and simple. Because of this, hydrazine sulfate was given to the chemotherapists to evaluate. In general, the chemotherapists were far less receptive or enthusiastic about innovative approaches, especially those advocated by mavericks such as Dean Burk.

Hydrazine sulfate was immediately put into clinical trials, an unusual step since most other drugs have first been subjected to extensive animal testing at Sloan-Kettering itself before human tests have been started. A meeting was held between Gold and his colleagues and the Memorial Sloan-Kettering leaders in September 1973. Shortly afterward, the public affairs department at MSKCC issued a press release stating that a "joint effort" was being undertaken by the two institutions (MSKCC and Syracuse Cancer Research Institute) to test the new substance in terminal patients. It appeared to many as if the two camps were finally coming together for serious study, for the benefit of all cancer patients.

However, according to Gold, SKI immediately reneged: "Once the study began, no person at Sloan-Kettering responsible for this study ever got in touch with me. No information was released. No data were volunteered. No questions were asked" (Gold, 1974).

Thirty-two patients were given hydrazine sulfate, patients on whom no other form of therapy any longer had any positive effect. Several of these patients died before the test could ever begin, in violation of the agreed-upon protocol that each patient put in the study have a life expectancy of at least two months. An SKI chemotherapist later claimed that hydrazine had failed to have an effect in these patients—literally true, since they were already dead at the time the test began (ibid.).

The two research centers had agreed at several meetings that the patients would start with a dosage of 60 milligrams a day. Instead, Gold said, the Sloan-Kettering chemotherapists took it upon themselves to change this to 1 milligram on the first day, then 2 milligrams on the second day, and so forth, until they reached a dosage of between 20 and 30 milligrams per day—still a fraction of the adequate amount (ibid.).

An emergency meeting was convened between Gold and Memorial Sloan-Kettering doctors Lewis Thomas, Robert Good, Lloyd Old, Raymond Brown, Irwin Krakoff, and Manuel Ochoa, who was supervising the clinical trial. The latter agreed—for the third time—to abide by the optimal dosage: 60 milligrams for the first three days, 60 milligrams twice a day for the next three days, and 60 milligrams three times a day thereafter "with the option of allowing the patient to remain on 60 milligrams [twice a day] if there was a continuing good response" (ibid.).

After hearing nothing from his Sloan-Kettering collaborators, Gold came to New York and paid a surprise visit to the cancer clinic, accompanied by Raymond Brown, then an aide to SKI vice president Lloyd Old. Four of the seven patients' records they examined showed strong subjective responses to the new therapy, Gold claimed; the patients were eating more and feeling more alert and stronger. This was documented in the progress reports and the nurses' notes (ibid.).

At this point, instead of going on the twice-a-day schedule as agreed upon, however, the chemotherapists gave each patient a massive, single dose of approximately 120–190 milligrams, "which quickly wiped out whatever good response they were beginning to show," according to a letter of protest that Gold sent to SKI's Ochoa (ibid.).

The SKI chemotherapist told a relative of one of the first patients that he had "no enthusiasm or interest in" hydrazine sulfate and that the drug was "worthless" in the treatment of cancer, Gold said (ibid.).

After treating the patients in this way, the chemotherapists then concluded not only that hydrazine sulfate 'was not effective but that it caused dangerous side effects, such as "serious central nervous system toxicities." Ochoa brought up these alleged shortcomings at an open discussion of Gold's paper at the March 1974 meeting of the American Association for Cancer Research in Houston. "You should know by virtue of your training," Gold told Ochoa, "that in critically ill patients it is quite easy to produce serious toxicities with any anticancer drug by overdosing" (ibid.).

In response to repeated public requests for information on the new drug, the author drew up the following statement in mid-1974 for the public affairs department of MSKCC:

> In September 1973 MSKCC began clinical trials on the drug hydrazine sulfate, after published reports indicated that it seemed to have effectiveness as an anticancer agent.
> This project was carried out under the directorship of Dr. Manuel Ochoa, Jr., M.D., Associate Member at Sloan-Kettering Institute and Attending, Solid Tumor Service at Memorial Hospital.
> Dr. Ochoa now reports that he has adequately treated 29 patients at Memorial with this drug. The results have been that (1) *none* of these patients responded positively to hydrazine sulfate and (2) some of the patients developed neurotoxicity [nerve damage], apparently due to the administration of this drug.
> Based on these findings, therefore, MSKCC is no longer treating patients with hydrazine sulfate, nor are we conducting any further experiments with it at the present time (Moss, 1974).

Gold strongly disputes this statement. First, he says, Sloan-Kettering never *adequately* treated twenty-nine patients, or even one patient: the correct dosages, which were worked out over a period of years, were never used. Second, the statement fails to mention the subjective responses of patients to initial treatment with the drug. These subjective effects are included in the published paper of the Sloan-Kettering group (Ochoa, 1975). Third, the nerve damage mentioned occurred only when the patients were overdosed.

In reviewing his experience with SKI, Gold has said: "I've heard of cancer politics, but I've never seen anything like this in my entire life. In fact, I wouldn't believe it, if I hadn't seen it with my own eyes." He feels that there are "several different Sloan-Ketterings," since while the official statements on hydrazine were as negative as the one above, several top officials at SKI have privately conveyed to him their continuing interest in the compound and their inability to influence the actions of the chemotherapists (Gold, 1975b).

The "failure" at Sloan-Kettering was one in a number of setbacks for hydrazine within the cancer establishment. Dr. William Regelson of the Medical College of Virginia also claimed to see no benefit in patients using hydrazine in a double-blind study. But neither did he see any toxicity. It was, in his view, totally inert. However, Regelson's study was never published. It was rejected by *Cancer Treatment Reports* (an NCI publication), says Gold, because of the paucity of patients and because the limited data were impossible to interpret (Gold, 1979).

Another doctor reporting negative results was Dr. Harvey H. Lerner of the Department of Surgery at the Pennsylvania Hospital in Philadelphia (Lerner, 1976). His negative one-page article was published in *Cancer Treatment Reports* despite the fact, says Gold, that the referees, who read the paper for accuracy, argued that it should not be published unless *all* the data upon which the conclusions were based were included.

Gold objects to the Lerner study on the grounds that it used only outpatients, who may have been using alcohol, tranquilizers, and barbiturates at the same time as receiving hydrazine. Any of these substances is incompatible with and inhibits the action of the anticancer drug.

The Syracuse physician soon countered with a clinical report of his own, published in the international cancer journal *Oncology*. In it he analyzed data gathered by many doctors under the IND granted to Calbiochem, Inc., the California drug company that was once interested in hydrazine (Gold, 1975c).

Gold found that out of eight-four advanced patients treated adequately, 70 percent had subjective improvement, such as increased appetite, weight gain or cessation of weight loss, increase in strength, and decrease in pain. In addition, 17 percent also showed objective improvement, including tumor regression, disappearance of cancer-related disorders, or more than a year-long stabilization of their condition. The length of time this improvement lasted varied from patient to patient, but in some cases it had lasted years and was still continuing when the paper was published (ibid.).

Under treatment with hydrazine sulfate, a dentist with Hodgkin's disease who had not responded to either radiation or chemotherapy was able to return to work after only two weeks on hydrazine. He remained working, in good health, for a number of years (Wayne Martin, 1977).

A forty-five-year-old man with prostatic cancer that had already spread throughout his body, and who was racked with pain, was freed from his agony and enabled to resume a normal life (ibid.).

A sixty-two-year-old woman with cancer of the cervix, in the last stages of cachexia, began to gain weight, got out of bed, and was finally discharged from the hospital, to the amazement of her doctors. Most remarkable was the complete disappearance of a secondary tumor the size of an orange (ibid.). Hydrazine sulfate appeared to be relatively nontoxic when given correctly, but at its worst the side effects were transient and mild, especially when compared to the harrowing effects of standard chemotherapy. Some individuals (about 2 percent, after long-term high-dosage administration) did experience a feeling of pain or weakness in their limbs, but this condition was quickly controlled by reducing the dosage and administering vitamin B_6. A few others experienced nausea, dry skin, dizziness, and drowsiness. Most importantly, in no cases did hydrazine therapy depress or destroy white blood cells or bone marrow, as standard chemotherapy often does. This is important because the bone marrow produces many of the cells that comprise the patient's immune system, which many scientists believe is crucial in the fight against cancer (Gold, 1975c).

Gold's paper concluded with a plea to his medical colleagues to keep an open mind on the new therapy:

> Hydrazine sulfate therapy is a new type of chemotherapy. Its clinical use at present represents a *beginning*. Whether a study with any new drug is positive or negative, it must always be evaluated in terms of the "state of the art." Hydrazine sulfate represents the *first* of a class of new agents designed to interrupt host participation in cancer. Other agents in this class now in development may prove to be far superior to hydrazine sulfate. . . . It must be emphasized that the clinical potential of hydrazine sulfate–like drugs in cancer has only just begun to be explored (ibid.).

Gold's plea fell on deaf ears within the establishment. Even Calbiochem, Inc. soon dropped out of the picture. A spokesperson for the company attributed this action to the fact that hydrazine was in the public domain and thus unpatentable. "We saw absolutely no place to go with it," he allegedly remarked (quoted in Rorvik, 1976).

In March 1976 the establishment made its condemnation official: the American Cancer Society added hydrazine sulfate to its unproven methods list.

The ACS spoke only of the negative results with hydrazine sulfate, such as the Sloan-Kettering study, and included tests that had been rejected by a scientific journal. On the other hand, it failed to mention Gold's positive clinical data or the important foreign data that were then emerging. So erroneous were the statements attributed to Sloan-Kettering's chemotherapists that they were later retracted by Sloan-Kettering itself under threat of "troublesome repercussions" by Gold's lawyer (Grauer, 1975).

The ACS also made what appears to be a personal swipe at Gold himself: it claimed that he was in "full-time practice" in Syracuse. This seemed to imply that cancer research was a sideline avocation in which he dabbled. The opposite is the case: Gold has been involved in cancer research since graduation from Upstate Medical Center of the State University of New York in Syracuse in 1956. He has published numerous papers on the disease and is anything but a dilettante.

After the ACS condemnation was made public, however, many newspapers automatically reprinted the thumbs-down verdict with stories entitled, for example, "Tests Show Drug Useless for Cancer" (*Long Beach* [Calif.] *Independent,* May 19, 1976).

Gold's funding dried up. From 1973 to 1976 the Syracuse group received NCI support for its basic scientific research. "Once hydrazine became clinical, and once it was placed on the ACS unproven list," he has said, "we could not get a renewal by hook or by crook" (Gold, 1979).

Despite this, hydrazine sulfate's prospects have hardly been diminished. First, as Dean Burk noted, hydrazine sulfate is so readily available that it is virtually impossible to stop anyone from taking it, or marketing it. It is extremely inexpensive. Burk once estimated that one year's supply of the drug, in pill form, would cost between $25 and $50, mainly "to cover the expense of the man who makes the pills" (Burk, 1974a). And, indeed, in 1989 the wholesale cost of 60 mg. pills was still only $6.00 per hundred and $20.00 per hundred on the retail level—a fraction of the cost of conventional chemotherapy agents (Michaelis, 1989).

Second, Soviet researchers appear to be impressed with hydrazine sulfate and the rationale behind its use. Workers at Lenigrad's N. N. Petrov Research Institute of Oncology of the USSR Ministry of Health, a large Soviet cancer center, were part of a joint U.S.-USSR cancer program and have supported Gold's concepts.

Soviet scientists seemed to grasp the philosophical basis of Gold's new approach better than his own countrymen. They wrote:

> Almost all research in the field of experimental and clinical chemotherapy of malignant neoplasia [cancer] up to the present time, one way or another,

reflects the principles of a direct . . . attack on growth and multiplication of cancer cells. However, there may well be other means of medicinal influence on the progress of neoplastic growth. One of these includes Gold's hypothesis (Seits et al., 1975).

The Soviet team then went on to confirm the following claims for hydrazine therapy:

Hydrazine stops the growth of animal cancers: Soviet scientists found that hydrazine definitely retards the growth of cancer in experimental animals. In Walker carcinosarcoma in rats, for instance, they were able to demonstrate a 97.4 percent inhibition of tumor growth with a high dose of hydrazine given orally. Other types of experimental cancer also showed moderate responses to the drug (ibid.).

Hydrazine works by stopping gluconeogenesis: This, at least, was the most likely explanation of the drug's action. Microscopic examination of tumor remnants in cured rats showed "well-preserved tumor tissues." This means that hydrazine destroys tumors without directly poisoning cancer cells by some "indirect mechanism of inhibition of tumor growth" (ibid.).

Hydrazine is relatively nontoxic: In animals, there was no damage to the liver of the treated animals, and little weight loss, especially at lower dosage levels. Most important, in humans there was no damage to the blood-making cells, although in a minority of patients the Soviet doctors saw the same minor side effects as Gold noted, such as limb weakness and nausea (ibid.).

Hydrazine controls cancerous growths in humans: This is of course the bottom line of any cancer therapy. Forty-eight patients were given hydrazine as a last resort "in all cases after exhausting possibilities of surgical, X-ray treatment or other types of chemotherapy." In other words, these were patients on whom nothing else would work—patients with debilitated bodies, doomed to die within a few months (ibid.).

The Soviet scientists carefully followed Gold's suggestions for dosages. They noted that the usual criteria for evaluation of the effectiveness of a drug—especially tumor shrinkage—may not be applicable in this case "in view of the unusual action of hydrazine sulfate." Nevertheless, in these forty-eight very sick, terminal patients the Russians achieved the following results:

Objective anticancer effects in over one-third of the patients tested: This included "objective regressions of tumor mass" in 20 percent of the cases and an additional 15 percent whose cases were stabilized; i.e., whose cancers stopped progressing.

Subjective anticancer effects in 58 percent of the patients: This included complete disappearance or marked reduction of bone pain, increase in appetite, and an unexpected desire to get out of their beds and walk around. In short, there was a "sharp improvement of general well-being" in over half the terminal patients (ibid.).

The Soviet scientists found that hydrazine was not simply a painkiller in the ordinary sense, but induced a sense of euphoria in many patients. Suddenly people who were in the doldrums, waiting to die, became active, cheerful, optimistic, wanting to live. The Soviet doctors noted hydrazine sulfate's "peculiar influence on the psyche," particularly a "sharp improvement of mood in a significant portion of the patients . . . to the point of euphoria" (Danova et al., 1977). This was so even in cases where no objective regression of the cancer could be seen.

The Leningrad researchers singled out two cases treated in 1974 with the new therapy. The first was a man of forty who was suffering from the last stages of Hodgkin's disease. He had already been through a succession of ten treatment sessions with practically every known anticancer agent, such as steroid hormones, cyclophosphamide, vinblastine, and Leukeran.

Several times these drugs had succeeded in putting him into remission for a year or more, but each time the cancer had returned. The last time his doctors attempted to treat him with a combination of vinblastine and a hormone, but with no effect.

Since his symptoms were progressing, the doctors decided on hydrazine therapy. "After one week," they report, "the first indications of curative effect were noticed in the form of diminution of weakness, lowering of temperature." Remarkably, after one and a half months, "the symptoms of malignant disease completely disappeared." The lymph nodes and the liver decreased in size and "there was noticed a gradual but steady improvement in the blood picture."

This lasted four months, and then moderate signs of cancer began to reappear. At this point the specialists took him off hydrazine and put him back on vinblastine and the hormone. Unlike before, these treatments were now successful, and the patient went back into complete remission of his cancer (Seits et al., 1975).

This case indicates not only the value of hydrazine itself but its possible use in conjunction with standard forms of chemotherapy. In some cases, as in the animal studies, hydrazine sulfate appeared to make the cancer more vulnerable to the cellular poisons.

Another case the Petrov Institute scientists reported in depth was that of a sixty-three-year-old woman with cancer of the lungs as well as secondary growths in the lymph nodes. This patient had difficulty swallowing food due to the progressive growth of the tumor, loss of appetite, and a coughing-up of blood. She was losing weight steadily.

On July 22, 1974, the Soviet doctors started her on hydrazine sulfate and within two weeks "a pronounced subjective effect was observed—marked diminution of weakness and coughing, restoration of appetite, disappearance of hemoptysis [spitting of blood]" (ibid.).

X rays revealed that the tumor was shrinking in the left lung, and there were other signs of cancer regression. The woman continued to improve as of the date of the report. Neither she nor any of the other patients showed any signs of damage to the vital immune system.

The Soviet report emphasizes that these observations were not flukes "but rather typical in those cases in which hydrazine sulfate was basically effective and as a rule did not cause side effects."

How has the American cancer establishment reacted to these Soviet studies? In general, quite negatively. NCI published an abridged and, Gold feels, watered-down version of one of the Soviet papers in 1976. But they coupled it with a negative American study. ACS editorialized about them both as follows:

> The July issue [of the NCI publication] contains two important reports on the lack of clinical effect of hydrazine sulfate. This compound received considerable publicity in the lay press prior to confirmation of clinical utility. Lerner and Regelson report no clinical effects in 25 evaluable cancer patients, and Gershanovich et al. (Petrov Research Institute of Oncology, Leningrad, USSR) report a minimal objective effect (greater than 50 percent tumor regression) in two of 95 evaluable patients. . . . Thus, the weight of clinical evidence has failed to confirm the early enthusiastic reports by Gold (ACS, 1976).

That ACS officials could consider the Soviet studies, summarized above, to be reports "on the lack of clinical effect of hydrazine sulfate" certainly defied logic. But such a version maintained the line that there are three—and only three—proven forms of cancer therapy, and that chemotherapy must be highly toxic to be effective.

Despite this type of official negativism, the interest in hydrazine sulfate continued to grow in both the United States and the Soviet Union.

In the United States in 1978, Gold estimated that about 5,000 patients were being treated with hydrazine sulfate by hundreds of physicians (*Medical Tribune*, October 4, 1978). Many of these doctors had written or telephoned their favorable impressions of hydrazine. In many cases, hydrazine sulfate lacked cell-killing ability but promoted subjective effects. Gold bristled at those who criticized his compound on these grounds.

"This is like faulting Babe Ruth for being a poor football player," Gold observed. "Baseball was the Babe's game—subjective response is hydrazine's game" (ibid.).

Many doctors were unwilling to allow their names to be mentioned in the same breath with hydrazine sulfate lest their professional standing suffer. But others told of positive experience with the drug.

Timothy P. Ahmadi, a Mobile, Alabama, internist, reported favorably on Gold's work in *Medical Tribune*. He had used hydrazine sulfate to treat his wife, who had a form of brain cancer; she had already undergone brain surgery and treatment with radioactive cobalt. Mrs. Ahmadi had a rapidly growing tumor of the type which the patient usually survives for only several months after diagnosis. "Following the use of hydrazine sulfate," he said, "my wife felt better, her headaches decreased. She survived for two and a half years, as against the usual few months" (ibid.).

Dr. R. O. Bicks, clinical professor of medicine, University of Tennessee, and chief of gastroenterology, Baptist Hospital, told *Medical Tribune* he had used hydrazine sulfate in the treatment of two male patients with inoperable cancer of the pancreas:

> I had the clinical impression that they survived longer than expected. In my experience these patients usually last four or five months. They survived nearly a year, with objective changes in the size of liver metastases, and with relative well-being. There were no cardiologic, renal, or hematologic side effects (ibid.)

"And then," the Memphis physician recalled, "the FDA got in touch with me and was very upset. They said the drug causes bone-marrow toxicity [a statement that has no basis in fact, Gold counters]. We'd have continued using hydrazine if the FDA hadn't raised hell" (ibid.).

In September 1978 the National Cancer Institute announced that it was looking for research into "host/tumor competition—cachexia metabolism" as part of its expanded Diet, Nutrition and Cancer Program. The description of the project in the National Institutes of Health's *Guide for Grants and Contracts* sounded remarkably like Gold's work:

> Further work is required in the area of carbohydrate, lipid, protein and overall energy metabolism of the cancer patient. Mechanisms of accelerated protein and fat depletion in these patients require further elucidation. Ineffec-

tive utilization of dietary carbohydrates with energy wasting metabolic pathways must be further clarified with the eventual aim being therapeutic intervention. . . . (National Institutes of Health, 1978).

Gold, who had had his grant renewal application turned down after the ACS unproven-method story appeared, wrote again to NCI and suggested that his work might qualify for a new NCI grant.

Daniel L. Kisner, M.D., special assistant for nutrition at the Institute's Division of Cancer Treatment, wrote back saying that "more extensive human biochemical work would be required before the Division of Cancer Treatment could invest the considerable sums of money necessary to test hydrazine sulfate as an anti-cachexia agent."

What sort of information was needed?

> There is no information with regard to dietary intake in the patients treated. Hydrazine sulfate may have been an appetite stimulant. There is no information as to whether the weight gain was in the form of body muscle, fat, or fluids. The meaning of this weight gain then is also left open to question. The exact metabolic effects of the drug in humans are unknown. . . . More basic biochemical rationale is not presented. Without that biochemical rationale, I believe the existing empirical data would be inadequate (Kisner, 1978).

Such an investigation would tax the resources of a major laboratory, of course, and the Syracuse Cancer Research Institute is a relatively small operation. It would also require "considerable sums of money"—but NCI was requiring Gold to perform this work *before* it would give him any financial support. This appears to be a classic double-bind situation: one must do more research before getting a grant—but in order to do that research, one must have a grant.

This is similar to NCI's treatment of Linus Pauling, who was also told he must do more laboratory work before his method could be tested in humans, but then was turned down five times in his request for funds to do that research (see chapter 11).

Yet, surprisingly, at the end of his letter NCI's Dr. Kisner had some encouraging words for Gold:

> Please do not misread my comments. As I have stated to you in prior correspondence and phone conversations, we are indeed interested in hydrazine sulfate as a potential anti-cachexia agent. The section on cachexia metabolism in the grants program announcement published September 25 [cited above]

was written with hydrazine sulfate specifically in mind. I will continue to try to stimulate grant proposals that will answer the basic metabolic questions surrounding this agent in humans. I, too, would like to see the development of a chemotherapeutic approach for interrupting the aberrant metabolism of the cancer patient (ibid.).

Hydrazine sulfate obviously had some friends, then, in high places. Even more encouraging was the fact that NCI, in early 1979, invited Dr. Michael L. Gershanovich, director of medical oncology, Petrov Research Institute of Oncology, Leningrad, to come to the United States and describe his four-year study of hydrazine sulfate.

Dr. Saul A. Schepartz, deputy director, Division of Cancer Treatment, stated, "We have an interest in seeing Dr. Gershanovich's report," which detailed positive results with 225 patients in the Soviet cancer center. In addition, in a cable to the Soviet scientists, NCI offered "to arrange for seminars" at which Gershanovich could present his data (*Medical Tribune,* May 16, 1979).

In March 1979 Gershanovich arrived at NCI headquarters in Bethesda, Maryland, as part of the annual meeting between Russian and American scientists under the U.S.-USSR Cancer Agreement.

In addition, Gershanovich was scheduled to speak at the American Association for Cancer Research (AACR), which met in New Orleans in May 1979. A summary of his paper, "Hydrazine Sulfate in Late-Stage Cancer: Completion of Initial Clinical Trials in 225 Evaluable Patients," was duly printed in the *Proceedings* of the American Association for Cancer Research as abstract #969. Gold was scheduled to introduce the Soviet scientist.

Suddenly, however, the cancer research group denied Gershanovich a place on the program. AACR chairman, Dr. Bayard Clarkson, a Memorial Sloan-Kettering chemotherapist said:

> Dr. Gershanovich's abstract was reviewed like any other, and, as I recall, it did not receive a high enough rating from the review committee. In any case, the important way to present data to the profession is through publication (*Medical Tribune,* May 16, 1979).

Asked by a reporter whether consideration should not have been given to the fact that the Soviet trial was the first large-scale test of this controversial agent and claimed to show significant benefits from its use, Clarkson replied, "Our decision is final. The Gershanovich paper is not going to be presented, and that's it."*

Since the abstracts had already been printed, however, Gershanovich's summary remained in the AACR *Proceedings*. It not only gives the relevant statistics cited above, but concludes that "initial studies thus indicate hydrazine sulfate to be clinically effective in reversing cachexia and producing disease stabilization in late-stage cancer patients" (Gershanovich, 1979).

A schism appeared to develop within the top circles of cancer orthodoxy on how to deal with hydrazine sulfate. On the one hand, certain forces within orthodox medicine in the late 1970s seemed to favor developing hydrazine. This group consisted principally of those within NCI who were most responsive to public pressure. As *Medical Tribune* noted:

> A turn of events began shaping up for Dr. Gold's concepts as pressures from Capitol Hill forced the NCI to take a closer look at the role of nutritional factors in cancer (May 16, 1979).

On the other hand, there were powerful forces who wished to maintain the ban on hydrazine sulfate. These included those conservative groupings more isolated from such pressure, including conservatives at the American Cancer Society, which had already committed themselves through the unproven methods list; Memorial Sloan-Kettering chemotherapists, whose own work was directly contradicted by the Soviet studies; and apparently the leadership of AACR, who were committed to the highly toxic forms of chemotherapy.

In late January 1979 an NCI official told a United Press International reporter that the Institute was

> interested in the research and would consider supporting additional tests in humans if the Soviet results—*which have not yet been officially reported to the scientific community*—show that the drug has an effect against cachexia (Frank, 1979).

The AACR's refusal to allow the Soviet scientist to present those results at its meeting therefore blocked NCI-sponsored testing of the drug. It still had "not yet been officially reported to the scientific community," al-

---

*According to MSKCC *Center News*, shortly before this conference Dr. Clarkson and another researcher received grants totaling $123,000 from the American Cancer Society (March 1979).

though twenty-five papers reporting positive results had been published by Gold and the Soviet scientists and many physicians' reports were available for analysis.

Had Gershanovich been allowed to present his paper at one of the most prestigious forums in the cancer field, however, it would have become nearly impossible for the conservatives to continue their blind opposition to hydrazine sulfate's use.

The crack in orthodoxy's solid front on the hydrazine sulfate question was significant. It accompanied similar divisions on laetrile, vitamin C, the treatment of breast cancer, and the nutritional and environmental approaches to cancer.

Nevertheless, Gold cautioned against premature optimism:

> As of now, hydrazine sulfate seems to be swinging toward the realm of being accepted. However, one mustn't delude oneself. I think the effect of the Russians' seminars and presentations has been not to decrease opposition to the drug, but rather to polarize it. There is still a long row to hoe (Gold, 1979).

The history of hydrazine sulfate in the 1980's could be subtitled "The Perils of Success."

In 1981 the Russian team, headed by Gershanovich, finally found an American outlet for their complete pro-hydrazine results. They reported in a new journal, *Nutrition and Cancer,* that the drug had a marked and dramatic effect on the symptoms and disease progression of cancer patients (Gershanovich, 1981).

Two hundred and twenty-five patients were evaluated. All of them had exhausted other possible therapies, including surgery, radiation, and toxic chemotherapy. In every case at least six weeks had passed since the patient had stopped conventional therapy (to preclude the charge that benefits were the result of the delayed effects of conventional treatment). Then the patients were given hydrazine tablets—working up to one 60 mg. capsule three times a day.

A remarkable 65.2 percent of these advanced, refractory patients experienced what was called subjective response. This included improvement of appetite; weight stabilization or weight gain; disappearance of the severe weakness seen before treatment; reduction or even *complete elimination* of pain, respiratory deficiency, coughing of blood, and fevers.

None of these advanced patients was cured. But four did experience dramatic recoveries, with greater than 50 percent regression of their tumors.

One woman, for instance, had a massive, metastasized tumor reduced to "only a cord on the pelvic wall." Her life-threatening complications disappeared. Another patient, a man suffering from high fevers, inability to breathe, and coughing fits, improved dramatically.

As Gershanovich wrote, "in terms of criteria adopted for the evaluation of cytostatic therapy, the efficacy of hydrazine . . . appears low. However, such an approach to the evaluation of hydrazine sulfate may be inadequate, due to this drug's peculiarities of action detected both experimentally and clinically (ibid.). In other words, in late-stage patients, subjective responses are a more realistic way of looking at hydrazine's benefits.

In addition, Gershanovich reported on the peculiar mood elevation associated with hydrazine even when the tumor continued to progress. So marked was this phenomenon that the Russians suspected it may be due to some as yet little-understood effect of the drug on the nervous system. To the Soviet scientists this indicated the need for a study specifically on tumors of the brain and spinal cord.

"A clear-cut statement for hydrazine sulfate as an anticachexia agent can be made," the Russians concluded (ibid.).

In the wake of such studies, in November 1979 the American Cancer Society removed hydrazine from its unproven methods list. Dr. G. Congdon Wood of the ACS was quoted as saying that hydrazine sulfate "shows great promise as a tool doctors can use to ease the symptoms of cancer" (*Miami Herald,* November 23, 1981).

Behind the scenes, however, continued a fierce struggle on how to deal with the drug. In fact, the cancer world split, not just over hydrazine sulfate, but over the value of anti-cachexia agents in general. Some scientists, like Gold, put their focus on restoring the health of the patient's metabolism. His drug was a way of helping the body fight its cancer and, in so doing, slow down tumor growth. Others were fixated on dramatic cures, the elusive kind of breakthroughs symbolized at that moment by much-heralded interferon. It was a profound philosophical divide.

"I believe that cachexia is a major problem in dealing with oncology today," said Dr. Gio Gori. Gori had left NCI because of its neglect of nutritional issues. He became founding editor of *Nutrition and Cancer* (Moss, 1983).

"In a sense, nobody ever dies of cancer," said Dr. Harold Dvorak, chief of pathology at Beth Israel Hospital in Boston. "They die of something else—pneumonia, failure of one or another organs. Cachexia accelerates that process of infection and the building-up of metabolic poisons. It causes death a lot faster than the tumor would, were it not for the cachexia" (ibid.).

Considering the importance of cachexia as a medical problem and the lack of effective anti-cachexia agents, one would think the National Cancer Institute would have jumped at a chance to extend the Russian findings.

But Dr. Vincent DeVita, then director of the NCI, remained hostile. He told Geraldo Rivera of ABC News's "20/20" that hydrazine research was "a very low priority thing" and "unexciting." Pressed on the significance of the Soviet studies, he emphasized, "I'm very unexcited—we throw away drugs that are better than hydrazine sulfate" ("20/20," 1981).

One of the scientists who was present in New Orleans when the Russians were barred from the podium was a young California researcher named Rowan T. Chlebowski, M.D., Ph.D. As a traditionalist, Chlebowski had never even heard of hydrazine and paid scant attention to the flap over the Soviet scientists. That was soon to change.

Chlebowski is a bright, serious, and, by his own admission, loyal member of the cancer establishment. In 1980 he wanted to perform blood-chemistry tests on cancer patients. Not surprisingly, few patients wished to volunteer for tests that did not hold out some hope of therapeutic benefit. At the same time, people were calling the hospital where he worked, pleading for hydrazine sulfate. Chlebowski and his colleagues therefore decided to undertake a double-blind clinical trial of the drug while at the same time getting a chance to study blood chemistry.

(The original IND for a double-blind study of hydrazine had been granted to Solomon Garb, M.D., a well-respected Denver oncologist, who himself died tragically of cancer before the test could get under way.)

The double-blind trial was to evaluate three things: the effect of hydrazine on *glucose tolerance,* on *glucose turnover,* and on *weight loss.* Each patient was given capsules to take—starting with one 60 mg. capsule and working up to three a day after eight days. After their in-hospital workup, they were treated as outpatients for the next thirty days. Each week they were contacted by Chlebowski's staff to make sure they were taking their capsules and were not using barbiturates, tranquilizers, or alcohol, any one of which could interfere with the drug's action.

When, after a final three- to four-day inpatient workup, the code was finally broken, the UCLA team found there was a statistically significant improvement in the hydrazine-treated group as opposed to the placebo-treated group in all parameters of the study. There was a statistically significant improvement in glucose turnover and in slowing of mean weight loss. The placebo-treated group had already lost on average 17–18 percent of their body weight, and they kept losing—almost eight more pounds in one month. The hydrazine-treated group lost, on average, less than two pounds in the same period (Chlebowski 1984).

Remarkable results—but isn't hydrazine supposed to stop or even reverse the cachexia process? Yes, it is. But not everyone responds to hydrazine. Therefore, much of this *average* weight loss was due to a few nonresponders in the hydrazine group who brought the average down.

"We have confirmed the rationale which Gold originally proposed for testing hydrazine," Chlebowski told the author after his historic presentation at the American Society for Clinical Oncology (ASCO) meeting in St. Louis, April 1982 (Moss, 1983).

Chlebowski followed this up with other double-blind studies.

In 1982, for example, he and University of California at Los Angeles (UCLA) scientists showed that hydrazine sulfate administered to terminal cancer patients had a dramatic effect on progressive weight loss and other factors that may influence survival (Moss, 1983).

In February 1987 he (and eleven coauthors) summed up their findings in *Cancer,* a medical journal of the American Cancer Society. "After one month," they reported "83 percent of hydrazine and only 53 percent of placebo patients . . . maintained or increased their weight. . . . Appetite improvement was more frequent in the hydrazine group—63 percent versus 25 percent. . . . Hydrazine toxicity was mild" (Chlebowski et al., 1987a).

In March 1987 Chlebowski reported to the ASCO meeting that he had found hydrazine "significantly increases survival in patients with non–small cell lung cancer" in another four-year study. Median survival was 292 days in the hydrazine-treated group and only 173 in the placebo. In the less severe cases, hydrazine did even better—a more than 50 percent increase in median survival (Chlebowski et al., 1987b).

In August 1987, the well-respected British medical journal *Lancet* published another double-blind study by the UCLA group. Twelve malnourished patients with lung cancer were given either placebo or hydrazine sulfate. The patients in the hydrazine group suffered less amino acid loss, or "flux." In other words, hydrazine helped cancer patients hold on to their protein (Tayek et al., 1987).

This is important since "it has not proved possible to replace the lost lean body mass in cancer patients with supplementary protein and energy, whether given in adequate or very large amounts. . . . [T]he metabolic changes induced by the hydrazine group may prove clinically beneficial" (ibid.).

In a 1987 article Gold eloquently summed up the potential of this agent for which he had fought for over 20 years:

> The devastating aspects of this disease are due to two principal causes: invasion of tumor into vital organs with consequent destruction of their func-

tion; and decay of the body by virtue of cachexia and its resultant effect on the integrity of all body systems.

Each of these processes has its own metabolic machinery, each is amenable to its own therapy, and each is to some degree functionally interdependent on the other. In the interest of treating the totality of malignant disease, each of these processes warrants intervention (Gold, 1987).

In 1988 Dr. Gold was invited to give a presentation to the American Cancer Society's Science Writers Seminar. For those who follow the alternative field, the sight of Joe Gold at this ACS meeting was a bit astounding, as was the ACS news release on his work (ACS, 1988b) and the positive write-up in the normally orthodox *Oncology Times* (May 1988).

"That went very well," said the Syracuse researcher. "But the ACS officials were awfully afraid I would get into politics and they were chewing their nails during the presentation" (Gold, 1988).

They needn't have feared. Gold spoke about his science in a noncontroversial way. While his natural style is to be extremely frank, over the years he has avoided confrontations with the cancer establishment. For example, he followed ACS's lead in pulling out of a New York City "Cancer '80" conference when orthodox scientists became afraid the meeting roster was stacked against them (*New York Times,* October 13, 1980). He has taken pains not to associate himself with other unorthodox cancer treatments. And although an M.D., he has assiduously refused to treat cancer patients with the new drug.

Chlebowski, too, has behaved in just the ways required of a good member of the cancer community. He has not sought to publicize his work, has performed rigorous double-blind studies, and has been published in some of the best medical journals in the world. And what has been the result?

Nearly twenty years after it was first proposed, despite numerous positive tests including three positive double-blind studies—hydrazine is still unaccepted by the mainstream.

Dr. Vincent T. DeVita, the official who "throws away better drugs than hydrazine," has even included hydrazine in a new chapter on unproven-methods in the second (1985) edition of his influential textbook *Cancer: Principles and Practice of Oncology.* The chapter, written by NCI Deputy Director Jane E. Henney claims, "Hydrazine sulfate, like laetrile, has been subjected to clinical testing and found ineffective" (Henney, 1985). Astoundingly, from internal evidence DeVita's book can be dated to at least April 1, 1984—two months after the first full-length paper from UCLA proving hydrazine's benefits against abnormal cancer metabolism in a double-blind study.

In the fall of 1987 Chlebowski submitted a grant application to NCI for a phase III* study of hydrazine sulfate, involving his institution (UCLA) and several other prestigious centers. He was not funded. Nor could he get funded by ACS, even after the UCLA team had demonstrated their results in double-blind studies (Chlebowski, 1989).

By April 1989 Chlebowski was simply finishing old work with the nontoxic drug. There are no new cancer studies on the drawing board. He would like to get back into this research, to which he has devoted ten years of his life, but cannot get funding to do so. He does have a grant from another NIH agency, however, to study the effect of hydrazine on Kaposi's sarcoma among AIDS victims, where weight loss is also a major problem (Chlebowski, 1985).

"I still don't know whether hydrazine will be fairly evaluated or not," Chlebowski said. He himself feels he has gained professionally by his association with the drug because of his recent entry into AIDS research. "It's turning out okay for me," he added, "but I don't know if it's turning out as okay for hydrazine" (Chlebowski, 1989).

It is often said that the person who discovers an effective treatment for cancer would have his or her statue in every town square in America. Gold may not have found a sure-fire cure, but he certainly seems to have found a highly useful, nontoxic approach to cancer—something that would decrease the pain and suffering of millions of people.

But there are no statues.

"NCI is up to its usual tricks," Gold reflects. "What it couldn't do in the scientific arena, it is trying to accomplish through politics" (Gold, 1988).

On June 7, 1989 agents of the Food and Drug Administration raided the offices of Great Lakes Metabolics of Rochester, Minnesota and A-O Supply Company of Millersport, Ohio, distributors of hydrazine sulfate. They seized not only supplies of the drug but all the writings pertaining to it, including the earlier edition of this book and the author's newsletter, *The Cancer Chronicle* (Spykerman, 1989).

At this writing, the Syracuse Cancer Research Institute is once again facing financial hardships. There is not enough research funding to do the necessary work. Why? Gold played by the rules. He did not profiteer from

---

*Under FDA regulations, experimental drug trials have been conducted in three phases: Phase I sets a safe dose and schedule; Phase II gives the drug to a small group of patients (15–20) with a rigidly defined kind of cancer; if that trial is successful, Phase III determines *how* effective the drug is and whether it is more effective than the state-of-the-art treatment (Laszlo, 1987: 195–96). In early 1989, however, the FDA started to allow the use of some drugs without their formal completion of the three-phase testing process (Young, 1989a, 1989b).

patients. During the 1980s, the cancer establishment simultaneously tried to neutralize hydrazine sulfate while grabbing credit
for its open-minded acceptance of new ideas.

1996 Update: By 1990, Dr. Chlebowski had shown that there was a
survival advantage from the addition of hydrazine sulfate to a cytotoxic
regimen in patients with advanced lung cancer (*JCO* 1990;8:9-15).
Following this, however, NCI funded several studies purporting to show
that hydrazine sulfate had no benefit for lung or colorectal patients.

Between July 1989 and February 1991, a team headed by Dr.
Michael Kosty treated 291 patients with advanced non-small-cell lung
cancer. They all received cisplatin and vinblastine; but half received
either hydrazine sulfate or a placebo. An analysis of most of these
patients showed that survival of patients also receiving hydrazine sulfate
was only slightly better than those receiving chemotherapy plus placebo.

There was also no differences in degree of wasting or weight gain.
The authors concluded that "this study suggests no benefit from the
addition of [hydrazine sulfate] to an effective cytotoxic regimen."
(Kosty, M. et al., *Proc Annu Meet Am Soc Clin Oncol,* A982, 1992). This
meeting report was followed by a volleys of papers concluding that there
was "no benefit from the addition of hydrazine sulfate" to chemotherapy
JCO 1994;12:1113-1120; 1121-1125; and 1126-1129).

Opponents rejoiced. Dr. Victor Herbert published an editorial in
the same journal entitled, "Three Stakes in Hydrazine Sulfate's Heart,
but Questionable Cancer Remedies, Like Vampires, Always Rise Again"
(1994;12:1107-1108). He called Dr. Gold a "well-meaning zealot" whose
treatment "has been lucratively promoted for two decades by 'alternative' practitioners." (*Note:* retail cost of the drug is $20 for 100 tablets.)

A blistering counter attack came from reporter Jeff Kamen, whose
reply to NCI appeared in the April, 1993 *Penthouse.* There were full-page
ads for the article in the *Washington Post* and the *New York Times;* the
National Cancer Institute then responded with complaints about the
advertisements which, it said, would raise false hope among patients.

Much of the criticism of the NCI-funded studies focuses on the so-
called "incompatible" substances. After an investigation was launched by
the General Accounting Office, Kosty and colleagues admitted that they
had not controlled for all the incompatibles, but claimed that upon
reanalysis this fact did not have any effect upon the outcome of their
studies (*JCO* 1995;13:1529-30).

Gold strongly disagrees, and believes that hydrazine sulfate was
tested unfairly, and that in fact allowing patients to take any incompatible substances entirely vitiated these efforts to test his non-toxic drug.

« 11 »

Vitamin C and Other Nutritional Approaches

In 1976 readers of the *Wall Street Journal* were startled to see, amid the Amex reports and notices of bond offerings, an unusual advertisement. Dr. Linus Pauling, professor emeritus at Stanford University and the only person ever to win two solo Nobel Prizes (chemistry, 1954; peace, 1962), was offering to sell "1,000 mice with malignant cancer" to readers of the *Journal* for $138 apiece in order to raise funds.

> Our research [the ad read] shows that the incidence and severity of cancer depends upon diet. We urgently want to refine that research so that it may help to decrease suffering from human cancer. The U.S. government has absolutely and continually refused to support Dr. Pauling and his colleagues during the past four years (Von Hoffman, 1976).

What was behind this unprecedented public appeal from an eminent researcher, a man who is generally considered one of America's greatest chemists and one of the outstanding scientists of this century?

Basically, Pauling had stepped over that invisible but very real line separating orthodoxy from heresy. He was to suffer for his sin.

For decades the California scientist had made contributions to chemistry, especially those chemical processes underlying life. He had helped

211

elucidate the nature of DNA and proteins, including hemoglobin and anti-bodies, and had played a major role in deciphering the riddle of sickle-cell anemia.

Despite the fact that Pauling was a political activist, who won his second Nobel Prize for initiating a massive peace petition during the cold war, he had never lost the support of the scientific establishment. This was because his research work was abstract and, to most laypersons, arcane. In April 1966, however, Pauling entered the field of medical controversy. Since he was not a medical doctor, some of his critics implied that he was un-qualified to speak on the subject of cancer or even disease in general.

A century before, Pasteur suffered a similar fate. A biographer has written that "at every incursion on the domain of medicine, he was looked upon as a chemist . . . who was poaching on the preserves of others" (Vallery-Radot, 1924).

The campaign against Pauling culminated in 1973, when one of his papers was rejected by the *Proceedings of the National Academy of Sciences* even though he was a member of the Academy. Pauling has commented that "it was the first paper with a member as an author that had been rejected in the fifty-eight years that the *Proceedings* had existed" (cited in Null, 1979).

Pauling's involvement came about initially because of a letter from biochemist Irwin Stone. Stone had done pioneering work with ascorbic acid, otherwise known as vitamin C, and had evolved a theory that mammals require very large amounts of this vitamin every day in order to maintain optimal health. Because of a genetic mutation, he said, humans are unable to synthesize their own supplies of this vitamin, as almost all of the earth's animals can. We therefore have to obtain our supply from outside, from our food (Stone, 1972).

A study of other mammals revealed that they produced substantial quantities of vitamin C, especially when they were under stress. These quan-tities, translated into human dimensions, meant that we needed *grams* of ascorbic acid. However, the National Academy of Sciences had declared that humans need only a tiny fraction of that amount—about 75 *milligrams* (thousandths of a gram) a day to remain healthy.

The reason for the glaring discrepancies between the conventional be-lief and Stone's is that it takes only milligrams to prevent the clinical signs of scurvy. Scurvy, a disease marked by fatigue, anemia, and bleeding gums, had been a scourge of Europe until scientists discovered that fresh fruit and vegetables could prevent and cure it.

But, argued Stone, vitamin C does more than just prevent scurvy. In fact, the scientific literature was filled with reports of vitamin C having a beneficial effect in other conditions, including, Stone believed, the common cold.

Pauling and his wife decided to pursue Stone's high ascorbic acid regimen for a while. They had both been particularly susceptible to colds. "We noticed an increased feeling of well-being," Pauling said later, "and especially a striking decrease in the number of colds that we caught, and in their severity" (Pauling, 1971).

Pauling began to tell others about this personal finding and soon was being quoted in the press as "pro–vitamin C." This brought a quick response from established figures in nutrition, especially Frederick J. Stare, a Harvard nutritionist.

Stare declared, "Vitamin C and colds—that was disproved twenty years ago." He then cited a 1942 study claiming that vitamin C did not prevent colds whereas, says Pauling, the study showed the opposite. Pauling comments:

> I gradually became aware of the existence of an extraordinary contradiction between the opinions of different people about the value of vitamin C in preventing and ameliorating the common cold. Many people believe that vitamin C helps prevent colds; on the other hand, most physicians deny that this vitamin has much value in treating the common cold (ibid.).

Medical men, in general, refused even to consider the possibility that vitamin C had this effect. Pauling proposed two reasons for their refusal.

First, doctors, drug companies, and government bureaucrats are looking for drugs that are uniformly effective in treating an ailment, such as the antibiotics. "In the search for a drug to combat a disease the effort is usually made to find one that is 100 percent effective," Pauling says.

"Another factor," he adds, "has probably been the lack of interest of the drug companies in a natural substance that is available at a low price and cannot be patented" (ibid.).

Pauling found a discrepancy between the facts and the medical opinions on vitamin C and the common cold. For example, researchers who achieved *positive* results in preventing colds with vitamin C sometimes reported those tests as *negative* in their summaries.

These inaccurate summaries were then reported uncritically in news articles, editorials, and reviews, which both laypersons and doctors depended upon for information and opinions.

When Pauling's book *Vitamin C and the Common Cold* appeared and

sold briskly, this seemed to sharpen the resistance of the medical conservatives, despite the many arguments and detailed analyses of data in that slim
volume. Apparently these doctors had made up their minds about vitamin
C. "The negative attitude of the medical establishment has continued to the
present time," Pauling noted in the second edition of his book (Pauling,
1976).

The commissioner of the Food and Drug Administration now launched
an attack, calling Pauling's arguments "ridiculous." Pauling wrote several
letters to the commissioner, Charles C. Edwards, and finally this official
telephoned and invited the California scientist to a meeting in Washington.
But when Pauling informed Edwards he was ready to come, Edwards withdrew the invitation.

A double standard was used to attack Pauling's arguments. These critics, wrote Abram Hoffer, a well-known Canadian physician,

> use two sets of logic. Before they are prepared to look at Dr. Pauling's hy-
> pothesis, they demand proof of the most rigorous kind. But when arguing
> against his views, they refer to evidence of the flimsiest sort for the toxicity
> of ascorbic acid (Pauling, 1971).

But Pauling's troubles with orthodoxy were only beginning. To be
sure, the common cold can be a serious health problem. But when Pauling
turned his attention to cancer, he entered an area of medical controversy
unprecedented in its bitterness.

It is difficult to say exactly where or how the belief that vitamin C
might benefit cancer patients originated. Juices containing vitamin C have
long been used as folk remedies. Its use may have originated among North
American Indians, who drank brews made from ascorbate-containing plants
as a kind of miracle drug to treat a variety of ailments (Bailey, 1972:14). A
sailor on the ship of the English explorer Captain James Cook, who introduced the use of limes for the British "limies," wrote exuberantly:

> We were all hearty seamen, no colds did we fear
>   And we have from all sickness entirely kept clear.
> Thanks be to the Captain, he has proved so good
>   Amongst all the Islands to give us fresh food.
>   (Quoted in Pauling, 1971:10).

Over the years a number of prominent doctors have abandoned surgery and radiation and introduced nutritional therapies for cancer (Morris, 1977). In retrospect it can be seen that many of these dietary regimens were high in vitamin C.

From the time of its discovery by Albert Szent-Gyorgyi in 1932 (Moss, 1988), in fact, vitamin C has been studied in relation to cancer. Early experiments were not promising. One of the first investigations on the effect of ascorbic acid on experimental animals was carried out by Kanematsu Sugiura and K. Benedict in the 1930s. They reported that "the vitamins A, C, D and E are not essential for the growth of transplanted neoplasms" (cited in Hoffman, 1937).

In the 1930s German physicians began to use vitamin C in one- and two-gram doses in the treatment of human cancer. Irwin Stone has indicated that W. G. Deucher (1940), Von Wendt (1949), and L. Huber (1953) all had some success with this method (Stone, 1972).

Richard Passwater noted in his book *Cancer and Its Nutritional Therapies* that researchers found cancer patients to have "lower than average amounts of vitamin C in their blood plasma and white blood corpuscles" (Passwater, 1978). This laboratory finding supported epidemiological studies which seemed to correlate a lack of vitamin C with a high death rate— including a high cancer death rate. A study was initiated in 1948 when 577 older residents of California's San Mateo County were interviewed. When scientists followed up these interviews eight years later, they found that the death rate for those receiving the highest amount of dietary vitamin C was only 40 percent of that for individuals with much smaller amounts of the vitamin (ibid.).

In 1954 the Canadian physician W. J. McCormick found that "the degree of malignancy is determined inversely by the degree of connective tissue resistance, which in turn is dependent upon the adequacy of vitamin C status" (ibid.). McCormick's work received little scientific attention but was widely reported by the health food movement. All this research pointed in the direction of an attempt at using large doses of the vitamin in a systematic study of cancer. A few years later, in the mid-1960s, Ewan Cameron and Linus Pauling entered the investigation.

Settling the question would not seem to be very difficult, since vitamin C is a chemically well-defined substance, unlike some other proposed anti-cancer agents such as Krebiozen, Coley's toxins, or Burton's vaccine (see chapter 12). Instead the investigation has turned into a bitter controversy.

To understand the reason for this, it is necessary to look at the broader context of the debate. Orthodox spokesmen have always reserved their greatest scorn for the "quacks" and "food faddists" who put "great stress on the special dietary value of various 'wonder' foods" (Young, 1967). Since 1929 the Food and Drug Administration in particular has kept up a running battle with the health food movement (ibid.:336).

"There is no diet that prevents cancer in man," Dr. Morris Shimkin wrote in an NCI primer. "Treatment of cancer by diet alone is in the realm of quackery" (Shimkin, 1973:112).

"To stress the nutritional approach to cancer," historian Nat Morris has written, "eventually became the surest way to become branded a quack" (Morris, 1977:44).

The biggest battle of the 1940s and 1950s raged over the work and theories of Dr. Max Gerson. In 1946 the German-born Gerson was called to testify before a United States Senate committee investigating cancer. Gerson brought with him five patients who had had some of the most common forms of cancer in the United States. He also came armed with X-ray photographs, pathology reports from leading hospitals (including Memorial), and testimonials from many other patients and relatives of cancer victims.

Gerson's credentials were respectable. He had graduated from a prominent German medical school between the wars and had studied with noted neurologists and physiologists. At the time of his appearance before the committee of Senator Claude Pepper (D.-Fla.), Gerson was affiliated with Gotham Hospital in New York and had a private practice on Park Avenue. He was the author of approximately fifty articles in medical journals (Haught, 1962).

What made Gerson controversial was his method—entirely dietary and natural. This included fresh fruit and vegetable juices, a vegetable broth, fresh liver juice, and foods high in potassium to counterbalance what Gerson considered the oversalting of modern foods. One unusual aspect of Gerson's regimen for cancer patients was a daily coffee enema to cleanse the body. This eventually became a source of jollity within the establishment—"With cream or sugar?" they invariably asked.

But Gerson's patients were articulate witnesses, and Senator Pepper's committee was not unfriendly to the unorthodox physician.

The Pepper hearings were convened at the request of the American Cancer Society. Pepper himself was politically in the ACS's debt.* Although Gerson received much favorable publicity because of his Senate ap-

---

*The *Miami Daily News* had supported Pepper for the Senate in 1944 in exchange for his support for holding hearings on medical research. Mrs. Daniel (Florence) Mahoney, Mary Lasker's friend and colleague in the ACS, was an owner of the newspaper. Mrs. Lasker chose and briefed many of the witnesses before the Pepper hearings, including C. P. Rhoads (Strickland, 1972).

pearance, Pepper's committee did not follow his recommendations for a dietary-preventive approach to cancer.

Gerson and his dietary method were gaining in credibility and prestige just at the moment that chemotherapy was seeking public acceptance. Orthodox forces in the cancer field were not slow in responding to this challenge. Their ire was heightened by the publicity given Gerson in the newspapers and on radio, and in John Gunther's best-selling memoir, *Death Be Not Proud*, in which Gerson's method is credited with a temporary remission in his son's brain tumor (Gunther, 1949).

Gerson was reviewed twice in *JAMA*, the journal of the American Medical Association, and both times it was concluded that his method of treating cancer "was of no value" (ACS, 1971b).

In 1947 a committee of the New York County Medical Society reviewed the records of eighty-six patients but claimed to be unable to find any scientific value in Gerson's treatment. Gerson was not allowed to defend himself before these investigative boards (Haught, 1962).

Gerson's medical privileges at Gotham Hospital were revoked, and he was unable to find an affiliation with any other hospital in the city. In 1953 his malpractice insurance was discontinued. Refusing to give up his innovative approach after the authorities had ruled it invalid, he opened a sanatorium of his own. On March 4, 1958, he was finally suspended for two years from the New York Medical Society. The leaders of the surgery, radiation, and chemotherapy approaches to cancer gathered at the New York Academy of Medicine and condemned a colleague who claimed to live by Hippocrates's dictum "Above all, do no harm." Gerson died a year later, and his method (documented in 1958 in the book *A Cancer Therapy*) was never subjected to the kind of double-blind test that could have established its true worth.

Upon Gerson's death, Albert Schweitzer, the Nobel Prize-winning physician and missionary, and a patient of Gerson's, issued the following statement:

> I see in him [Gerson] one of the most eminent medical geniuses in the history of medicine. Many of his basic ideas have been adopted without having his name connected with them. Yet he has achieved more than seemed possible under adverse conditions. He leaves a legacy which commands attention and which will assure him his due place. Those whom he cured will now attest to the truth of his ideas (Haught, 1962).

Gerson's daughter, Charlotte, has kept her father's ideas alive. She runs the Gerson Institute in Bonita, California, is a consultant at the Pacifico

Hospital de Baja in Tijuana, Mexico (the latter employs the Gerson method in the treatment of cancer) and frequently speaks at health-food conventions on her father's approach (*Cancer Control Journal* 3(1–2), 1975). A popular book on Gerson's work (*Has Dr. Max Gerson a True Cancer Cure?*) has reputedly sold almost a quarter of a million copies. Some physicians today have quietly incorporated Gerson's ideas into their practice: a number of the latest developments in cancer research appear to owe a debt to Gerson "without having his name connected with them."

But to the cancer establishment, Gerson is still the refugee quack with the coffee enemas.

It was controversies such as this over "food faddism" that set the stage for Linus Pauling's entrance into the cancer controversy. In 1971 Ewan Cameron, M.D., at the Vale of Leven District General Hospital in Loch Lomondside, Scotland, working with Pauling, began to give terminal cancer patients high doses of vitamin C on the theory that ascorbic acid was not (in Pauling's words) "a special anticancer wonder drug" but could "bolster up the body's natural protective mechanisms."

Most of these patients had first received standard methods of treatment—surgery, radiation, and hormones; only a few had received cytotoxic drugs. When at least two doctors decided these methods had failed and nothing further could be done—in other words, when the patients were terminally ill—high-dose vitamin C therapy was begun.

Dr. Cameron had arrived at vitamin C therapy by a different route from Pauling's. A clinician as well as a cancer researcher, Cameron had studied the biochemistry of cancer cells and found that cancer spread by invading healthy, normal tissue in its vicinity. To do so, it was known, the cancer cell produced an enzyme, hyaluronidase. This enzyme attacked the intercellular ground cement, the material that holds cells together in tissues. In 1966 Cameron published this theory in a book called *Hyaluronidase and Cancer*. From that point on, the Scottish surgeon searched for a substance—he thought it would be a hormone—that could strengthen the intercellular cement and slow the growth of the tumor. Success came not from a hormone but from vitamin C, which other researchers had shown was a powerful builder of this cement.

Cameron was well situated to undertake a large-scale study of cancer. Scotland had the dubious distinction of being the cancer capital of the world—more people died of the disease, per hundred thousand, than in any other country. In fact, the Scottish cancer death rate was more than *nine times* that of some countries, such as the Dominican Republic or Mexico (ACS, 1971a). The exact reasons for this are not known but it is generally assumed

OTHER NUTRITIONAL APPROACHES

to have a great deal to do with environmental factors, including diet (Fraumeni, 1975:206).*

In the Loch Lomondside area near Glasgow, about 90 percent of the cancer patients were sent to the Vale of Leven hospital, whose surgical unit was under Cameron's control. Cameron's clinical research work was supported financially by Scotland's Secretary of State and the Linus Pauling Institute.

The vitamin testing began in 1971 and, as Pauling related, the doctors were startled by the results:

> Dr. Cameron first noticed that the patients felt well when they received 10 grams a day or more of vitamin C. They developed good appetites, increased energy, got up from the hospital, went home, went back to work and got along much better than with conventional therapy. Patients who were on morphine for pain could be taken off their morphine in five days (quoted in Newbold, 1978).

In order to put these results into a scientifically provable form, the doctors began a detailed study of one hundred terminal cancer patients—terminal being defined as a situation in which continuance of any conventional form of treatment would offer no further benefit, according to two independent physicians.

A biostatistician, Dr. Frances Meuli, went through the records of cancer patients at Vale of Leven and matched each experimental subject with ten other patients who had the same kind of cancer and were of the same sex and approximately the same age (plus or minus five years). In the records of each there was a notation that treatment had been abandoned because the patient was considered terminal. Meuli then computed the survival time for each of these one thousand patients, who had been treated by conventional means, and compared this to the patients receiving vitamin C under Dr. Cameron's care.

The results were striking. Patients receiving 10 grams a day of vitamin C lived, on the average, four times as long—after having reached the terminal state—as those who received only conventional therapy. They also experienced the improvements in life quality already mentioned. What was even more interesting, a minority of the vitamin C patients—about 16 percent—experienced a dramatically marked increase in survival time. While

*In a 1982–83 survey, it was still first in lung cancer, second in female cancers of all sites, and sixth in cancer among males. Luxembourg now holds the dubious distinction of being number one among men (ACS, 1988).

the mean control group survival was only fifty days, these individuals all lived more than a year. Some of them, declared terminal in the early 1970s, were still alive over five years later (Passwater, 1978).

One woman who had been terminally ill with breast cancer was said to be healthy and free of cancer. Another patient, a truck driver on the Glasgow–London route, was cleared of all visible signs of cancer within four to five days of starting on vitamin C. As with many patients, however, once he was cured his physician stopped his medicine—the vitamin supplements. His fever returned, and soon he was back in the hospital with cancer. It took somewhat longer the second time, but after vitamin C therapy the cancer disappeared again. The trucker remained in good health (ibid.).

Cameron continued to treat terminal cancer patients with vitamin C, and he soon had 4,000 cases in his records. The results appeared to be better when the treatment started earlier, however. "We surmise," Cameron and Pauling wrote in their 1976 *Proceedings of the National Academy of Sciences* article, "that the addition of ascorbate to the treatment of patients with cancer at an earlier stage of development might chang[e] life expectancy . . . from, for example, 5 years to 20 years" (Pauling and Cameron, 1976).

"With the proper use of vitamin C for cancer," says Linus Pauling, "we could cut the death rate by 75 percent. It is probably wise for every cancer patient to receive vitamin C" (Passwater, 1978).

In some cases Cameron used 20 or 30 grams a day on patients, by intravenous drip. "The results were really quite astounding," says his California colleague (quoted in Newbold, 1978).

In the United States the cancer experts responded with suspicion and hostility to Pauling, Cameron, and vitamin C therapy.

They refused to accept foreign clinical accounts and insisted that animal work be started from scratch before clinical trials in the United States could begin. This could take years, but Pauling consented to do it and applied for a modest $30,000 grant from NCI. The government then refused him the money.

Five times this well-known scientist, author of more than four hundred scientific papers, requested funds from NCI, and five times he was rejected. In fact, in some ways the lines seemed to be hardening. When Pauling first applied for funds the application was technically approved, but with "low priority," and it was never funded. But after the 1976 National Academy of Sciences paper came out, the chief of diagnosis and treatment at NCI wrote in his summary statement, "Based on evaluation of scientific merit of this application, disapproval must be recommended" (Passwater, 1978).

Pauling replied:

> The National Cancer Institute is not operated in such a way as to favor
> the discovery of new methods of controlling cancer. . . . In my opinion the
> NCI does not know how to carry on research nor how to recognize a new idea
> (cited in Houston, 1978).

Instead of funding Dr. Pauling, the NCI set up a study of vitamin C
at the Mayo Clinic in Rochester, Minnesota. Terminal cancer patients received vitamin C while others received only a placebo. According to an NCI
press handout:

> Subjective data about relief of symptoms is being collected from all of
> the patients, and survival times are being recorded. Results are expected to be
> available in 1979. In addition . . . NCI has tested vitamin C in animal models
> used to screen drugs for anticancer activity. These tests are continuing, how-
> ever, results thus far have not been encouraging (Cancer Information Service,
> 1978).

In September 1979, Mayo Clinic researchers announced that they had
found large amounts of vitamin C ineffective in curing cancer or in alleviat-
ing pain in patients with advanced cancer (Creagan, 1979). The majority of
these patients had first received chemotherapy and radiation. The researchers
themselves granted that it was "impossible to draw any conclusions about
the possible effectiveness of vitamin C in previously untreated patients"
(*New York Times,* September 27, 1979).

In a press release dated September 28, 1979, Pauling disputed the
validity of the Mayo test, claiming that the results of the study had been
"misrepresented by the Mayo Clinic investigators and in newspaper articles" (Hoefer-Amidei, 1979).

The release stated that the Mayo test was intended to be closely mod-
eled after the work of Dr. Ewan Cameron. But Pauling earlier, on August
9, 1978, had warned the Mayo scientists that the "patients studied by Dr.
Cameron had not received chemotherapy. The cytotoxic drugs damage the
body's protective mechanisms, and vitamin C probably functions largely by
potentiating these mechanisms. . . . You should be careful to use only patients who have not received chemotherapy. . . . Otherwise, the trial cannot
be described as repeating the work of Cameron" (ibid.).

Furthermore, the Mayo oncologists claimed that 50 of the 100 ascor-
bic-treated patients in the Scottish study had received chemotherapy and

high-energy radiation, "whereas in fact," says Pauling, "only 4 had received chemotherapy and only 20 had received high-energy radiation" (ibid.).

Pauling and Cameron called on NCI to do another controlled clinical study on patients with advanced cancer who had not received treatment with chemotherapy.

In 1981, on his eighth try in as many years, Linus Pauling was finally awarded an NCI grant of $204,000 to study the effects of vitamin C on breast cancer in mice. The grant was the work of a "special action subcommittee" of the National Cancer Advisory Board; the ad hoc group was headed by Dr. Bruce Ames. The purpose of the group was to consider oddball ideas that had been proposed to NCI and had been rejected routinely in the past.

In 1982 Pauling published several studies of malignant skin tumors in hairless mice which had been subjected to ultraviolet light. All the animals received a standard diet with either 0 percent, 0.3 percent, 5 percent, or 10 percent vitamin C throughout the length of the study. No skin lesions developed in the unirradiated control group. In the mice which were exposed, the numbers of tumors varied. After analyzing the data, using statistical methods recommended by the International Agency for Research on Cancer, Pauling and his colleagues concluded that vitamin C had in fact prevented malignancies in this system:

> A pronounced effect of vitamin C in decreasing the incidence and delaying the onset of the malignant lesions was observed with high statistical significance (Dunham et al., 1982).

Another animal study involved feeding different amounts of vitamin C to hundreds of RIII mice, a type of rodent which spontaneously develops breast cancer. In a report published in the *Proceedings of the National Academy of Sciences* Pauling and thirteen colleagues found a significant delay in the time of appearance of the tumors in the vitamin-treated group:

> The rate of appearance of the first palpable tumor decreases significantly with an increase in the amount of ascorbic acid in the food, with the median age of appearance increasing as an approximately linear function of the amount. The conclusion that increased intake of ascorbic acid decreases the rate of tumor appearance has extremely high statistical significance (Pauling et al., 1985).

Over the years there has been talk that vitamin C might itself be carcinogenic in large amounts. A disgruntled associate of Pauling, Arthur Robinson, even claimed that Pauling had surpressed the link between vitamin C and skin cancer in mice (Richards, 1988:660). But Pauling's research confirmed that of independent scientists (Douglas et al., 1984) whose work showed an absence of new cancers in rodents which had ingested high doses of ascorbic acid.

These animal studies were overshadowed, however, by developments at the Mayo Clinic. In 1979 Pauling had challenged the first double-blind study carried out by Charles G. Moertel and his colleagues at the Rochester, Minnesota, medical center. In particular, he complained that many patients had first been treated with cytotoxic chemotherapy before being given the vitamin. This, he said, could have compromised their immune systems.

Moertel unexpectedly responded to this criticism by arranging a second randomized, prospective double-blind controlled study, funded by the National Cancer Institute. In January 1985 the results were announced to the world in the pages of the prestigious *New England Journal of Medicine*. They were devastating.

This time Moertel studied one hundred patients with advanced colorectal cancer who "were in very good general condition, with minimal symptoms. None had received any previous treatment with cytotoxic drugs" (Moertel, 1985).

Half the patients were randomly assigned to take 10 grams per day of vitamin C; the other half got a placebo sugar pill. According to Moertel, when the code was broken, "among patients with measurable disease, none had objective improvement." If anything, the vitamin C–treated group did a bit worse than the controls.

Moertel's sweeping conclusion was that "high-dose vitamin C therapy is not effective against advanced malignant disease regardless of whether the patient has had any prior chemotherapy" (ibid.).

In an accompanying editorial, Robert Wittes of the National Cancer Institute drove the point home. After first paying homage to Pauling's "legendary reputation for being right about all sorts of things" and his "awesome intuition," Wittes concluded: "It is difficult to find fault with the design or execution of this study."

Meanwhile, in a "well-orchestrated publicity campaign," (Richards, 1986) Moertel appeared on the main television networks to denounce vitamin C as "absolutely worthless" in cancer treatment. Pauling knew nothing about the impending paper and was left speechless, upstaged by his Mayo Clinic adversaries. It was a coup, and seemed to augur an abrupt end to the long and bitter controversy.

Within days, however, Pauling struck back. At a meeting sponsored in part by the Fresno chapter of the American Cancer Society, the two-time

Nobel laureate charged that the latest Mayo Clinic paper was based on "a false and misleading claim that they had repeated the work of Ewan Cameron . . . medical director of the Linus Pauling Institute . . . on the response of cancer patients to large doses of vitamin C" (Linus Pauling Institute, 1985).

Examination of the paper led most impartial observers to conclude that the test was fair. At first reading, in fact, it appeared that the Mayo researchers had exactly duplicated the Pauling-Cameron protocols. Yet according to the California chemist,

> the Mayo Clinic paper was written in such a way that in his opinion it would give nearly every reader of the paper the impression that the Mayo Clinic patients had been treated in the same way as Dr. Cameron's patients, which is false (ibid.).

As the dust settled, three significant problems with the Mayo study emerged.

The first was a deviation in the length of time the vitamin was administered. In the Cameron study, ascorbic acid was given throughout the life of the patient, regardless of temporary ups or downs in the case. All patients received the optimal dose even if they appeared to be dying.

Yet in the Mayo study one can read in the small print that "therapy was continued as long as the patient was able to take oral medication or until there was evidence of marked progression of the malignant disease" (Moertel, 1985). Progression was defined as

> an increase of more than 50 percent in the product of the perpendicular diameters of any area of known malignant disease, if new areas of malignant disease appeared, if there was substantial worsening of symptoms or performance status, or if there was a loss of body weight of 10 percent or more (ibid.).

In other words, at any sign of worsening, even of subjective symptoms or "performance status," the treatment with vitamin C was discontinued.

Because of this odd departure from Cameron's protocol, patients in the treatment arm of the experiment received vitamin C for a median time of only ten weeks. None of the Mayo patients died while receiving it. Their deaths occurred after the vitamin had been taken away from them.

To understand the implication of this, imagine a patient who receives vitamin C and then experiences a downturn—a new tumor, an increase in pain, or a loss of ambulatory ability. The logical thing might seem to be to maintain, or even increase, the dose. Instead, however, the Mayo Clinic at that point would cut off the treatment! They would then put the patient on toxic chemotherapy. When that didn't work, and the patient worsened and died, this was registered as a failure—for vitamin C.

What the Mayo Clinic was measuring was "the impact on life span of taking vitamin C only for the period up until the tumor began to grow again" (Richards, 1986).

A second objection was that this sudden withdrawal of vitamin C might have actually accelerated the decline in these patients. One of the drawbacks of vitamin C therapy is the *rebound effect*. Persons taking high doses of vitamin C cannot be suddenly removed from it without suffering an adverse bodily reaction. Put simply, this is because the body has built up a high level of enzymes that digest the vitamin. When the high-dose supplement is suddenly removed, these enzymes go to work on the small amount of the vitamin that is left. This can leave the patient with a dangerously low concentration of vitamin C in his bloodstream—or possibly even a case of scurvy.

Pauling did not invent this for the occasion. He and Cameron had discussed this principle at length in, for instance, their 1979 book *Cancer and Vitamin C*. They warned:

> There is some evidence that during the period of the rebound effect the susceptibility to infections is increased; the control of cancer might also be less at this time. It is accordingly recommended that a high intake of vitamin C not be suddenly stopped, even for one day; instead it should be gradually decreased, over a period of several days, if a decrease is deemed to be necessary (Cameron and Pauling, 1979:118).

Is it possible the Mayo researchers were unaware of this effect? Oddly, it is not even mentioned in the paper, much less taken into account in the protocol. And according to Pauling, "it is likely that some of the Mayo Clinic patients died as a result of the rebound effect when their high-dose vitamin C was taken away from them" (Linus Pauling Institute, 1985).

The third problem concerned the integrity of the control group. Some of them may have surreptitiously been taking vitamin C. If so, that would have thrown off the calculations about the merits of the vitamin and possibly rendered the test statistically invalid.

Healthy individuals with a balanced diet normally excrete around 30 milligrams of vitamin C in 24 hours. For cancer patients not taking supplements this figure ranges from around 0 to 10 milligrams. But of six patients whose urine was tested, two excreted over 550 milligrams; the other four excreted an unspecified amount less than this. Thus, of the controls, a third of those tested excreted amounts ten to one-hundred times greater than normal.

Moertel stated that one of these patients was diabetic and that this may have led to the discrepancy. Another possibility, however, is that some of these advanced cancer patients were making sure they didn't wind up in a dead-end placebo group and joined the estimated 100,000 cancer patients already medicating themselves with the vitamin.

"Some of the controls were clearly taking vitamin C independently of the trial," Evelleen Richards concluded in the *New Scientist* (Richards, 1986).

Another peculiarity of the study was the role of chemotherapy. In the past, Dr. Moertel had been an outspoken critic of the indiscriminate use of chemotherapy in advanced cancer cases (Gastrointestinal Tumor Study Group, 1984). In this paper as well he writes that "there is no known form of chemotherapy for colorectal cancer that has been demonstrated to produce substantive palliative benefit or extension of survival." In fact, there is evidence that patients on this drug do *worse* than those getting nothing (Richards, 1986). Yet after being taken out of the experiment, more than half the patients were given fluorouracil, a toxic chemotherapeutic agent.

For Pauling, the publication of this paper and its manner of presentation came as a great shock. The misrepresentation seemed deliberate. The Mayo doctors had promised to let him see a prepublication copy of the study so that he and his colleagues could make constructive criticisms. Instead they dropped it like a bomb, without warning, with the clear intention of blowing the vitamin-C-and-cancer controversy off the medical map.

Powerful mass media, medical journals, and government agencies cooperated in this. The *New England Journal of Medicine*, which has garnered unprecedented power in the last decade, not only approved of the study but refused to give Pauling space to criticize its faults. At that moment they were holding Cameron's latest clinical report, which they refused to print (Richards, 1986).

There was much that could have been cleared up if all the facts in the experiment were made known. But Dr. Moertel ignored Pauling's request for the raw data on which the paper was based, and the National Cancer Institute turned down all bids for a new trial (ibid.).

In the *New Scientist* Evelleen Richards, an Australian sociologist of science, concluded that the vitamin C debate was a triumph of politics over science. She contrasted the harsh treatment of vitamin C with the uncritical acceptance of toxic drugs such as fluorouracil:

Most chemotherapies for cancer, including fluorouracil, have been widely applied in practice without previous evaluation by randomized controlled trials. . . . [B]ecause of its uniquely privileged and powerful status, the medical profession has been able to obscure with ethical and scientific rhetoric its self-interested double standards in the evaluation of therapies . . . (ibid.).

We are led to believe it is truth that governs scientific evaluations. But surveying the vitamin C fiasco, Richards arrived at a chilling conclusion: "The success of a therapy has less to do with its intrinsic worth than with the power of the interests that sponsor and maintain it" (see also Richards, 1988).

Some doctors began vitamin C megadoses along with other nutrients in the treatment of cancer. One such nutrition-oriented doctor is H. L. Newbold of New York City. Trained as an internist and a psychiatrist, Newbold treated many ailments with nontoxic approaches. With cancer he favored the use of vitamin C.

For skin cancer Newbold used a combination of about 15 grams a day by mouth and a topical vitamin C ointment applied to the tumor itself, five or six times a day. In other kinds of cancer he tried to get the dosage up as high as possible but "by mouth you can seldom go to more than 50 or 60 grams a day." He also generally gave 50 grams by the intravenous route—in one case "for two months, six days a week. There were no serious complications" (Newbold, 1979).

"If I had cancer, that's what I would do," he added. "I'd take that for three months, and as much as I could get by mouth also" (ibid.).

One patient with a deadly oat cell carcinoma of the lung received an extraordinary 105 grams a day of vitamin C starting in December 1977. More than a year later this woman was back on her job and feeling fine, even with the tumor still there (ibid.).

To put this in perspective, the Food and Drug Administration says adults need only 60 milligrams of this nutrient (*Merck Manual,* 1987). Newbold was therefore giving almost *two thousand times* the government's recommended dosage.

Other forms of nutritional therapy are also generating interest after many years of neglect. For example, there is increasing evidence that vitamin A has anticancer properties. In 1976 the NCI announced clinical trials with a chemical substance related to vitamin A. But the empirical use of vitamin A-containing foods for cancer goes back much further than the NCI—in fact, it goes back at least to the eighteenth century.

Bernard Peyrilhe (1735–1804), professor of chemistry at the École Santé and professor-royal at the College of Surgery in Paris, who is remembered as the winner of a 1773 prize from the Academy of Lyon on the subject "What Is Cancer?" (Shimkin, 1977), advocated the use of carrot juice in the treatment of cancer. Carrot juice is one of the best sources of vitamin A; it figured in Gerson's diet as well.

The rationale for the use of vitamin A in cancer is that this oil-soluble vitamin nurtures and protects the epithelial (lining) cells of the body. A lack of vitamin A will lead to night blindness as well as to many kinds of skin diseases, retarded growth, and a susceptibility to infection.

In the 1920s Japanese scientists showed that stomach cancer could be produced in rats simply by depriving the animals of this life-sustaining nutrient (Hixson, 1976b).

In the 1930s scientists in Cambridge, England, showed that vitamin A was essential for the proper differentiation—or maturation—of epithelial cells. A majority of lung cancers occurred when these same cells in the bronchi of the lungs failed to mature (ibid.).

Experiments at Memorial Hospital in the 1940s showed that there is often a deficiency of this vitamin in the blood of cancer patients. (The same observation has been made for vitamin C.) At the time, this deficiency was related to an impairment of the liver, which stores and distributes vitamin A throughout the body (*New York Journal-American,* November 17, 1941).

Although heralded at the time as a discovery of "capital significance," vitamin A was forgotten or scorned when chemotherapy came to the fore. During the 1960s some interest in vitamin A was revived. Dr. Umberto Saffioti, now a government cancer researcher, found that vitamin A inhibited the development of lung cancer in experimental hamsters. Unsupplemented animals, however, developed lung cancers "remarkably similar" to the human kind when they were dosed with a by-product of cigarette smoke (Hixson, 1976b).

This discovery, too, was widely heralded as a breakthrough that could "possibly lead to results of practical significance for the prevention of lung cancer," according to the scientist (ibid.). Ten years later, however, Saffioti resigned in protest as head of NCI's entire prevention program, charging that there was "inadequate support for . . . cancer prevention" (*Cancer Letter,* May 7, 1976).

But NCI's stance did not stop some clinicians from using vitamin A against cancer. To increase their resistance to the disease, Newbold gave his patients this vitamin in dosages tailored to their individual needs. To some patients he gave as much as 200,000 International Units (I.U.) of the vitamin. Vitamin A in high doses can be toxic; if this dose produced signs of toxicity, he lowered it. By orthodox standards, this was a very high amount, since 100,000 I.U. is supposed to be the threshold for toxicity (*Merck Manual*, 1987).

Some German cancer specialists have long been using a special form of vitamin A called A-mulsin as part of an overall treatment for cancer. They have found a way to emulsify it so that it is supposedly no longer harmful, even when given daily in colossal (up to 3,000,000 I.U.) dosages.

In early 1976 *Esquire* magazine prepared to publish a controversial story on cancer by science writer Pat McGrady, Jr. Son of the former ACS official, McGrady hailed the use of this therapy at Germany's Robert Janker Clinic (now headed by Dr. Wolfgang Scheef). Using a combination of agents unavailable in the United States, the Janker Clinic, he said, got full or partial remission in 70 percent of the 76,000 patients it treated from 1936 to 1975. Yet the Food and Drug Administration had banned A-mulsin, the NCI was uninterested in it, and the ACS "prides itself on keeping the Janker techniques out of the United States" (McGrady, Jr., 1976).

In March 1976, as the *Esquire* article approached publication date, the National Cancer Institute suddenly announced a clinical trial with a vitamin A-like compound of its own. The "breakthrough" was given wide publicity and made banner headlines across the country. Yet, as Joseph Hixson pointed out, "The timing of the . . . revelation was curious. It came while the April issue of *Esquire* was still on the presses" (Hixson, 1976b).

The NCI did not choose to use carrot juice or plain vitamin A for its trial, much less the "unproven" A-mulsin. It chose instead a synthetic variant, a chemical called the 13-cis isomer of retinoic acid. This form of retinoic acid is manufactured by the Swiss pharmaceutical giant Hoffmann–La Roche. Actual clinical trials did not begin until the summer of 1978, and only about a dozen patients were studied initially, all of them with premalignant lesions that had the possibility of developing into bladder cancer.

This and many other studies have demonstrated the protective effects of beta carotene, which is converted into Vitamin A in the body. In 1986, for instance, scientists at Johns Hopkins School of Public Health and Hygiene in Baltimore confirmed that smokers with low levels of beta carotene in their blood were about four times more likely to develop squamous cell carcinoma, a comon type of lung cancer, than those with normal levels. In addition, they found that low blood levels of vitamin E increased the risk of cancer by two and a half times (*New York Times*, November 13, 1986).

"There appears to be something in the diet that is protective," said Dr. Marilyn Menkes, the epidemiologist who headed the study.

Supplements of vitamins A, C, and E had long been advocated by holistic health practitioners as a way to "ACE the cancer." It certainly is not difficult to see the connection between such therapy and the Gerson method, which for fifty years has advised daily ingestion of carrot juice to fight cancer (Gerson, 1958). Perhaps for this reason the Johns Hopkins researchers were quick to warn the public *against* vitamin supplements because in large amounts "they can be toxic," according to the report in the *Times* (November 13, 1986). They recommended a balanced diet instead. The American Cancer Society, which had belatedly jumped on the diet-and-cancer bandwagon, agreed.

"Our feeling is that if you eat a good, balanced diet you get all the beta carotene you need," added Dr. Lawrence Garfinkel of the American Cancer Society (ibid.).

Such statements ignore the fact that many people do not get even the government's recommended daily allowance (RDA) for vitamin A or other nutrients. This is especially true of smokers and hard drinkers, who sometimes suffer serious depletion of vitamins due to their habits (Merck, 1987: 932).

Linus Pauling points out that the Committee on the Feeding of Laboratory Animals of the U.S. National Academy of Sciences–National Research Council recommends far more vitamin C for monkeys than the Food and Nutrition Board of the same organization recommends for people!

> I am sure that the first committee has worked hard to find the optimum intake for the monkeys, the amount that puts them in the best of health. The second committee has not made any effort to find the optimum intake of vitamin C or of any other vitamin for the American people. In its Recommended Daily Allowances . . . the committee rations the vitamins at not much above the minimum daily intake required to prevent the particular deficiency disease that is associated with each of them (Pauling, 1987).

Vitamin A has also proven useful in therapy of oral cancer. Vancouver scientists have found that large supplemental doses of vitamin A or beta carotene could cause the shrinkage of precancerous lesions, called oral leukoplakia, and also prevent new lesions from forming. Weekly ingestion of 200,000 international units (IU) of vitamin A caused leukoplakia shrinkage in 12 of the 21 participants in the study. Both vitamin A and beta carotene prevented the development of new leukoplakia during a year of treatment of Indian betel quid chewers (*Science News*, June 11, 1988).

The U.S. recommended daily requirement of vitamin A is only 5,000 IU's. Afraid of potential toxicity, the Canadian scientists are looking for ways of delivering the vitamin or its precursor with greater assurance of safety (ibid.).

The same team, headed by Dr. Hans F. Stich, has also found a possible rationale for the vitamin's effectiveness. Studying bovine papilloma viruses in mouse-cell cultures, they discovered that a vitamin A relative, retinoic acid, reduces viral DNA inside cells. Papilloma viruses have been implicated in some forms of human cancer. This suggests that some of vitamin A's anticancer effects may be due to reducing the devastation of cancer-causing viruses in human patients as well (ibid.).

Many people have heard of the Harvard study of 22,000 physicians, aged 40 to 84 years, which has demonstrated that an aspirin every other day could cut in half the risk of a first heart attack. Although the aspirin portion of the study has terminated, most of the doctors continue with a lesser-known aspect of the same study: to assess the benefits of beta carotene in reducing the risk of cancer. Half the group is taking 50 mg. of beta carotene; the other half a placebo. Results of this study should be available soon (*Science News,* January 30, 1988).

Not long ago the cancer experts rejected any suggestion of a link between food and malignancy, and generally pointed with pride at the "great American diet." Because of this attitude, throughout the 1960s and much of the 1970s NCI spent virtually nothing on nutrition research. The same held—and still holds—true of other centers, such as Memorial Sloan-Kettering, which avoid the topic almost entirely.

In 1974, under pressure from the parents of children with cancer, Congress forced NCI to devote a part of its budget to nutrition. Even so, this amounted to just 1 percent of its total funds, and even this amount was not always spent (Chowka, 1978b).

A turning point came, however, when Senator George McGovern's (D.-S.D.) Senate nutrition subcommittee issued a report, "Dietary Goals for the United States," which indicted the fatty, overprocessed American diet for the high incidence of cancer and other degenerative diseases. Despite screams of "insufficient evidence" from the AMA and other bastions of cure-oriented medicine, McGovern's report was influential (*Los Angeles Times,* January 24, 1978).

Federal health officials depend on Congress for their jobs and appropriations; they could not afford to ignore what McGovern was saying. National Institutes of Health director Donald Frederickson testified before McGovern's committee that of the estimated 75 percent of human cancers due to environmental causes, *most* may be related to food. The NCI director at the time, Arthur Upton, Ph.D., declared, "A large fraction of the cancer burden may be related to diet" (quoted in Houston, 1978).

Upton hastened to add, however, that this is "still only a hypothesis and the leads must be nailed down."

"To a cross," added Robert Houston sardonically.

Even so, in the last ten years there has been an increasing openness to nutritional approaches.

"After years of resistance," wrote critic Peter Chowka, "the cancer establishment today is admitting the value of—and even promoting—progressive concepts such as preventing the disease through diet" (Chowka, 1987).

The American Cancer Society, he says, is inching toward a recognition of the role of nutrition in the *treatment* of cancer (once the very hallmark of quackery), and the long-neglected use of herbs "seems destined to be rediscovered and popularized" (ibid.).

The stage was set for this turnaround by three official reports: the aforementioned *Dietary Goals* (1977); the National Institute of Health's *Dietary Guidelines* (1979); and the National Academy of Science's *Diet, Nutrition and Cancer* (1982). "All of [these] unequivocally confirm the importance of nutrition in the prevention of cancer," Chowka wrote (ibid.).

Particularly important was the statement of Senator George McGovern, co-chair of the U.S. Senate committee that issued *Dietary Goals,* that the link between diet and disease was "an idea whose time has come."

In February 1984, for the first time in its history, the ACS issued specific dietary recommendations for the prevention of cancer. Following what it calls a "common sense approach," the ACS began advocating the following measures: (1) avoid obesity; (2) cut down on total fat intake; (3) eat more high-fiber foods such as whole grain cereals, fruits and vegetables; (4) include foods rich in vitamins A and C in your daily diet; (5) include cruciferous vegetables (such as cabbage, broccoli, brussel sprouts, kohlrabi and cauliflower) in your diet; (6) eat moderately of salt-cured, smoked and nitrite-cured foods; and (7) keep alcohol consumption moderate, if you do drink (ACS, 1988).

At the 1987 Science Writers Seminars in San Diego there was almost no talk of chemotherapy. Presentations centered on immunology and nutrition. ACS Vice President Diane Fink, M.D., trained as a chemotherapist, expressed her enthusiasm about the change: "New ideas on nutrition," she said, "are incredibly hot right now with both the public and the health profession" (cited in Chowka, 1987).

According to a National Cancer Institute publication:

> A large-scale study of lung cancer among white men in New Jersey showed a protective effect of vegetables and fruits, especially those high in beta-carotene. In Louisiana, a study of lung cancer showed fruit intake to be protec-

tive, while a small study of mesothelioma suggested that vegetable and carotenoid intake lowers the risk (NCI, 1988).

The National Cancer Institute also announced that it had awarded over half a million dollars to the New York Botanical Garden to undertake a worldwide search for natural plant substances that might fight cancer. At the same time, NCI has established a Cancer Nutrition Laboratory and worked out elaborate plans to study "dietary factors associated with cancer risk" (ibid.).

This turnaround on diet and nutrition, while belated, is one of the most welcome and unexpected developments in the cancer field in the last decade.

1996 Update: Linus Pauling passed away on August 19, 1994, at the age of 93. He remained active and productive until the very end. In addition to several recent biographies of Dr. Pauling, a scholarly book, *Vitamin C and Cancer: Medicine or Politics?* by Evelleen Richards, appeared in 1991 (St. Martin's Press). Ms. Richards had access to Dr. Pauling's manuscripts in writing her work and it is indispensable reading for any serious student of this controversy.

« 12 »

Burton's
Immunological Method

Since the early 1970s, immunology has been one of the great hopes of cancer research. The basic principle of cancer immunology is to find natural factors which will attack cancer cells in the same way that our native immune system attacks bacterial, viral, or parasitic invaders.

The existence of such immune mechanisms was postulated in the 1950s by such prominent scientists as Sir MacFarlane Burnet and Dr. Lewis Thomas. They argued that cancer cells are different from normal cells. Ordinarily the immune system recognizes these cells as foreign, and destroys them before they reproduce and get out of control. But if the defense mechanisms are weak, they cannot do away with the mutant cancer cells. They therefore run wild, invade normal tissues, and ultimately, if they are not destroyed, kill the host (Burnet, 1970).

Animal experiments to corroborate this thesis were encouraging. But when scientists attempted to carry this work into the human, clinical situation, they ran into a number of problems. In 1976 Dr. Peter Alexander, head of tumor immunology at the Chester Beatty Research Institute in Surrey, England, said that cancer immunotherapy had been on the wrong track for at least a decade (*Medical World News,* November 1, 1976).

No procedure, he told a combined American Cancer Society–National Cancer Institute meeting, has proved clinically effective against human cancers. The reason for this "failure to translate immunotherapy from mouse to man" was that researchers were unable to simulate in their laboratory the actual human situation, in which patients die most often of secondary growths.

Dr. Donald Morton, chief of oncology at the University of California, Los Angeles, agreed with Alexander's assessment. In recent years, he said, "over-enthusiastic" newspaper reports raised hopes that immunotherapy might provide a cure for cancer. "It was doomed not to live up to that type of expectation," he said. "With present-day knowledge it is unlikely immunology will reverse the tide and make the patient disease-free" (ibid.).

Yet, as fund-raising time rolls around each spring, newspaper reports about immunology's great promise begin to pick up once more. This leads to an upsurge of hope among the desperate and, probably, an increase in donations to the cancer fund-raising agencies. More often than not, however, these reports speak of distant promises and vague hopes rather than the concrete achievement of present-day clinical accomplishments.

At least one unorthodox immunologist has attempted to break out of the confines of the laboratory and directly apply his mouse techniques to suffering, often dying, human patients. This scientist is Lawrence Burton, Ph.D. In doing so, he has incurred the wrath of his former colleagues and the medical profession, and alienated himself from the established centers of power.

Burton's background seems orthodox enough. Born in the Bronx, New York, in 1926, he attended Brooklyn College and New York University, from which he earned a Ph.D. in 1955. Burton held various research and teaching positions at the California Institute of Technology, New York University, and St. Vincent's Hospital, where he was a senior investigator in the Hodgkin's Disease Research Laboratory.

In the mid-1950s Burton and another researcher, Frank Friedman, Ph.D., managed to extract from the larvae of fruit flies a factor that induced tumors in noncancerous insects. Burton and Friedman, fresh out of graduate school, published this work in *Science* and then went together to the California Institute of Technology for postdoctoral research (Burton and Friedman, 1956).

Back in New York in the late 1950s, Burton and Friedman joined with Dr. Antonio Rottino, M. L. Kaplan, and Dr. Robert Kassel in extracting, through trial and error, a tumor-inhibiting factor. The original purpose of these experiments, says Burton, was not to find a treatment for malignancies but to speed up cancer experiments and thus save money. The group received research grants for this purpose from the Damon Runyon Memorial Fund for Cancer Research and from the National Cancer Institute (Kassel et al., 1963).

The group now extended these fruit-fly findings to mice. Using similar techniques, they extracted a factor from mouse blood that caused long-term remission of cancer in mice (Burton et al., 1959).

Actually, this prosaic description cannot convey the excitement of the St. Vincent's group at what they had discovered. The animals' cancers would begin, within a matter of hours, to *disappear*. According to Rottino, it was new, original, and dramatic (Rottino, 1978). Eventually the cancer would return, but an exciting empirical observation had been made about the relationship between normal blood and the defense against malignancy. The tumor-inhibiting factor could also cross species lines. Thus, a factor derived from fruit fly or mouse could trigger anticancer effects in human cells, and vice versa. This finding "strongly suggests that the inhibitor system in the human may be directly comparable to that demonstrated in the mouse," the scientists wrote later in the *Annals of the New York Academy of Sciences* (Kassel et al., 1963).

In the early 1960s the St. Vincent's team came to the attention of the cancer establishment. Sloan-Kettering Institute dispatched Dr. John J. Harris to Burton's laboratory to learn the new techniques. After several months, Harris coauthored a paper with the St. Vincentians in which his name, quite properly, was listed *after* those of the original discoverers (ibid.).

Burton claims that the SKI administration put pressure on Harris for this. For example, Harris received a reprimand from Frank Horsfall, the director of Sloan-Kettering Institute, for publishing with the St. Vincent's team; Horsfall told him that Sloan-Kettering scientists never allowed their names to be listed in papers after those of scientists at "lesser" institutions.

Harris died on April 17, 1978, at the age of fifty-four, but his widow confirmed Burton's account of the episode. According to Mrs. Harris, when her husband published with his name listed fourth on the 1962 article,

> Horsfall couldn't take this. If anything, Sloan-Kettering should be first. But my husband didn't see it that way. He and Horsfall had several disagreements.
>
> My husband was enthusiastic about what Burton and Friedman were doing, and pushed them along. Horsfall tried his best to hamper my husband in every way. He finally left. He had had it. They pressured him quite a bit (Bertha Harris, 1979).

It was Harris, or possibly another Sloan-Kettering scientist, who was given what Burton called "the office treatment":

> They put him in a room—no telephone, no lab, no work. "You're here nine-to-five, you can bring all the newspapers you want. No secretary, no

visitors." He lasted about a year and a half and then he couldn't take it anymore (Burton, 1978).

"But they weren't through," Burton recalled heatedly. "They sent us contracts. They said they'd give us all the wonders of the world, all the credit, if we would work with them." The St. Vincent's scientists turned down the offer. "What the hell do we need them for?" they asked (Burton, 1978). "Then the fun started," Burton said. "We were on a Public Health Service grant. Termination. We had the largest Damon Runyon grant at St. Vincent's. Termination. We couldn't understand what hit us. We were naive" (ibid.).

Brought to their knees financially by this sudden withdrawal of their support, the researchers decided to offer their techniques to Sloan-Kettering after all. SKI now dispatched the late Dr. Aaron Bendich, one of its senior scientists, and a person as outspoken and blunt as Burton himself. When the SKI scientist heard the offer, Burton recalls, he told the young researchers, "It's got to be a pile of crap if you're offering it to us for nothing" (ibid.).

The St. Vincent's group desperately started reapplying for government grants. Each time, however, they were turned down, on the recommendation of a Sloan-Kettering chemotherapist who was sent to make a site visit for the National Cancer Institute.

On the advice of another scientist who said, "Let 'em look at bumps," the St. Vincent's team switched from leukemic mice to animals with spontaneous breast cancers, similar to those used in Sugiura's laetrile experiments. The type of mouse they chose was designated $C_3H(t)$, (t) for Dr. Albert Tannenbaum, director of the Department of Cancer Research at Michael Reese Hospital in Chicago, who supplied the strain.

Injecting their mouse-derived tumor-inhibiting factor into animals with rock-hard breast tumors, the St. Vincent's scientist watched in amazement as the growths became soft, spongy, and disappeared within a day or two. "We achieved tremendous results," Burton says, with no false modesty. "It was dramatic to see how the tumor would undergo necrosis," says Rottino, a scholarly research physician not given to overstatement. "That is important, and it is something very fundamental that should be studied" (Rottino, 1978).

In 1966 Patrick McGrady, Sr., happened to be a patient at St. Vincent's. He asked Burton for an on-the-spot demonstration of his techniques. "I saw him perform miracles on these mice," McGrady recollects. "He'd make the tumors disappear while you watched. There's no question in my mind that this was authentic" (McGrady, Sr., 1979).

McGrady was well aware that no form of orthodox treatment had an equivalent effect on such tumors. Since he had originated (and controlled the selection list for) the annual ACS Science Writers' Seminar, he invited Burton and Friedman to Phoenix that March to demonstrate their new technique.

As prominent scientists and reporters watched, Burton picked up four mice with big, bulging tumors and injected them with what he called a deblocking agent. An hour later the assembled doctors and writers, many of them skeptical of the whole procedure, approached the demonstration table.

According to David Cleary, science writer for the *Philadelphia Bulletin* who was present at the meeting, "The two gentlemen from St. Vincent's Hospital demonstrated before our very eyes that injection of a mysterious serum . . . caused the disappearance of massive tumors in mice within a few hours" (cited in Houston, 1979b).

Here was the stuff scoops are made of. Reporters suddenly rushed from the room and fought for telephones to be the first ones to break this story. By the end of the day, banner headlines in Los Angeles and other major cities proclaimed, "15-MINUTE CANCER CURE FOR MICE: HUMANS NEXT?" (Anderson, 1974). Burton since claimed that the American Cancer Society made $4 million from the public as a result of favorable publicity generated by his work (Houston, 1979b).

Many of those present reacted with hostility and suspicion. A rumor even began to spread: "The mice were switched!" Five top scientists, including a leading New York cancer virologist, formed a committee and scheduled a news conference to denounce Burton as a fraud and his method as quackery. At the last minute, McGrady and others at the ACS managed to dissuade them (Burton, 1978).

Within a year there was a repeat performance at the conservative New York Academy of Medicine. Burton once again injected the mice with the "de-blocking" factor and once again the tumors began to melt away. "The immediate reaction was that it was a fake," Rottino recalls (Rottino, 1978).

One researcher said, "That's very interesting, but since I didn't do it, I can't really say that it works" (Anderson, 1974).

Rottino shrugged it off with philosophical comments about "human nature." But Burton lashed out publicly at his accusers and detractors. With obvious sarcasm, he told the gathering that he had hypnotized them en masse during the performance and then substituted fresh, healthy mice for the tumorous ones.

By the early 1970s the researchers, principally Burton and Friedman, had elaborated a theory on how the mysterious injections worked. It involved the interaction of *blocking protein, de-blocking protein, tumor antibody,* and *tumor complement.*

These terms are foreign to the public, and it is beyond the scope of this discussion to greatly elaborate on their meaning. They are fairly familiar to orthodox cancer researchers (see Maugh and Marx, 1975:58–61). Tumor antibody is Burton's term for a form of gamma globulin (IgG) as well as related proteins (IgA and IgM). Blocking factors are now common scientific concepts. Similarly, unblocking, or de-blocking, factors, such as the alpha-2-macroglobulin, which Burton claims caused the sensational remissions in mice, have also been frequently posited by scientific researchers (ibid.).

Unorthodox cancer scientists are sometimes accused of inventing outlandish scientific vocabularies simply in order to amaze and befuddle the nonprofessional. The American Cancer Society has suggested that "the proponents of new or unproven methods of cancer management . . . are often inclined to use complex jargon and unusual phraseology to embellish their writings" (ACS, 1971b).

Needless to say, the orthodox medical profession is not famous for its verbal clarity, and many cancer patients have been totally befuddled by their doctors' language. Open a cancer textbook at random and you will find a jumble of terms incomprehensible to the average layperson: "radioimmunoassay . . . melanocyte-stimulating hormone . . . pheochromocytoma . . . hypercalcemia . . ." (Rubin, 1983:113).

All scientists use (and some of them abuse) technical terms. In Burton's case, at least, the novelty does not lie so much in arcane terminology as in the way the terms are put together to formulate a theory of cancer.

The greatest challenge for a research scientist is to see his work applied to the human situation. As Dr. Peter Alexander indicated, this is often the moment of greatest disappointment as well. Laboratory conditions are usually far different from clinical conditions.

In 1974 Burton was offered a chance to test his approach on human patients. With the help of wealthy supporters, he and Friedman left St. Vincent's after more than fifteen years and founded the Immunology Research Foundation in Great Neck, New York.

Burton administered an immuno-competence blood test to determine the levels of blocking protein and other factors, and medical doctors affiliated with the new foundation began to treat cancer patients with a sequence of the various blood components.

In July 1974 *New York* magazine ran a front-page story on the two Long Island researchers entitled "The Politics of Cancer—Why Won't the Medical Establishment Pay Attention to These Two Men?" The cover of this widely read magazine showed Burton and Friedman, in full color, holding out a $C_3H(t)$ mouse for the inspection of the general public (Anderson, 1974).

Suddenly Sloan-Kettering seemed interested again. This was the period of liberalism toward unorthodox approaches at the New York cancer research institute, the period of laetrile and hydrazine sulfate. According to nutritionist Carleton Fredericks, Ph.D., Sloan-Kettering even sent a small number of patients to Burton's clinic for treatment at this time. (A relative of Fredericks was treated with Burton's method and apparently underwent a remission of his cancer, but he died of other causes.) (Fredericks, 1978).

For a brief period the following year, it looked as if Burton and Freidman were about to be accepted back into the establishment fold. They applied for an Investigational New Drug permit from the Food and Drug Administration. Dr. William Terry and other National Cancer Institute officials visited the Great Neck laboratory and told *Modern Medicine,* a magazine for doctors, "Anything that can control tumor growth is significant" (Yasgur, 1975).

Modern Medicine also reported that

> eleven New York-area doctors, including some physicians at Downstate Medical Center, have expressed great interest in participating in a clinical protocol if the IRF [Immunology Research Foundation] request is approved, and it is possible that trials may have begun by the time this article appears (ibid.).

That was January 1, 1975. But trials never began. There are radically different versions of why human tests of Burton's method did not come to pass. According to an official National Cancer Institute release, Burton was simply asked to answer several questions by the Food and Drug Administration. "No response to these questions was ever received. Consequently, Immunology Research Foundation's IND application was not accepted by the FDA and was withdrawn at the request of IRF on March 8, 1976" (NCI, 1978).

Burton tells a different story: First the FDA sent back his request with three questions. Burton answered the questions and then prepared for trials to begin. But the FDA responded with more questions, three pages of them, single-spaced. "It became apparent that the FDA regulations and the National Cancer Institute (NCI) protocols would take too long" (Cameron/Friedlander, 1979).

Furthermore, Burton considered the kind of clinical trial proposed by the NCI to be unethical. According to a press release prepared for him,

The NCI protocols would have required Dr. Burton to treat a certain number of terminal patients—half of which would have to be a control group and would in actuality receive no treatment. "It's not humane to keep human controls. Why should some people get the 'good' treatment and others get none?" (ibid.).

Burton therefore took a very radical step for a laboratory scientist: in 1977 he moved to the Bahamas and established a research-treatment center at the Rand Hospital, Grand Bahamas. The clinic was a new, one-story building within the grounds of the hospital, with a modern waiting room, treatment rooms, and several spacious laboratories where the blood fractions were prepared and animals were tested.

Burton's method in the Bahamas, renamed Immuno-Augmentative Therapy (IAT), is basically the same as it was in Great Neck, but on a larger scale. During the early years Burton administered the blood tests using a computer to keep track of the patients' blood profile. A physician colleague, initially Dr. Frederick Weinberg, then administered blood fractions, derived from normal human blood (serum) flown over from the mainland. (Friedman did not join Burton in his Bahamian venture.) Burton has claimed that he offers these fractions "only after they [had] been fully tested for toxicity and efficacy in the strain of spontaneous tumor mice" (ibid.).

How successful has Burton been in the Bahamas?

It is impossible to give a definite answer to this question. Burton's follow-up of his nearly 3,000 patients is understandably poor, since patients come from—and return to—places all over the United States, and even the world. What is more, Burton has not published any clinical results; in fact he has not published any scientific papers since the mid-1960s, a point to which we shall return.

Burton claims to be having success with his treatment, however, and a number of other physicians and patients back him up on this. A follow-up report on 227 patients who were treated at the clinic in 1977 showed that at least 18 percent had survived in good health five years later. The expected survival rate was one percent (cited in Houston, 1987a). Burton calls some of these effects "miracles." He modifies this by adding that he does not have all the answers. "We don't have a cure-all," he hastens to add (Burton, 1978). The author visited him nearly two years after he established his clinic (1978) and again a decade later. The clinic had moved to a new building and employed 26 people, including three medical doctors (Wiewel, 1989).

As of the late seventies the best results had been claimed in cases of prostate cancer, malignant melanoma, bladder cancer, and some head and neck tumors. Burton claimed, for instance, that nine cases of metastasized prostate cancer "have improved and gone home." A person who came at the same time that Hubert Humphrey was dying, with the same diagnosis and the same prognosis, "is completely free of the disease according to an oncology center in Atlanta, Georgia" (Burton, 1978).

Of the 186 patients treated between 1974 and 1977 (presumably in Great Neck), Burton claimed that 30—or 16 percent—had what he calls "miracle remissions—they exhibit no sign of cancer." Some 80 others experienced tumor regression, and there was at least a partial stoppage of tumor growth in 60 percent of those treated. Only 8 of these 186 individuals were *not* deemed terminally ill at the time of treatment with Burton's method.

Twenty advanced patients were sent to Burton by John Beaty, M.D., of the Greenwich Hospital, Greenwich, Connecticut, who also taught medicine at Columbia University's College of Physicians and Surgeons. Beaty told science writer Robert Houston that ten of the twenty underwent tumor regression. "All ten," he stated, "owe their very survival to Dr. Burton's treatment. . . . They also show tumor shrinkage, appetite improvement, weight gain, and loss of pain. I believe this is a breakthrough in the treatment of cancer—the single best frontier in cancer therapy today" (cited in Houston, 1979b).

A number of other individuals familiar with Burton's work concurred. One of these was Dr. R. J. Clement, president of the Bahamian Medical Association. Clement was born in England and studied at London's St. Thomas Hospital. He practiced medicine for five years before going to the Bahamas in 1965.

This physician spoke highly of Burton and his work. He claimed to see many of the American's patients for their non-cancer-related problems. "I'm all for it," he said, simply, in an interview. "I go by the patients I've seen." He then recounted many anecdotes of Burton's apparent success. "If I get cancer, I know where I'm going," he added (Clement, 1989). By the late 1980s Clement had become medical director of Burton's clinic, and had written a paper on the success of IAT in producing a number of unusual remissions in mesothelioma, an often deadly form of lung cancer (Clement, 1987).

Others complain that Burton's treatment is inordinately expensive. In 1978 Burton requested a $7,500 donation to his not-for-profit foundation, called Immunology Researching Centre, Ltd., before treatment could begin. In 1979 this was lowered to $300 for an evaluation, $2,220 for the first four weeks of therapy, and $300 for each week thereafter (Immunology Researching Centre, 1979). Today the costs are $5,000 for four weeks of therapy and $500 a week thereafter. Home maintenance is $50 for each week's supply of serum (IAT, 1987). Patients must also come with a companion and make their own living arrangements on the island. Burton justifies the expense by the cost of the treatment itself and the difficulty in obtaining research support (Burton, 1978).

Burton's most serious problem concerns publication or, rather, his lack of it. From 1956 to 1963 Burton and his colleagues published regularly in prestigious journals such as *Cancer Research, Science,* and the *Annals of the New York Academy of Sciences.* Between November 1962 and February 1963 they published four papers on their work and methods. At that point they began to experience great difficulty in getting their work published. After one last attempt to publish, in a South American pathology journal, Burton simply gave up in disgust on his critical colleagues. He has published nothing since that time.

In *Modern Medicine,* Burton invoked the authority of Dr. Sidney Farber, who had been one of the most prominent cancer chemotherapists, for his decision not to publish:

> We visited Sidney Farber at his laboratory, and he said, "Look, you're 10 to 20 years ahead of your time. You've got three options. First, you can keep repeating the same work over and over.
>
> "Or, second, you can keep rewriting and resubmitting your papers. Or, third, you can keep chopping wood—just keep working and forget what's going on around you." Contrary to what our peers would have advised, we chose the last one (cited in Yasgur, 1975).

Critics offered a less charitable explanation of Burton's reticence. "By nature he's secretive and paranoid," Rottino said. "His great fear was that other people would steal his ideas and he wouldn't get the credit for it" (Rottino, 1978). (A sign on the bulletin board in the Bahamas clinic at that time read "Even paranoids have enemies.")

Others maintain that Burton is less than candid about the way he derives his blood factors, that for all his apparent openness, there may be some secrets to the method Burton is reluctant to part with.

In the 1960s, for example, a prominent Israeli researcher sought to duplicate Burton's methods. According to one account,

> There were a few steps that puzzled him, but he thought it was an exceedingly interesting project and definitely worth pursuing. He even asked for a flow chart to try running their program in his own lab in Jerusalem (Anderson, 1974).

But Burton and Friedman refused to send him instructions for isolating the fractions of blood serum—apparently the key step in the whole process and the one most difficult to arrive at empirically. "What if something went wrong?" Burton asked. "We'd be hung without a trial" (ibid.).

Instead of staying in the United States, attempting to publish his ideas, and battling with the government—a process that would almost certainly take years—Burton attempted to shortcut the entire process by going to the Bahamas.

In the summer of 1978 Burton tried to gain the cooperation of the new director of the National Cancer Institute, Dr. Arthur Upton. Wealthy sponsors, he wrote, had agreed to put up $1 million for Burton to treat 1,000 patients. The patients would be chosen by NCI itself and certified by them to have advanced cases of cancer. They would then be sent to the Bahamas and after their treatment would return to NCI for evaluation. NCI-appointed scientists could then decide for themselves whether these patients had benefited from Burton's techniques.

But NCI rejected the offer, once again hammering at Burton's weak spot, his conspicuous lack of publications, especially relating to his clinical work. In a letter dated August 11, 1978, Upton replied:

> The question of collaboration is not as simple as it may appear. . . . In other words, we cannot force our intramural staff to work on a problem in which they have no interest.
>
> In order to determine possible interest, I believe it will be necessary for you to provide us with written reports of the studies already carried out . . . (Upton, 1978).

Almost a year later Upton confirmed his stand on Burton's proposal. "Since we have never received the reports of Dr. Burton's studies that I have requested, I would state that our position at this time is the same as it was one year ago. . . ." (Upton, 1979).

If NCI scientists had "no interest' in Burton's techniques, Sloan-Kettering researchers appeared to be working on a similar research project with great enthusiasm.

In 1977 Sloan-Kettering announced that it had assigned several of its most experienced researchers to investigate a substance called tumor necrosis factor (TNF). This was described as "a substance, derived from animal's blood, which has the ability to swiftly and dramatically destroy some animal tumors." They claimed it was discovered by accident at Sloan-Kettering in 1971. "One afternoon we injected this serum into mice growing transplants of Meth A tumors. When we walked into our laboratory the next morning, we couldn't believe our eyes. All the Meth A tumors had turned black, had just shriveled and died" (cited in Moss, 1977).

One of the two scientists who made this discovery was Robert Kassel, Ph.D., at the time a Sloan-Kettering researcher, but from 1953 to 1963 a member of Burton's team at St. Vincent's (ibid.).

In March 1979, amid much fanfare, another Sloan-Kettering researcher, Saul Green, Ph.D., announced the discovery of a similar substance in human blood. Green called this substance NHG, or normal human globulin. NHG destroyed human cancer cells in the test tube as well as human tumors growing in mice. Green made his announcement at the American Cancer Society's annual Science Writers' Seminar in Daytona Beach, Florida, and the discovery was promptly announced to the world and carried by the wire services and the tabloid *National Star* (April 17, 1979).

Green drew an enthusiastic picture of NHG's potential. If his experiments were correct, he said, and the human factor does have antitumor effect, then large-scale tests in humans would be justified. It also might be possible to increase the normal production of NHG by the liver, the apparent site of its synthesis. Also, a test might be devised to detect deficiencies of NHG in the blood of individuals with a high risk of developing cancer (Cameron/ Friedlander, 1979).

Shortly thereafter, Burton hired the public relations firm of Cameron/ Friedlander, Inc., Fort Lauderdale, to issue a press release on his work. Not surprisingly, the release claimed that "experimental evidence announced at an American Cancer Society seminar during March corroborates" Burton's work and that "Dr. Burton is now a man whose early work has been vindicated by this latest paper delivered by Dr. Green before the American Cancer Society seminar" (ibid.).

Some scientists would undoubtedly turn up their noses at a scientist who publishes through a press release. Burton's defenders charged, however, that Green also did not publish his work before announcing it, in dramatic fashion, at the American Cancer Society affair.*

Burton's work appeared to have reached an impasse. In the Bahamas, he may have had the freedom to treat cancer patients, but he was almost completely isolated from his scientific colleagues as well as the general public. Having been stung by what appeared to him to be unreasonable rejection in the past, he refused to publish his methods or his results on principle.

---

*Green subsequently left Sloan-Kettering. He has become scientific director of Emprise, Inc. and a leading crusader against Dr. Burton's methods (Green, 1989).

Although his facilities on the island were modern, it was questionable whether any single individual could develop both a new scientific concept and a methodology for treating cancer on his own. As Rottino explained,

> He can't see it through because he doesn't have the physical capabilities nor the knowledge of the basic sciences. He's a biologist, but the basic science is very deep and broad. No one man can encompass it all. You need a National Cancer Institute to take a concept like this and really go into it in depth (Rottino, 1978).

But the National Cancer Institute had "no interest" in the matter, as Dr. Upton said. Sloan-Kettering, on the other hand, while displaying no official interest in Burton's technique, pursued research projects strikingly similar in their basic concepts and goals.

Bad Blood: Lawrence Burton, Part Two

> "The stuff is junk. I wouldn't give it to a dog."
> —Dr. Gregory Curt, former NCI official

> "The purpose of 'exploiting the negatives' is to get everybody bloody-minded, purple in the face, and fighting mad by calling the other side very inferior citizens, not to say pimps, 'card-carrying members' of monstrous conspiracies, and human rats."
> —Russell Baker

On Sunday evening, May 18, 1980, tens of millions of viewers settled down to watch a "60 Minutes" presentation, "The Establishment vs. Dr. Burton." It was highly favorable. The ever-reasonable Harry Reasoner called Burton "a prickly, fiercely independent, rejected cancer researcher." He continued:

> Fifteen years ago . . . he believed immunology offered promise in treating cancer, but the leaders in cancer were convinced viruses were the answer. Now viruses are out, immunology is in, but Burton is still out, and out of the country.

With his first words Burton tried to put to rest the oft-repeated claim that he was promoting a cancer cure:

I don't think there's a cure. There is no such thing. We'd rather talk about a control. The patients control their own cancer, because the odds are it will return. . . . [It's] called a symbiotic relationship: The body is living with the cancer.''

Various physicians testified to the remarkable results they had seen in some of Burton's patients. A New York internist, for example, called one such case "a most incredible thing."

The author was interviewed and quoted as follows:

I'd say that the problem is basically in the cancer establishment's attitudes and interests rather than in Lawrence Burton himself. I think there's a tendency in the big places to think that they are going to find the cure for cancer, and to resent an upstart, such as a man from St. Vincent's or from the Bahamas, who tells them anything about cancer. The field itself has its own limitations built in, and people who go outside the limitations become the heretics and mavericks, such as Burton ("60 Minutes," 1980).

Shortly after the show, Burton changed the name of his treatment to Immuno-Augmentative Therapy, or IAT. This is because it is intended to "augment" the deficient immune system of cancer patients.

The "60 Minutes" interview generated a great deal of attention. There was a flurry of legislative activity on behalf of his method. In Washington, HR 7936 was introduced in the second session of the 96th Congress to exempt for five years the blood fractions used in IAT from the Federal Food, Drug, and Cosmetic Act. This would have taken his sera out of FDA's hands long enough to have them freely tested in the United States. The bill, however, was defeated.

The following year Florida House Bill Number 747, the Cancer Therapeutic Research Act of 1981, did pass, overriding the veto of Governor Robert Graham. This act authorized a Patient Qualification Review Board to permit "qualified" patients to obtain unconventional therapies for the "control and cure of cancer." (This act was repealed in 1984.)

On March 2, 1982, House Bill Number 1633 was passed in the State of Oklahoma House of Representatives. This specifically legalized the prescription and administration of IAT by licensed physicians for "the treatment of any malignancy, disease, illness, or physical condition," provided patients had signed a "written informed request." The act still stands, and there has been an ongoing effort, unsuccessful so far, to open an Oklahoma IAT clinic.

Lobbying and letter writing had an effect on the establishment as well. On December 1, 1982, Vincent DeVita, Jr., M.D., director of NCI, wrote to Burton asking for samples of his materials "in response to numerous inquiries that the National Cancer Institute continues to receive regarding the work carried out by your organization. I am hopeful," De Vita added, "that we can find a working arrangement for a clinical study that is acceptable to both of our institutions and benefits all cancer patients" (DeVita, 1982).

Five days later, at DeVita's request, Bruce A. Chabner, M.D., the director of NCI's Division of Cancer Treatment, also wrote to Burton. The tone was encouraging:

I would be interested in knowing whether you would like to participate in a collaborative effort to test the efficacy of the Burton therapy in a carefully conducted, prospective trial. Among various alternatives, we would consider the possibility of referring patients to your facility following NCI workup and then evaluating them here after their treatment (Chabner to Burton, December 6, 1982.)

For some reason DeVita's letter was sent unsigned, and Burton insisted on receiving a signed one before he would respond. When he did, it was on June 2, 1983, and was dictated through IAT Communications, Inc., Burton's support group in Olathe, Kansas. (Correspondence with the Bahamas is always difficult because of irregular mail service.)

Burton raised some technical points about the kind of trials proposed but quickly got down to his real objections. There had recently been a spate of attacks on him and his method, one of them by Richard Block (the *R* of the tax firm H&R Block) at a forum also addressed by Dr. DeVita himself. Burton asked the NCI Director, ". . . How am I supposed to stake my life's work, and our patients' hopes for continued success, on the integrity of people who (1) put Richard Block on a public podium in Palm Beach, Florida, to slanderously . . . refer to our therapy as blood washing; and (2) send Helene Brown to audiences and newspaper interviews to falsely, ignorantly, and slanderously imply that I am a 'quack' and that Immuno-Augmentative Therapy is a 'fake cure' and a 'fraud?' (Burton, 1983)

DeVita replied that "the Palm Beach Round Table put Mr. Block on the podium. He and I did not discuss our presentations. He certainly has earned the right to speak his mind on these issues. You apparently attribute any bit of adverse publicity you get to the National Cancer Institute." Helene Brown, also, "is not a member of the staff of the National Cancer

Institute and does not contact us before she makes appointments to speak.
. . . We should not let these issues get in the way of a detailed discussion
of what it is you use, how you prepare it, and how we might go about
setting up a clinical trial" (DeVita, June 13, 1983).

DeVita's tone was reasonable; Burton's unpleasant. Yet one wonders
what DeVita's response would have been if an NCI colleague had been
similarly vilified at a public forum as a "blood-washing" fraud. His very
silence in the face of this quack-baiting seemed, to Burton, to indicate DeVita's
secret complicity with his friend Richard Block. (Block, a lung cancer patient, was a chief supporter of the PDQ computerized cancer information
system for physicians, one of DeVita's pet projects while at NCI. See *Washington Post,* August 10, 1988.)

On June 22, 1983, Burton wrote the director of the NCI that he found
his letter "extremely evasive and regrettably unscientific. In order to put an
end to the political charade, no further communication with you can continue until you personally, not a staff member, answer my previous letter's
questions punctually, factually, and succinctly." It was the kind of reply
that makes a public-relations person cringe. But Burton was not doing PR.
He was addressing himself—in the only way he knew how—to what he felt
was the underlying *reality* of NCI's proposal. The price for naiveté could be
the death of his lifelong quest. He had seen how the establishment had
treated other unconventional therapists. Not surprisingly, Dr. DeVita did not
write back.

One of the many who saw the "60 Minutes" broadcast was a Long
Island businessman named Irwin Peck. Some time later a close relative developed cancer and was specifically told by doctors not to go to Freeport.
Peck became intrigued. He contacted both Burton and NCI and was dis-
mayed to learn that negotiations had broken down.

"Being a private citizen and a layman," he wrote in an open letter to
both sides, "my intent and suggested program may seem presumptuous. I
see no other way, however, to try to foment movement. . . . My conclusion is that only a bold course will prove of value" (Peck, open letter of
July 11, 1983).

Peck volunteered to play honest broker. There followed over a year of
letters and lengthy phone calls back and forth to Bethesda and Freeport.
Burton eventually authorized Peck to be his legal representative in the negotiations, and for a while it appeared that real progress was being made.
An agreement was drawn up, Burton gave his verbal assent, and Peck read
it to NCI's Gregory Curt over the phone. According to Peck, Curt's reaction
was, "The agreement will be difficult to live with, but if we want to evaluate IAT we will have to live with it."

But NCI refused to sign. In fact, after February 1984 there was a decided toughening in NCI's tone. The earlier letters had been, on the whole, conciliatory. Yet suddenly all sorts of querulous complaints were raised on the government's side.

Peck was reluctantly forced to conclude that the difficulties were the result of NCI intransigence. Seeing the abrupt change, he wrote Curt:

> It is my opinion that you are under pressure from your superiors. It is further my opinion that you are a man of open mind and good will, and would, as an individual, help lead the way to an evaluation of IAT. Unfortunately, it has become apparent that you cannot do that.
>
> Every solid effort for evaluation has come from Dr. Burton's camp—and it continues this way. He is in earnest.
>
> We have brought this so close to fruition, yet the NCI continues to waltz away by sheer repetition of issues already obviated. . . . The charade indeed must stop. Is IAT of value? Do you wish to find out? The means is being provided, intelligently and fairly. . . . There is nothing more we can do—and NCI can do no less than proceed (April 9, 1984).

But NCI showed no intention of proceeding. In fact, the whole negotiating process quickly broke down. NCI denied Peck's charges, putting all the responsibility for the failure on Burton. NCI had apparently decided that the agreement was not something that they could, or would, live with.

While Dr. Curt was negotiating in seemingly good faith with Peck, he also was preparing a statement on Burton for the Birmingham, Alabama, Cancer Information Center. Despite his apparent openness during the negotiations, this statement was a rehash of the same old charges—Burton failed to publish, failed to cooperate, etc.

In addition, behind Burton's back NCI had gotten hold of "four samples of IAT blood fractions that were obtained from a physician in the United States":

> The fractions were found to be dilutions of proteins normally found in human serum, the clear portion of the blood that remains after the blood cells have been removed. The principal protein in these samples was albumin, which is found in many plant and animal tissues (directive of April 24, 1984, approved by Dr. G. Curt, April 16, 1984).

Curt finished his statement with a plea for patients to visit his own institution instead of that of Lawrence Burton:

> The NCI strongly urges cancer patients to remain in the care of qualified physicians who utilize proven methods of treatment. . . . Patients interested in experimental forms of treatment should ask their physicians to determine whether they are eligible for one of the clinical trials supported by the NCI or other medical institutions (ibid.).

Since these samples came to NCI in an unauthorized manner, there was no way of knowing whether they were in fact identical to what Burton was using. And since IAT serum had to be kept frozen until use, the materials in question may have decomposed before analysis (Houston, 1988).

Most importantly, in April, while negotiations were proceeding, NCI was quietly developing a set of charges about the alleged contamination of Burton's sera by microorganisms (Curt, 1986).

In June 1984 Dr. Chabner gave an interview to the *Cancer Letter*, an industry newsletter, which was similarly hostile to Burton. Peck's efforts at conciliation were over. He wrote—but never sent—a letter to Dr. Curt which summed up his feelings:

> The record is now complete. The NCI attitude toward, and resistance to, Dr. Burton and IAT have remained unchanged since the '70s. Our telephone conversations of June 1, 1984, and your directive of April 24, have closed the circle . . . (Peck, July 15, 1984).

From the time of this breakdown of communication, NCI and its allies followed a different approach. From a tactical point of view, it was brilliant—so brilliant, in fact, that within one year Burton's entire operation would be thrown into a state of total disarray.

The intervening years had only strengthened the case for immune augmentation. The idea that the body had its own defenses against cancer lay behind Coley's toxins. It was also the basis of the notorious Krebiozen, a serum driven out of use by the concerted effort of the American Medical Association and its allies (Bailey, 1958).

At Sloan-Kettering, researchers working under Lloyd Old pretreated mice with *Bacillus Calmette-Guérin* (BCG) and then injected them with lipopolysaccharide (LPS). The result was a dramatic destruction of tumor in the mouse, due to the action of tumor necrosis factor (TNF) (Carswell et al., 1975). This discovery led to the removal of Coley's toxins from the ACS *Unproven Methods* list, where it had languished for ten years (1965–75).

In 1978 three officials of M. D. Anderson Hospital and Tumor Institute declared that immunotherapy, "now in its eariiest stages of development, should be considered the fourth modality of cancer treatment" (cited in Ward, 1988a).

In 1981 NCI created the Biological Response Modifier Program due to "a combination of intense political pressure and scientific readiness" (ibid.). These substances, which include TNF, interferon, interleukin-2 (IL-2), and various other agents, became the hottest research topic at NCI and the object of almost frenzied interest on Wall Street.

In 1982 Helen Nauts reported that in a randomized trial of Coley's toxins (now called mixed bacterial vaccine, or MBV) at Memorial Sloan-Kettering, advanced non-Hodgkin's lymphoma patients receiving MBV had a 93 percent remission rate, as opposed to 29 percent for controls receiving chemotherapy alone (Nauts, 1982:8–9).

In May 1988 Lloyd Old outlined the history of immunotherapy in a cover story on tumor necrosis factor in *Scientific American*. Old ended his article eloquently:

> We are just beginning. If we are fortunate, the new treatments will consistently arouse the body's natural anticancer forces and produce the tumor regressions that have fueled the imagination of generations of cancer researchers. The forces exist; the task ahead is to find ways to unleash them (Old, 1988).

Not surprisingly, there is no mention of Burton in this or in any of the other articles. Once again Burton has claimed that this work is derived from his own—carried from his laboratory to Old's when Dr. Kassel moved to Sloan-Kettering in 1963. He believes that tumor necrosis factor is practically identical with his own tumor antibody, one of the four substances he uses in the diagnosis and treatment of cancer (Burton, 1988).

Be that as it may, the fact is that by the mid-eighties the *kind* of work Burton was doing had become quite respectable. TNF and other biological modifiers had begun to be produced in large quantities by several biotechnology companies, including Genentech, Inc. and Biogen S.A. (Old, 1988).

On a theoretical level, by 1985 Burton found himself practically in the mainstream of thinking—except he had had twenty years experience *treating* cancer patients with immunotherapy. But from another point of view Burton also became more dangerous, since he now had direct competitors at powerful, major centers.

In mid-1985, Steven Rosenberg, M.D., a researcher at the National

Cancer Institute, began treating cancer patients with interleukin-2. To Burton partisans, the procedure sounded suspiciously similar to the multistep approach of IAT. As described in a front-page article, entitled "Cancer Breakthrough," in *Fortune:*

> Rosenberg's secret is to give patients massive doses of an immune system activator called interleukin-2, IL-2 for short, together with a patient's own activated cancer-killing cells. He first withdraws about 10 percent of a patient's white blood cells and mixes them with IL-2. Then he injects the cells and large doses of IL-2 back into the patient. The IL-2 multiples the killer cells in the patient's body, which start attacking the tumor (November 1985).

To proceed with testing such substances as IL-2 requires willing patients to take part in NCI clinical trials. Getting such patients is one of the most difficult tasks for NCI, however, since patients fear they are merely guinea pigs in the researchers' game (see DeVita interview, *Washington Post,* August 10, 1988). In addition, IL-2 is toxic. Side effects include fever, chills, malaise, and sometimes a swelling of the spleen (*Fortune,* November 1985). Patients experience fluid retention "that can cause them to gain 10 percent or more of their body weight and may result in fluid accumulation in the lungs." Moreover,

> One patient . . . apparently died as a result of the therapy, although the individual had widely disseminated melanoma.
> The death was not mentioned either in the *New England Journal* report or in a press "update" sent out by NCI's Office of Cancer Communication (*Science,* December 20, 1985).

Burton's treatment is virtually free of side effects. And every patient gets the experimental therapy—not a placebo or a dose of traditional chemotherapy. From NCI's point of view, IAT was siphoning off seventy to eighty patients a week, those daring patients who were willing to undergo experimental therapy. It thus presented a serious competitive challenge to NCI, which cannot proceed without human subjects for its Phase II trials.*

Unable to bring Burton himself into the process of prolonged clinical trials, NCI officials began to make moves to put him out of business entirely.

*For explanation of "Phase II" see footnote on page 324.

The Bahamas are only fifty miles from Florida; but in Freeport, with its palm trees, casinos, and postcolonial airs, the frenzy of American cancer politics sometimes seemed nonexistent—a distant rumble.

On July 2, 1985, a small delegation from the Centers for Disease Control (CDC), the Pan-American Health Organization (PAHO), and the Bahamian Health Ministry showed up at Lawrence Burton's clinic in Freeport. They stayed a matter of minutes, but the exchange was acerbic. Through the closed door of the conference room, patients could hear the shouting.

Two weeks later, on Wednesday, July 17, the results of this visit appeared in the Miami *Herald*. The news was not good. A mood of apprehension hung over the low-lying clinic across the road from the Rand Memorial Hospital. Rumors of an impending, if unspecified, disaster were in the air.

On the 19th it became clear what was happening. When patients appeared for their 7 A.M. "blood pulls," the routine diagnostic test that preceded each day's therapy, they were told that "the Doctor" wanted to talk to them.

Normally Burton remained ensconced in his office, puzzling over a mass of patient data on two linked computer screens—reclusive as the Wizard of Oz. (On the rare occasions he did appear, the bearded immunologist risked a mob scene. Everyone wanted fresh information on the most important case in the world; others simply wanted to express their thanks.) Above his office desk was a hand-drawn cartoon of a feisty mouse, a.k.a. Lawrence Burton, holding up his middle finger to an ACS eagle. The eagle, terrified at this exorcism, was frantically trying to reverse direction midstream.

That morning, the eagle had finally landed—on him. Normally a voluble raconteur, Burton was ashen and at a loss for words. He soberly announced that he had received an order from the Bahamian health authority directing him to padlock the clinic doors and not allow any treatment until further notice. The charge: contaminating patients with AIDS and hepatitis.

The warning was dramatic. The night before, a police car had shown up at Burton's house. Island constables, their eerie blue lights flashing, had driven him to the Freeport jail and shown him the lock-up. Three or four reprobates stared out from a cell so small they could sleep only by taking turns. "That's where you're going," the police chief told the bearded New York scientist, "if you defy this order and try to treat patients."

Burton was shaken. For five years things had been looking up, and life in Freeport had become quite pleasant. Although the focus of his life was still the esoteric branch of immunotherapy he had developed, he had learned how to enjoy himself. He had come through a messy divorce and found a new love, an eternally grateful brain cancer patient named Betty Abernathy. For several years, in fact, there had been signs of a new attitude from the National Cancer Institute, including friendly letters from its director. But now Burton's life work stood on the brink of extinction.

Other alternative clinicians hired top lawyers and lobbyists to defend them at the slightest hint of trouble. But Burton himself, his doctors, and clinic workers were so thunderstruck when the closure order came that no one even called NCI or PAHO to find out exactly what was happening. Details of the order finally appeared July 19 in the *Freeport News*, a daily newspaper on Grand Bahama Island. There were 98 IAT patients in Freeport at the time; for weeks the front-page stories in the *News* were their main source of information.

Burton's clinic, the paper reported, had been declared a serious health hazard. Patient serum was contaminated with AIDS (HIV, formerly called HTLV-III) and hepatitis B viruses.

In addition, the papers repeated 1984 charges that patients were subject to an exotic infection called nocardia at the injection puncture sites.

The AIDS charge hit particularly hard. The summer of 1985 was when the world finally woke up to AIDS. On the same day as the shutdown, Rock Hudson collapsed at his home in Los Angeles and was rushed to Paris for treatments. His agonizing decline was the lead item on the evening news. "Just the possibility that Rock Hudson had AIDS electrified the nation," wrote Randy Shilts in *And the Band Played On*. "Suddenly, all the newscasts and newspapers were running stories about the disease" (Shilts, 1987).

The very word *AIDS* struck terror into the patients who, day after day, had been injecting themselves with what they were now told was contaminated serum. Many patients assumed that in addition to their manifold problems, they now had AIDS as well. Lester Maddox, former governor of Georgia, was a Burton patient at the time. "I'd rather go with straight cancer than AIDS," he told reporters. "There's more dignity with cancer" (ibid.).

The closing of a clinic because of HIV contamination was unprecedented. John Clement, M.D., who had become medical director of the IAT clinic, testified:

> I know of no other instance of the closing of a clinic, hospital, or blood bank in this manner; in similar instances, the institutions are simply informed of the problem, they correct it, and go on (Molinari, 1986).

After years of neglect, Burton was suddenly besieged by reporters. But almost without exception, the coverage was hostile. The New York *Daily News*, the largest-circulation paper in the country, informed its readers that Lawrence Burton was a "snake oil" salesman, a "zoologist" who was "not even a horse doctor." It was no secret that Burton had a Ph.D. in experimental zoology from New York University. This was a proper degree for the kind of research he was trained to perform. But some in the media used this fact to sow confusion in the public mind about zoology—linking it to zoos and veterinary science. Burton became hostile to all reporters, including those who had previously been friendly to him.

One of those present when the clinic was closed was Frank Wiewel, a 35-year-old recording engineer from Otho, Iowa. That mild description hardly does justice to his forceful personality. For years Frank had been a passionate rock-and-roller, the lead singer with bands that toured the Midwest ballrooms. John Lennon was his hero and music was his life. He had just signed a multirecord deal with CBS Records and seemed poised for the big time. Suddenly all that went by the wayside. Something in Frank was ignited by the Burton closure. The edge of a heavy curtain seemed to have been lifted. Something was happening that he didn't understand, but he intended to find out!

Frank was in Freeport accompanying his father-in-law, Robert Dallman, who had colon cancer, one of those malignancies with which Burton claimed a good rate of success. Out of the blue, Robert was cut off from his last-remaining form of treatment. A hastily scrawled sign on the door of the clinic informed patients that the center was closed until further notice. The two floundered around the next morning, talking in sober terms about an unseen conspiracy but unsure of what to do.

Once inspired, Frank is a man of tremendous determination. He began staying up night after night with his wife, Denise, with Burton, with patients, with anyone else he could find—talking, talking, talking. He "talks about cancer care with the fervor of a TV evangelist," the *Des Moines Register* later said (January 25, 1988). The phrase, however, hardly captures the earnest sincerity that even some of his opponents acknowledge.

Burton, a secular Jew, seemed to view this attack from the perspective of two thousand years of persecution. A knife in the back was no less than he expected. Wiewel, however, had a Midwesterner's directness in dealing with the government and a young person's optimism. He and Denise demanded answers. They acted with an implicit belief that because they were citizens, public officials worked for *them*. Why was the clinic closed? What would be needed to reopen it? When would the patients get their medicines again? They demanded answers.

Just before the closure, Frank and Denise had packed their bags for a return to the States. Frank now decided to stay with Robert at Lafayette Gardens, the ramshackle apartments where many of the 98 IAT patients in

Freeport at the time lived. Denise went home, and on the following Monday she was on the phone with all the principal players mentioned in the July 17 *Herald* article: Dr. Gregory Curt of NCI, Ronald St. John of the Pan-American Health Organization (PAHO), and Dr. Curran of the Centers for Disease Control. Curran, she says, was fairly neutral and nonjudgmental, but when she was finished talking to Deputy Director Curt she was "scared to death." Her own dad was taking "tainted" serum!

"These are convincing people," she told Frank by phone that night.

If the patients were in a panic, Burton was gloomy. A particular problem was his wife Betty. She had been diagnosed at the Mayo Clinic with brain cancer and given one to six months to live. In an act of desperation she had come to Burton, who at first refused to take her because she was so far gone. Nevertheless, he agreed to allow Dr. Weinberg to treat her. That was 1980, and she had made a remarkable recovery. (Betty's story, along with those of many other "best cases," has been detailed in the book *Diagnosis: Cancer—Prognosis: Life* by Jane Riddle Wright.) Burton was afraid she would relapse, however, if she did not get her shots. Late at night he would sneak into the darkened laboratory and, risking imprisonment, prepare medications for Betty and other critically ill patients.*

Further word on the status of the clinic would have to come from Bahama's prime minister, Lynden O. Pindling, or from his minister of health, Dr. Norman Gay. To facilitate this, Burton and his clinic head, Dr. Clement, met with Dr. Gay while a few of Dr. Burton's supporters flew to the capital in Nassau to meet with Pindling. The Prime Minister refused to see them. Another time they tried to see the long-time leader at an election rally in Freeport, but there was an assassination scare and he was bundled into a waiting car and whisked away.

All the while, Burton and his supporters were trying to make some sense out of the charges.

There *had* been an outbreak of nocardia infection in 1984. In fact, Burton himself had asked CDC's help in locating its source. Fifteen patients had become infected with the bacteria at their injection sites; all of them recovered, but it was disturbing. CDC had come but had been unable to root out the problem. Eventually Burton's staff had surmised that the source had to be the air vents connecting the clinic to the Rand Hospital. And so the old IAT clinic was shut down and a new one was built across the street. Each room in the new clinic had its own separate air system. There had been no subsequent incidents of this type of infection in over a year. The authorities were therefore rehashing a solved problem for political reasons.

*Betty Abernathy died of cancer while on a visit to Alabama in June, 1989.

The charge of widescale hepatitis contamination, too, proved exaggerated. The alarm first surfaced in 1984 when Dr. Curt published a letter in the *New England Journal of Medicine* alleging that the serum issued to four patients at the IAT clinic in Freeport had tested positive for antibodies to hepatitis B. No further specifics were provided.

If true, this was certainly a matter of concern, but hardly something over which one normally shuts a clinic.

A definitive article by the government's Centers for Disease Control, published in September 1985, put the matter in perspective. It reveals that an estimated 200,000 Americans, mostly young adults, are infected with hepatitis B each year. Although this disease is responsible for over 5,000 deaths annually, most cases are not serious, contrary to popular opinion (Gong, 1986). There are 500,000 to one million infectious carriers in the United States. And five percent of the U.S. population—one in twenty persons—will get the infection in the course of a lifetime (CDC, 1985).

Hepatitis B virus has contaminated much of the U.S. blood supply and blood products, not just IAT serum. For example, the CDC notes that "tests of immune globulin lots prepared since 1977 indicate that both types of antibody [to hepatitis A and B] have been uniformly present" (ibid.).

The exposure level in foreign countries, especially in the Third World, are much higher. "Travelers to developing countries may be at significant risk of infection," the government warns (ibid.). In some parts of the world "most persons acquire the infection at birth or during childhood," and 5 to 15 percent are active carriers. Where hepatitis B is only "moderately endemic," 1 to 4 percent of persons are virus carriers (ibid.).

In eleven years the CDC reported only two cases of hepatitis B among Burton's 3,000-plus patients. That would seem to be a remarkable record of safety, rather than failure (IATPA, October 1988).

A few months after Curt's letter appeared, however, a copy came to the attention of one of Burton's patients, Mary Anna Good of Tacoma, Washington. Frightened at the prospect of contracting hepatitis from her cancer treatment, she brought eighteen vials of the serum (her own and that of several other IAT patients) to the Tacoma–Pierce County Blood Bank for testing.

Dr. Sam Insalaco, medical director of the Tacoma–Pierce County Blood Bank, and Dr. Gale Katterhagen, director of oncology at the Tacoma Hospital tested the vials. According to the two Tacoma doctors, *all* of these samples were positive for hepatitis antibodies. Since the vials originated in the Caribbean, an allegedly high-risk area for AIDS, the doctors decided to also test them for AIDS antibodies: eight out of the 18 samples tested positive (Null and Steinman, 1986).

After these results were confirmed by the state laboratory in Olympia, Washington, Dr. Katterhagen, a member of the select National Cancer Advisory Board (NCAB), contacted both NCI and the Centers for Disease Control (CDC) in Atlanta. CDC in turn contacted PAHO, which helps oversee Caribbean health matters. It was their negative report on the clinic July 2, 1985, that led to the closure two weeks later.

In the face of this barrage of criticism, by August 1985 it seemed as if the clinic might never open again. But IAT's defenders were busy doing their homework. Probing with research, taped telephone interviews, and Freedom-of-Information revelations, they were able to refute nearly every charge originally presented to the world. In fact, when they were done there was not much left of NCI's case.

"The more we questioned them the more threadbare their story became," Wiewel reflected. "And the more threads we pulled, the more it came apart" (Wiewel, 1988). In the end, they were able to show that

(1) There had been no confirmed reports of IAT toxicity.
(2) There had been no reported cases of AIDS in IAT patients.
(3) There had been no reported cases of HIV antibody in IAT patients.
(4) There had been only two cases of hepatitis B reported by CDC in eleven years of IAT (IATPA, October, 1988).

No one has ever gotten seriously ill from taking IAT treatment. Cassileth (1987) reported that three percent of patients reported side effects and that most of these were minor or transitory. This is certainly an extraordinary record of safety for an anticancer drug.

As for AIDS and HIV, it turned out there was no factual basis to the charge that people were getting infected. When the clinic closed, fifty-six Burton patients volunteered to be tested during the period of the closure, including Mrs. Good (now deceased) in Tacoma whose questions had originally triggered the government action. None of these 56 came up positive for the HIV antibody, much less AIDS itself (Molinari, 1986).

This was confirmed by an October 1, 1985, IAT Patients' Association patient survey. In addition, four Canadian patients submitted their sera for HIV testing to the Canadian Centers for Disease Control in Ottawa. All these samples were also found to be negative (letter from IAT patient Mark Scanlon to IATPA, October 1985).

By January, 1988, even Helen Sheehan of the Committee on Unproven Methods of the American Cancer Society had to admit there was no evidence of confirmed AIDS cases among Burton's patients (*Des Moines Register,* January 25, 1988).

But as Burton's patients probed more deeply, they discovered even more shocking facts. It was hardly preposterous to suppose that some of Burton's blood sera were, in fact, positive for HIV antibodies. By 1985 such contamination was widespread in the U.S. blood supply and had led to numerous cases of full-fledged AIDS through transfusions.

Just how widespread the danger was emerged in February of the following year. At that time a letter in the *Journal of the American Medical Association* revealed that people who had received gamma globulin shots could test positive for HIV antibodies, even if they never became infected. As *USA Today* explained,

> Gamma globulin is made from blood collected from thousands of donors and is routinely given to millions each year as temporary protection against many infectious diseases. If just one donor has AIDS antibodies, the entire pool will test positive (February 7, 1986).

Although millions of people might have been affected, officials of the Food and Drug Administration's Blood and Blood Products Division did not release this information because "we thought it would do more harm than good, since we saw no risk to the public health whatsoever." The reason they saw no risk was that "in making gamma globulin, the AIDS virus itself is killed" (ibid.)

The mere presence of HIV antibodies was, by FDA's own admission, not something to worry about, since virtually the entire blood supply was contaminated with it. Why then the special treatment for IAT?

It is even more startling to find out, then, that the test results for Burton's sera were actually *negative* for HIV antibodies!

As most people are now aware, the test for HIV is twofold. First the blood is screened with an ELISA (enzyme-linked immunosorbent assay) test. If this proves positive, it is followed up with a more accurate test called the Western Blot. This is necessary because "the ELISA tests are not perfect: in populations with a low incidence of infection, the proportion of false positives (positive results in people who do not have antibodies against [the virus]) is relatively high" (Nichols, 1986). People who have received blood transfusions and women who have had several pregnancies "may have a false positive reaction to the ELISA test," according to another standard text (Gong, 1986:10). No reputable doctor would diagnose a patient as HIV-positive on the basis of just an ELISA test.

The ELISA tests on the Burton sera were only marginally positive. Lab reports of the Pierce County Blood Bank of Tacoma, obtained under the Freedom of Information Act by Washington attorney Bill Casselman read, "None of these are strong positives, only C-1 has any real strength and it's only .3 above the cutoff."

More significantly, the obligatory Western Blot follow-ups were *all negative*. The Western Blot test sheet even referred to the results as " a lot of junk" (Wiewel in Molinari, 1986). These were unguarded comments by the people actually performing the tests and, since they had to be obtained through FOIA, were never meant to be seen by outside observers.

Months later, after this data became public, even Burton's nemesis, Dr. Curt, reversed himself and acknowledged publicly, "We can't say it's a positive test" *(Birmingham News,* November 7, 1985). Similarly, Dr. Harold Jaffe of the CDC called the results "confusing and impossible to interpret" (Wiewel in Molinari, 1986). The JAMA report on IAT calls them "uninterpretable" (Immuno-augmentative, 1988). But all this backtracking took place *after* the damage had been done and the general public had been convinced that IAT spread AIDS.

It also seems significant that CDC made no effort to trace the distribution of the serum or to impound existing supplies. These are routine measures taken to prevent or control epidemics *(Health Consciousness,* August 1986). By failing to do so, said supporters, they "declared the absence of the very hazard that Dr. Curt used to obtain IAT clinic closure" (Link, 1985).

In fact, CDC seemed to lose enthusiasm for the case as time went on. In conversation with Frank Wiewel, CDC's Dr. Jaffe said, "I would not suggest testing the serum because it's very difficult to interpret the results. We can't tell people to take this stuff [i.e., IAT] or not. We just want people to be aware of a possible risk." Then he added as a personal aside, "Now it may be if I had terminal cancer, it might be more important to me to continue this therapy. I just can't say."

Since the twofold antibody test was turning up negative, CDC three weeks later attempted to culture the virus. If HIV could actually be grown from samples, this would be a more definitive proof of its presence.

CDC faced a procedural problem. The process for culturing HIV from blood was well-known. But IAT serum was not a substance normally tested, and the procedures CDC used for doing so are still not clear. Significantly, out of all the materials tested, in the end they were able to culture HIV from only one sample.

In a phone conversation with Curry Hutchinson of the IAT Patients' Association (IATPA), Dr. Donald Barreth of CDC is quoted as having said:

> The CDC doesn't know the magnitude of the situation. One out of nine vials has been found to contain the virus. It is not unusual to find AIDS virus in blood or blood products. If you look for it, you're probably going to find it when you look at a number of samples like that *(Health Consciousness,* August 1986).

A definitive test at CDC would have strongly bolstered NCI's case. Without the strong support of the government's own disease-controlling agency, there was little basis for shutting down Burton's clinic in the name of public health. Yet CDC was not impressed with the test results and refused to line up behind NCI's crusade. Instead, it sensibly declared that it was unable to make a risk assessment based on the finding of HIV in a single sample.

On August 12, 1985, Dr. Curt wrote to CDC's Dr. Jaffe, "I wonder whether you might reconsider your decision not to follow up on your discovery more vigorously." But CDC hung tough. IAT patients saw Curt's letter as a possible "attempt to coerce the CDC to assign a risk factor consistent with his own hysterical proclamations" *(Health Consciousness,* August 1986).

Just as the case against Burton was falling apart, however, the clinic sustained another direct propaganda hit. Virginia H. Knauer, Special Adviser to President Reagan for Consumer Affairs, spoke to the National Health Fraud Conference on September 11, 1985. Referring to the IAT Clinic, she said:

> This clinic was finally closed by the Bahamian government this past July and is being held accountable by many health professionals for at least several hundred cases of AIDS worldwide (Knauer, 1985).

Again the story was carried far and wide. Lawrence Burton, quack and horse doctor, was now Lawrence Burton, human rat—a kind of "typhoid Larry" of mythic proportions, spreading the most dreaded disease around the globe.

It was nonsense, of course, but the damage was incalculable. Where did Knauer get her information? From Feena McLaverty, her research analyst. She in turn told a Congressman Molinari staff member, Ed Burke, that Dr. Gregory Curt had actually reviewed the speech in question before Knauer gave it to the quack-busting conference in September (Molinari, 1986).

A single contaminated specimen, analyzed by methods unknown, became an international incident—"hundreds of cases worldwide"! One questionable sample, and an entire clinic is shut down, patients' lives are lost, thousands are thrown into a panic, and millions are dissuaded from seeking alternative treatments for cancer.

In the words of science writer Patrick M. McGrady, Jr. (son of the ACS official who first "discovered" Burton in 1965), this whole episode was a skillful "disinformation campaign" on the part of U.S. medical authorities to discredit an unconventional competitor (ibid.). The charges continued to be repeated long after they had been refuted. Mention Burton to the average doctor today and you are likely to get a lecture on AIDS. NCI may not be able to find a cure for cancer but they have certainly learned the art of medical politics. AIDS contamination was a tar baby, which stuck to IAT long after the charges themselves were refuted.

During the period of the closure, approximately sixty of Burton's patients died. Of course, many of these might have died even with uninterrupted treatment. But according to supporters, this was "an historically unprecedented rate of mortality," which they ascribed to "patients being denied full IAT clinic services" and "exacerbated stress borne of fear . . . associated with AIDS publicity . . ." (Health Consciousness, August 1986). Robert Dallman, Denise Wiewel's father, succumbed to his colon cancer during the period of the closure. He had thrived on the treatment but, Denise says, his condition began to deteriorate when the clinic was closed and he had to leave.

Although the patients energetically organized an underground network so that the serum was kept available to all, blood testing was not available to them. In addition, the psychological shock of the shutdown was enormous, which may have affected the mortality rate. This raises an interesting point about the psychosocial dimensions of Burton's therapy.

It is often said that any benefits of Burton's treatment are simply the result of the warm, inviting climate and relaxed atmosphere in the Bahamas. "Fun in the sun" is the usual derogatory dismissal.

Certainly, anyone who has experienced traditional cancer treatment knows how bleak it can be. One doctor has called Memorial Hospital's outpatient facilities "worse than the disease" (Goodell, 1989). "It's like a subway station in there," said a patient. "You feel like you've been buried alive" (ibid.). A stateside cancer clinic can resemble the scene in *Moby Dick* where the whalers and their families attend church services just before the sailing of the *Pequod*. "Each silent worshipper," Melville writes, "seemed purposely sitting apart from the other, as if each silent grief were insular and incommunicable."

Cancer puts an enormous burden on those afflicted and on their family members and caregivers. In one survey, 90 percent of the caregivers reported "psychoemotional burdens" (Mor et al., 1987). Family members have been known to desert their loved ones because of the hopelessness of the situation.

By contrast, the waiting room at the IAT clinic is like a party. To a large degree, patients have organized themselves for their own cure. A strong feeling of camaraderie seems to bind these people together. They have chosen a difficult course which involves taking responsibility for their own bodies. In doing so, they feel they have broken away from the inevitable path of disease, dismemberment, and death. If the mind can affect the outcome of cancer, this very atmosphere would seem to be therapeutic. As one of the rules of the clinic is that the patient must come with a companion, few feel abandoned. In her study of IAT and other alternatives, Barrie Cassileth wrote:

> This study shows that many patients receiving alternative care do not conform to the traditional stereotype of poorly educated, terminally ill patients who have exhausted conventional treatment. . . . Contemporary alternatives, unlike the pills and potions of the past, are long-term, lifestyle-oriented options that exist within a broad view of health and personal responsibility. Patients welcome the self-care role and the concomitant responsibility to attain health . . . (Cassileth, 1984).

In IAT, patients do their own injecting of serum. (Initially Burton had physicians do this but found the results were better when patients did it themselves.) In this and in other ways they are made active participants in their own treatment. This sharply contrasts to traditional, "allopathic" medicine, in which the patient is told to be almost entirely passive. In fact, the very word *patient* means one who suffers passively, without complaining. In orthodox medicine, it is the doctor who is heroic.

This is not to idealize Burton. There is no awareness of the role of tobacco, diet, or other environmental factors in his therapy. (The man himself smokes a pipe almost incessantly.) There is also a tendency among his patients to form a "cult of personality" around the mesmerizing scientist. But by and large they are brought into the healing process as participants. For this reason it was possible for patients to rally to his defense, because they truly felt that by doing so, they were rallying to their own defense as well.

Within days of the shutdown, IAT patients in Freeport and New York City began to form a patients' organization. In Freeport they took over an old motel room as makeshift headquarters, coordinating ideas for reopening the clinic. Eventually two businessmen-patients, Jack Link and A. T. La-Prade, as well as Nat Owen, the husband of patient Janet Owen, founded the IAT Patients' Association (IATPA) as a tax-exempt, public-benefit corporation.

In August 1985 they marched on Washington. Led by Board Member Joan Wickham, they lobbied Congress, demanding help. Simultaneously, legal proceedings were begun against the U.S. Department of Health and Human Services (parent agency of both NCI and FDA), aimed at compelling it to help reopen the clinic (IATPA, May 1988).

The patients got a warm reception on Capitol Hill. Representatives, like their constituents, also get cancer. And many have become frustrated by the snail's pace of progress against the disease. Others are concerned over the erosion of personal freedom, forcefully demonstrated by the closure of this unconventional clinic.

One of the Representatives who was especially responsive was Guy V. Molinari of Staten Island, New York. He had learned about Burton's treatments from Elaine Boies, a reporter for the Staten Island *Advance,* whose husband Jack was treated by Burton in 1984–85.

Jack, a college English teacher, died of metastatic prostate cancer in early 1985, but before he died he experienced an "amazing improvement" (Boies, 1988).

He had arrived in Freeport in a wheelchair. After a few weeks, as Elaine tells it, "He got rid of the wheelchair, and started using a cane. Then he got rid of the cane and would just walk holding on to me. And one day he kind of pushed me away and said, 'I don't need you.' " He had become fully ambulatory.

"There was no question that Jack lived longer than traditional medicine here expected him to," she asserted (ibid.). Despite her husband's demise, Boies remained an enthusiastic and articulate supporter of IAT. Just before the shutdown she wrote a series of articles for the *Advance* on their experiences.

Molinari listened to such stories and promised the patients that he would visit the clinic to investigate. "I was not espousing Burton's therapy at this point," Molinari said, "but was approaching it simply on a humanitarian basis" (Molinari, 1986).

Molinari travelled to the Bahamas on August 13, 1985—less than a month after the closure—to meet with Bahamian officials. Although he had followed State Department protocols for a visiting U.S. Congressperson, the Bahamians categorically refused to discuss the IAT clinic with him. He visited the shut-down center, however, to meet patients and Dr. Burton, and came away favorably impressed.

"After all," he said, "if patients were terminally ill from cancer and their doctors told them there was nothing further that could be done for them, then they should be allowed to pursue that last hope, whether the treatment worked or not" (ibid.).

On December 5, 1985, Congressman Molinari said in a statement to the House of Representatives:

> I visited the Burton clinic four months ago at the request of dozens of cancer patients around the country. . . . Many of these patients were diagnosed as terminally ill and evidenced some dramatic recovery. While I do not have the expertise to determine if Burton's treatment works, I do know that it did offer hope to many individual cancer patients .. . . . (quoted in IATPA "Resolution to the Congress," 1986).

On January 15, 1986, he held a congressional public hearing at Federal Plaza in New York. It was an epochal event in the struggle for freedom of choice in cancer. In his opening remarks Molinari stated, "In my investigation I have found inconsistencies, and in some cases actual untruths, on the part of the various agencies which I contacted, especially on the part of Dr. Gregory Curt of the NCI" (Molinari, 1986).

Burton himself testified that over five hundred previously terminal cancer patients were alive due to IAT, "significantly past the date of their terminal prognosis, many for periods in excess of ten years" (ibid.).

Of the twenty-nine people who spoke at the hearings, the most unusual testimony came from two South Salem, New York, veterinarians, Drs. Robert and Martin Goldstein. These brothers had been treating pets with IAT since 1983; 85 were under therapy at the time of the hearing. They had found, one vet testified, "that one out of two animals with serious or terminal cancer goes into remission and live normal lives with no side effects whatsoever" when treated with the serum. IAT was efficacious, they said, in precisely those types of animal cancer in which it seemed to work in humans. If true, this was significant, since "animals, unlike humans, don't respond to placebos," according to Robert Goldstein (ibid.).

No member of the establishment accepted Congressman Molinari's invitation to testify at the hearing that day. But the 433 pages of testimony and affidavits were distributed to all members of Congress, along with a cover letter soliciting their help. By early 1986 political opinion in Washington was beginning to turn in favor of Burton.

In addition, IATPA members canvassed congressional offices seeking support for Molinari's letter calling for an independent study. Virtually every congressional representative was contacted, and eventually forty (thirty-seven House members and three senators) signed. Representative John Dingell, chairman of the House Committee on Energy and Commerce, made the official request for the Office of Technology Assessment (OTA) to do a study (*The Choice,* Fall 1988). In September 1990 the OTA published a report that has become itself the center of a raging controversy between proponents and enemies of alternative approaches.

In addition, Burton has been attacked by the American Medical Association (AMA), which sponsored a "survey" of its members' opinions about IAT, and the American Society for Clinical Oncology (ASCO). The AMA survey was predictably negative. Not surprisingly, physicians with no direct experience of the treatment were by and large convinced it had no value (Diagnostic, 1988).

Similarly, ASCO members in the majority were against Burton. The chairman of ASCO's Committee on Unorthodox Therapies is Dr. Daniel S. Martin, the same Dr. Martin who figured so prominently in the attack on laetrile at Sloan-Kettering. Under Dr. Martin, the ASCO committee published a pamphlet called "Ten Ways to Recognize Ineffective Cancer Therapy." It states, among other things, that IAT claims "the need for special nutritional support when the remedy is used"—a sure sign, it says, of a phony-cure promoter. In point of fact, Burton is widely criticized in the alternative health community because he puts *no* emphasis on diet! (He even brags about eating eight eggs a day.) The publication of this pamphlet was supported by Adria Laboratories, Inc., manufacturer of the toxic chemotherapeutic drug Adriamycin.

Most of these "studies" of IAT were based on prejudiced opinion, not fact. Not so the 1986–87 study of IAT patients by Dr. Barrie Cassileth and colleagues at the University of Pennsylvania.

Cassileth is no friend of unconventional methods. She has coauthored articles with long-time California quackbuster Helene Brown. Cassileth shares NCI's "concern" over an "unproven or questionable cancer treatment" that "may be ineffective, toxic, or otherwise unsafe" (Cassileth, 1988). Nevertheless, she developed a reputation for being generally fair and adhering to scientific criteria of objectivity in her work.

With the enthusiastic cooperation of most IAT patients, Cassileth and her colleagues were able to study seventy-nine of Burton's long-term patients. They found them to be "younger and of higher socioeconomic status than are cancer patients in general" (Cassileth, 1987).

Thirty-three percent of the patients reported becoming more ambulatory; 29 percent reported appetite improvement. Most importantly, 50 of the 79 patients studied (or 63 percent) were alive an average of 65 months after diagnosis. Yet "the majority of subjects studied had an expected survival of 36 months or less, based on tumor site and stage alone." Thus, Burton's patients were living *about twice as long* as the maximum survival rate of conventionally treated patients.

In the prospective portion of her study, four out of fifty-four advanced patients died after six months of observation. This is an excellent result—far better than what would be expected in a random sample of traditionally treated advanced cancer patients (cf. Moertel, 1987).

Although Cassileth seemed especially interested in information about HIV and hepatitis contamination, her retrospective study did not confirm the charges of widespread viral contamination. The blood of four patients was found positive for hepatitis and one for the AIDS-causing virus before the first interview:

> This one HIV-positive patient is believed to be the same individual reported positive by the NCI. These data do not prove that the infections were acquired via the immune serum treatments (Cassileth et al, 1987).

Interestingly, while Cassileth encouraged the patients to seek hepatitis B and HIV testing, they were not impressed:

> In general, patients neither believed nor trusted the NIH warnings, feeling that they were simply part of a broad effort to discredit IAT and the Burton clinic (Cassileth, 1987).

Those few who heeded her warning were tested and proved negative for both viruses. Only 3 percent of patients reported any adverse side effects from the therapy.

In September 1987 Cassileth circulated prepublication copies of the paper for review. But after making these startling findings, she then refused to publish them. In fact, she repeatedly tried to debunk the implications of her own statistics. Over and over she repeated that "these survival data reflect the bias toward longer survival in this group," meaning the white, relatively better-off, more ambulatory, and "somewhat younger" population she found taking IAT. According to Cassileth "it is impossible to draw valid inferences from this dataset concerning treatment efficacy and safety." She called for "an appropriately designed study of IAT, conducted in a manner convincing to both conventional medical practitioners and to Dr. Burton and his colleagues" (Cassileth, 1987).

In response to Cassileth, medical writer Robert G. Houston pointed out several factors: that national statistics for cancer are generally given for whites only; that there is a lower percentage of nonambulatory patients at, say, M. D. Anderson Tumor Institute than at Burton's IAT clinic; that the mean age for Burton's patients, 62, is exactly the same as NCI's mean patient age (Houston disputes Cassileth's figures here); and finally, that while there is some influence of economic factors on cancer survival, it tends to occur at the bottom of the scale, i. e., between indigent and lower middle class, rather than between middle class and affluent (Houston, 1988).

As other studies have indicated, patients with advanced disease do not fare well—rich or poor, black or white. The main reasons poor people do worse is that they wait until the disease is more advanced before presenting themselves. "No matter how skilled the surgeon . . . how advanced the technology . . . we cannot cure people with advanced, widely spread cancer," said Harold P. Freeman, M.D., then Chairman of the ACS's Subcommittee on Cancer in the Economically Disadvantaged (ACS, 1986). (Dr. Freeman has since become President of the ACS.)

Houston praises Cassileth's milestone studies, yet he remarks that ". . . the Cassileth team appear to be genuinely embarrassed by the positive results of their survey" (Houston, 1988).

By 1986 Burton managed to establish contact with the Bahamian authorities. In private conversations they indicated they had no desire to harm Burton. A great deal of their involvement came down to economics. About 90 percent of the island's economy is based on tourism—cruise boats, hotels, casinos, and the like. If AIDS became associated with their small country they could be ruined (Null and Steinman, 1986).

At the same time, there is no doubt that IAT is good for the economic health of Freeport. Patients come for long stays and spend money. Burton expressed his willingness to overcome Bahamian objections to reopening. He installed ELISA and other equipment to screen the blood supply. Just as significantly, he finally realized the necessity of taking on a local businessman as senior partner. "Forty-nine percent of something," he said, with a resigned shrug, "is better than one hundred percent of nothing" (Burton, 1988).

On March 5, 1986, in response to a variety of factors, the clinic was finally reopened, seven and a half months after its dramatic closure. Burton tends to credit his own business acumen. Others see it as testimony to the power of grassroots organizing, of the efforts of hundreds of patients and their supporters as they lobbied, telegrammed, and picketed to bring their case to the American public. The Bahamian Ministry of Health is said to have imposed strict blood screening as a condition for the IAT Clinic staying open (Young, 1986).

Nevertheless, the war is far from won. Burton remains isolated in the Bahamas, far from the centers of medical power. (Two satellite clinics have opened, one in Dusseldorf, Germany, and the other in Playas, Tijuana, Mexico.) Judging from initial appearances, at least, the OTA study will not break the deadlock. And the various medical societies still seem determined to "get" Burton, even if they were frustrated this time. The man himself is uncooperative in publishing a detailed explanation of either his intriguing methods or his provocative results. This remains the biggest mark against him in the scientific community. The paper on mesothelioma by his colleague, Dr. Clement, which was rejected by a British medical journal, was published in an obscure journal, *Quantum Medicine* (Clement, 1988). It could still be rewritten and resubmitted to a major, peer-reviewed publication, however. The OTA failed to come up with a testing protocol.

On October 11, 1988, hundreds of AIDS patients were arrested blocking the entrances to FDA headquarters. A few days later, FDA Commissioner Frank Young announced that he was lowering the barrier to new drug acceptance by eliminating Phase III in the IND process. In practice, however, this seemed to augur faster approval only for traditional chemotherapy. So far at least, nontoxic therapies, such as those of Lawrence Burton, remain forbidden.

In fact, since August 1986 it has been illegal to bring Burton's serum into the United States. *After* the reopening of the clinic, when all alleged hazards had been overcome, the FDA issued an Import Alert against what it called a dangerous cancer remedy:

> In order to protect U.S. citizens from continued exposure to this dangerously contaminated blood serum, FDA is issuing an Import Alert directing U.S. Custom and Postal Service authorities to detain all quantities of these biological agents that are being brought into the United States (FDA Talk Paper T86-60, August 7, 1986).

The FDA Talk Paper is cleverly worded to suggest what the facts themselves will not support. For instance, it claims that the Washington State ELISA test was "strongly suggestive of the presence of the AIDS virus." No mention of the weakly positive ELISA or the negative Western

Blot. The NCI tests, it says, showed that "more than half were possibly contaminated." Possibly contaminated—not actually so. And the CDC reported "at least two cases of hepatitis." At least two? Doesn't the FDA know how many cases have been reported? The number is in fact two (out of approximately 3,000 people treated by Burton's method till then).

On such innuendoes does the government make its case. Yet the alert remains in effect. FDA warns its import program managers that "as agents require refrigeration, they may be smuggled in thermos bottles or similar insulated containers." One wonders if Florida custom inspectors, unable to stem the flow of heroin and cocaine into this country, will have more success seizing the thermos bottles of terminal cancer patients?

Since the "60 Minutes" program appeared, about sixteen million Americans have gotten cancer and about eight million have died of it. In that time a few thousand of them have broken with their orthodox oncologists and—often with their friends and family members—made the big jump to the Bahamas.

Burton's patients represent one-tenth of one percent of the cancer patients in America. Yet something about Immuno-Augmentative Therapy sticks in the craw of the American cancer establishment and will not let them rest. What could that be? Do they fear that in his uncontrollable way Burton has actually gone out and done what immunologists since the days of Coley have only dreamed of?

Sometimes it appears that the chief target of the "war on cancer" is not the dread disease itself but a feisty medical maverick by the name of Lawrence Burton.

It has been three decades since Burton and his colleagues at St. Vincent's discovered the growth-inhibiting factor, and almost two dozen since they demonstrated the effects of this factor at the American Cancer Society seminar. It has been many years since Burton branched out on his own and initiated the treatment of patients with blood components. Yet today the cancer establishment still shows little interest in giving Burton credit for anything more than troublemaking.

A great deal is said and written about immunology, which is struggling to become a fourth modality of cancer therapy, alongside surgery, radiation, and chemotherapy. In the eyes of some people, however, the orthodox immunologists are simply borrowing freely from the unorthodox innovators, and especially from Lawrence Burton.

1996 Update: Dr. Burton died of a heart attack on March 8, 1993. His clinic remains open under the direction of R.J. Clement, M.D. Please see the new preface for a description of the Office of Technology Assessment's failed attempt to evaluate Dr. Burton's method.

« 13 »

Livingston and the Cancer Microbe

In the late nineteenth and early twentieth centuries, it was widely believed that cancer was caused by a microorganism, a germ. In fact, this idea was as much a dogma as the belief today that it cannot be caused by a microbe. According to an NCI-sponsored history of cancer:

> It appeared to have been a question, not so much as to the infectious origin of cancer, but rather as to which of the many parasites was the real causative agent (Shimkin, 1977:176).

James Ewing, later medical director of Memorial Hospital, listed thirty-eight different kinds of bacilli, molds, spirochetes, and protozoa which were candidates for the title in 1907 (ibid.). The director of research at Roswell Park Memorial Institute, Buffalo, and many other prominent scientists were firm believers in the microbial theory. Scientific thinking changed rapidly, however. "By 1910," wrote the historian Michael Shimkin, M.D., "scientific consensus was for a noninfectious nature of cancer" (ibid.). Those who continued to believe in the role of an infectious organism were branded "quacks."*

In the 1922 edition of *Neoplastic Diseases,* Ewing summed up the controversy as follows:

*"The theory that cancer is of germ or infectious origin" was attacked on the grounds "that it was supported by 'quacks' who thrive on the gullibility of the public" (Coley, 1926).

The parasitic theory is the oldest hypothesis of the origin of cancer. It appealed to the ancients, was tacitly accepted throughout the Middle Ages, was definitely argued by modern observers, and reached the height of its popularity as a scientific theory around 1895, but during the last fifteen years it has rapidly lost ground, and today few competent observers consider it as a possible explanation (Ewing, 1922:13).

At an international cancer research conference held at Lake Mohonk, New York (September 20–24, 1926), Ewing went so far as to claim that the microbial theory itself was the greatest hindrance to progress in the study of the control of cancer, according to William B. Coley, who reported on the meeting for a medical journal (Coley, 1926).

Only "feeble voice[s]" were raised in defense of the theory. Yet the perceptive Coley warned his readers:

> Until it is settled beyond the shadow of a doubt that cancer is not due to a microorganism, we believe that every effort should be made to stimulate to the utmost cancer research along these lines rather than to attempt to hinder or to discredit it (ibid.).

One of those scorned by the establishment was Peyton Rous, a medical researcher at the Rockefeller Institute (now Rockefeller University). Rous claimed to have discovered an infectious agent in fowl in 1910, but his findings were ignored. Furthermore, Rous claimed that his agent would pass through the smallest filter known.

It was only with the development of virology—the study of submicroscopic organisms—that scientists took a second look at Rous's once-heretical theory. In 1966, at the age of eighty-nine, Peyton Rous was awarded a Nobel Prize for this work.

The discovery of viruses and the unraveling of the genetic code led to a new enthusiasm for the infection theory of cancer. The first director of the National Cancer Program, Dr. Frank Rauscher, was a young virologist, and hundreds of millions of dollars were spent on the search for a cancer virus.

While viruses have been shown to play a part in numerous animal tumors and to be involved in several forms of human cancer, including Burkitt's lymphoma and nasopharyngeal carcinoma, they do not appear to be the cause of most forms of the disease (*Immunology Tribune*, April 30, 1979).

Enthusiasm for the viral theory appears to be waning. Even Dr. Howard Temin, who won the 1975 Nobel Prize for his work on cancer virology, commented:

> We can now say that infectious viruses like those that cause many human diseases do not cause most human cancer. Therefore, we cannot hope to develop a vaccine against a virus to prevent most human cancer. . . . We do not have the fundamental knowledge to prevent or cure most human cancer (cited in Harper and Culbert, 1977).

At the same time, the bacterial (as opposed to the viral) theory of cancer has never died in this country or abroad (Boesch, 1960). In fact, some of the fiercest cancer controversies of this century have concerned proposed treatments for the cancer "germ" (ACS, 1971b:79 ff).

Today a small number of scientists keep alive this theory. The leader of this school of thought is Dr. Virginia Wuerthele-Caspe-Livingston-Wheeler—Dr. Livingston, for short—who believes that major breakthroughs have already been made in the cause, prevention, and cure for human cancer.

Scorned by the establishment for several decades, in more recent years some of Livingston's ideas have received surprising support from scientists at Rockefeller University, Princeton Laboratories, the University of Pittsburgh, and other well-known institutions.

Livingston was president of the Livingston-Wheeler Medical Clinic in San Diego, California. She died of a heart attack, June 30, 1990, at the age of 84. Dr. Livingston was a graduate of Vassar College and received her medical degree from New York University. She was the first woman to be a resident physician in a New York City hospital (the Contagious Disease Hospital), and in the course of her long career has been associate professor of biological sciences at Rutgers University, New Jersey, director of the Laboratory of Proliferative Diseases at Presbyterian Hospital in Newark, New Jersey, and a research associate at the San Diego Biomedical Institution. In addition to overseeing the Livingston-Wheeler Clinic, with its staff of thirty six, including three staff physicians, Livingston was also an adjunct professor of immunology at United States International University.

What makes Livingston controversial is not her background or credentials but her ideas: in essence, that a hitherto-unsuspected microbe is virtually the source of life (conception) and death (cancer) in many vertebrate species, including man.

Livingston's first encounter with this microbe was in 1946 when she treated a nurse in the New Jersey public schools for scleroderma, a condition sometimes called the hidebound disease. Orthodox medicine recognizes no known cause of this condition, but Livingston found a swarm of unidentified microbes deep inside skin specimens taken from this patient. With the help of a pathologist, she injected these microbes into laboratory chicks and guinea pigs. The chicks died, but the guinea pigs developed a scleroderma-like disease. "The involvement of a lifetime can start with a very simple observation," Livingston has said. "All of my life's work started with the desire to help a school nurse who had ulcers of her fingertips and a perforated nasal septum" (Livingston, 1977:8).

Livingston named this microbe *Sclerobacillus Wuerthele-Caspe* (*Sclerobacillus*, meaning the "scleroderma-causing organism"; *Wuerthele-Caspe* was then her surname). She published a paper on "a probable cause of scleroderma" with two other physicians in 1947 (Wuerthele-Caspe et al., 1947).*

At the same time, Livingston noted that some of the guinea pigs developed cancer, an exceedingly rare occurrence among these animals. Working with staining techniques utilized by Eleanor Alexander-Jackson, Ph.D., of Cornell University Medical College, Livingston began to examine cancer specimens from many animals, including man. In more than fifty tumors she found a particular microbe present. This microbe, which is now called *Progenitor cryptocides,* was similar to the *Sclerobacillus* organism she had identified a year before.

In fact, Livingston noted in 1947, "the disease entities of tuberculosis, leprosy, generalized sclerosis, and cancer have certain features in common. All four diseases are characterized by a simultaneous process of production and destruction of tissue and by a progressive, systemic involvement of the host" (Livingston-Wheeler, 1977a:18).

At this point Livingston invoked a concept also employed by Dr. Alexander-Jackson in her work on tuberculosis: pleomorphism. This means that the organism is not fixed eternally in a single size or shape, but can radically change both of these. Livingston now formulated a remarkably fluid and dynamic view of the microscopic world, a view perhaps too radical for her more conventional colleagues:

> Instead of a bacillus being a bacillus, *ad infinitum,* it can and does change into numerous other forms dictated by its need to survive or stimulated to greater productivity by an unusually favorable environment. Since man exists in a sea of microorganisms his ability to withstand them and their urge to

*Livingston's observations on the *Sclerobacillus* have since been given support by a number of research groups, including N. Delmotte and L. van der Meiren (1953) and Alan R. Cantwell, Jr., M.D., and Dan W. Kelso of Los Angeles (1971).

survive often leads to a stage of symbiosis, that is, they live together. This can be on a competitive basis where the human keeps the bugs in check so that they are latent or resting. In some cases the captive microorganisms may play a useful role (Livingston, 1972).

In the early 1950s Livingston appeared on the way to gaining acceptance for her ideas. She was appointed director of the Laboratory for Proliferative Diseases. She collaborated with prominent scientists at leading laboratories. She received grants from the Damon Runyon Fund, the Rosenwald Foundation, Reader's Digest Associates, Chas. Pfizer & Co., Lederle Laboratories, Abbott Laboratories, and even the American Cancer Society. Much basic work on the microbiology of cancer and other diseases was done at this time. For instance, the Newark researchers decided they were dealing with organisms that formed part of the Actinomycetales order, a family of germs which dates back to the Precambrian era, hundreds of millions of years ago (Livingston, 1972).

They attempted to fulfill Koch's four postulates, the four laws laid down by Robert Koch (1843–1910) for establishing the microbial origin of any disease. By the early 1950s they believed they had done so. They could show, Livingston says, that the cancer organism was present in every case of the disease which they examined; that it could be cultivated outside the host animal in an artificial medium; that inoculation of this culture produced the disease in a susceptible animal; and that the germ could be reobtained from the inoculated animal and cultivated once again.

At that time Virginia Livingston had a large tumor service at Presbyterian Hospital in Newark, where she cared for twenty to thirty cancer patients daily. She obtained her cancer specimens from these patients. Using cultures of human blood from cancer patients, the incidence of cancer among guinea pigs could be increased from the natural rate of 1 in 500,000 to 1 in 4 by injecting microbes derived from human patients into these animals. The "cancer microbe" crossed species lines, Livingston said. Animals could catch it from man; and man, she believed, could catch it from animals— specifically by eating the contaminated flesh of fowl and other animals. *

Livingston had not yet begun to *treat* cancer with any unusual methods. Nonetheless, her work came to the attention of the leaders of cancer research and began to meet resistance. This was at the time that chemother-

---

*Cancer in America's chicken flocks has been called a "nightmare" by the *Wall Street Journal* (cited in Livingston, 1972). Livingston claims to have found a large degree of infection with *Progenitor cryptocides* in chickens, and therefore considers them particularly dangerous. (See Livingston, 1972, and Livingston-Wheeler, 1977b for full discussion of this controversial point.)

apy was being promoted as *the* answer to cancer. Sloan-Kettering Institute dominated the drug-testing field, at least until 1955, and not surprisingly, the strongest opposition to Livingston and her Newark colleagues came from the leader of the Sloan-Kettering chemotherapists, C. P. "Dusty" Rhoads. In her autobiography Livingston recalls Rhoads and Sloan-Kettering in the early 1950s:

> Many of the large research centers, such as Sloan-Kettering . . . under Dr. Cornelius P. Rhoads, were dedicated largely to finding a chemical or group of chemicals that would destroy the cancer cell. He would brook no competition or interference from anyone who disagreed with his concepts. He considered us an upstart group. This included our collaborators as well. He was often heard to say, "When the cause and cure of cancer are found, I will find it." He died a disappointed man (ibid.).

Rhoads proved to be a determined and powerful opponent. For example, says Livingston, he opposed Dr. Irene Diller, a Philadelphia scientist who collaborated with the Newark group. His opposition seemed to increase after Diller's work was featured in a mass circulation magazine. (Rhoads himself had been on the cover of *Time,* June 27, 1949.) In 1950 Dr. Diller attempted to set up a symposium at the New York Academy of Sciences to present a number of papers on the infectious nature of cancer.

Rhoads managed to kill this meeting, says Livingston, by charging Diller with having "commercialized" her work. Diller had received several ultraviolet sterilizing lamps from a company, with no strings attached. But the charge appeared serious enough—and its source powerful enough—for the meeting to be canceled. This charge was ironic, Livingston noted, coming from the head of a center with millions of dollars in grants from giant corporations and individuals financially interested in the cancer field (see Appendix A). The meeting was not finally convened until twenty years later, well after Rhoads's death *(Annals of the New York Academy of Sciences* 174, October 30, 1970).

In her autobiography Livingston includes many other instances of the way in which Rhoads and other establishment figures attempted to block the free development of her research approach (Livingston, 1972). For example, in the early 1950s, amid much publicity, Livingston's laboratory at Rutgers was awarded a bequest of $750,000 from the Black-Stevenson Cancer Foundation for excellence in cancer research. These funds were never conveyed to the microbial researchers, however, but instead were used to build a new wing on Presbyterian Hospital in Newark to house a giant cobalt machine (Livingston, 1984). Among other factors, this misappropriation, as Livingston calls it, forced her to close the Laboratory for Proliferative Diseases. "Dusty" Rhoads appears to have been involved in convincing a trustee of the Black-Stevenson fund, then a patient at Memorial Hospital, to divert the money away from the "upstarts." "It was the long arm of Dr. Cornelius P. Rhoads that closed the Newark laboratory," says Livingston (Livingston, 1972).

In 1953 the Newark researcher and her colleagues traveled to Rome to present some of their findings to the Sixth International Conference on Microbiology. Livingston presented a summary paper, "Microbiology of Cancer: Neoplastic Infection in Man and Animals" (Livingston-Wheeler, 1977a:53). The expenses for this journey were paid for by Livingston's then-husband, Dr. Joseph Caspe, a chemist working as a consultant to the British leather and fur industries. Upon returning to the United States, however, they found that they had been attacked in the press by the president of the New York Academy of Medicine. Soon after this the Internal Revenue Service, acting on an informer's "tip," began to question Dr. Caspe about the source of his revenue and how he had paid for the European trip. Livingston was told that the informer was "someone high up in New York in cancer" (Livingston, 1972).

Eventually Caspe was cleared of all suspicion, but the experience was an embittering one. The couple decided to resettle in California. In the early 1960s Dr. Livingston did little work; she struggled with personal illness and problems, including a divorce, but she did manage to speak at a few conferences and pursue a small amount of research.

In 1966 Pat McGrady, Sr., invited Virginia Livingston and Eleanor Alexander-Jackson, who had joined her as a full-time researcher before the closing of the Newark laboratory, to speak at the American Cancer Society Science Writers' Seminar. This was the same Phoenix meeting at which Lawrence Burton demonstrated his "fifteen-minute cure" for mouse cancer. Livingston attempted to keep her presentation on a theoretical plane, but questions naturally arose about the practical application of her work: How did she *treat* cancer?

Actually, although both she and her second husband, Afton Munk Livingston, M.D., were practicing physicians, they shied away from cancer therapy:

> We were reluctant to enter the field of cancer therapy since we believed that present-day methods of treatment were seldom effective. In the past, observations on animal models led to the conclusion that the very methods used to treat cancer were carcinogenic in themselves, that is, that radiation and chemotherapy not only induced cancer but also destroyed immunity to cancer (Livingston-Wheeler, 1977a:9).

Nevertheless, Livingston conceded that some colleagues had begun to make attempts to immunize cancer patients, based on her earlier animal experiments with the microbes. Some reporters immediately blew this out of proportion and asserted she was claiming another "cure for cancer." The furor surrounding a different unorthodox technique—Burton's blood fraction—may have spilled over into the Livingston controversy.

When Alexander-Jackson returned to New York from this meeting, she discovered that she had been abruptly terminated from the Institute of Comparative Medicine at Columbia College of Physicians and Surgeons, where she had gone to work after the Newark laboratory had closed. Both women believe the American Cancer Society instigated the firing.

In 1968 the "Livingston vaccine" took its place in the ACS's *Unproven Methods* book. After "careful study," the American Cancer Society did not find evidence that "the treatment with the Livingston vaccine resulted in objective benefit in the treatment of cancer," nor that it could be used as a diagnostic tool.

An interesting fact about the so-called Livingston vaccine, evident from the ACS book, is that at that time Livingston herself had never used a vaccine to treat cancer. The "careful study" was a report of Livingston's speech at the aforementioned ACS seminar, at which she said that other doctors had treated approximately fifty patients with an anti-*Progenitor cryptocides* vaccine. Of these, Livingston said, thirty-seven had died, but the others had improved. In particular, ACS quotes her as having said, three patients "with far advanced cancer had received no treatment except the vaccine, and these were reported to have survived for more than eighteen months and to be still improving" (ACS, 1971b).

What sort of investigation was conducted of Livingston's method before it was included on the list? None—no examination of patients, materials, or methods, no study of case records, of objective or subjective effects, much less a single- or double-blind test. The "investigation" consisted of the fact that "at the Science Writers' Seminar, the findings of Drs. Livingston and Alexander-Jackson were strongly criticized" by a Sloan-Kettering scientist, among others (ibid:150).

The scientist, Dr. Jørgen Fogh, told the author, "You realize that the agents they [Livingston and Alexander-Jackson] claim to work with probably don't exist. I think they are imagining them" (Fogh, 1979).

The establishment's condemnation does not seem to have daunted Dr. Livingston. Perhaps it even goaded her into activity, for her California years have been among Virginia Livingston's most productive.

In 1968, under a Fleet Foundation grant at the Biomed Laboratory of San Diego, it was shown that the "cancer microbe," when filtered and put into tissue culture, produced the degeneration of cells under certain conditions and the proliferation of cells in others. The study of several hundred cultures showed that the specific microbes were sensitive to some antibiotics when they were outside cells, but markedly less or not at all when they nestled inside the human cells (Livingston-Wheeler, 1977a:12).

In 1970, working under Fleet and Kerr grants at the University of San Diego, Livingston showed that the cancer microbe produced an antibiotic (actinomycin) as well as toxic materials that enhanced the incidence of cancer in mice. In the same year the New York Academy of Sciences finally held a symposium to air the views of the microbial school. It was at this symposium that the microbe received its present name: *Progenitor cryptocides,* the hidden, ancestral creator and killer.

In 1972 Livingston reexamined the various phases of the microbe through the use of the dark-field microscope. The dark-field microscope has a special condenser and other attachments that make light scatter from the object observed, with the result that it appears bright on a dark background instead of the other way around. It is said to be a superior method of viewing *Progenitor cryptocides.* Using it, Livingston was able to describe the entire life cycle of this complicated, ever-changing germ, and name it according to modern usage.

This same year, Livingston made what some scientists now call a major breakthrough in the cancer field. She found that this organism is capable of producing what was previously thought of as a *human* hormone—HCG (human choriogonadotrophin)—in the test tube (Livingston-Wheeler, 1979).

For the average person, of course, this finding may not appear earthshaking. But there are several important features to the discovery. First, until this time, no microbe had ever been found to produce a human hormone. The implications were intriguing for scientists, especially those concerned with the topical field of recombinant DNA research.

Second, this particular hormone—HCG—has long been associated with cancer. The test for HCG is, in fact, not only the standard pregnancy test, but an accurate monitor of at least one type of cancer (choriocarcinoma) and a fair barometer of some other types as well. Many theories have been propounded to account for this unnatural—or "ectopic"—production of what is essentially a growth hormone by a cancer cell.*

---

*Technically, HCG (also called CG or CGH) is a glycoprotein with a carbohydrate fraction composed of galactose and hexosamine, and has traditionally been thought to be produced by placental trophoblastic cells. In pregnancy, it appears to stimulate the ovarian secretion of estrogen and progesterone required for the integrity and survival of the embryo during the first trimester of pregnancy. It plays an essential role in the trophoblastic theory of cancer propounded by Beard (1911) and Krebs (1970).

Livingston's lifelong research may provide a more fruitful explanation of why HCG appears in so many cancer cells and in the blood of many cancer patients. According to her theory, the cancer microbe produces it. The hormone, in turn, may "transform" (turn cancerous) normal cells when their immune functions are inadequate or when "essential nutritive elements become deficient" (Livingston-Wheeler, 1977a:11). Thus, HCG may be the hidden killer secreted by the ever-changing, mysterious microbe to kill the deficient cell.

Yet, Livingston emphasizes, this microbe has two names: one redolent of death, the other full of life. It is also a progenitor, a life-giver. Other experiments suggest that the microbe is also present in normal sperm and may enter the newly conceived human at the union of sperm and egg. Once inside, it multiplies and provides the embryo with its HCG, a hormone without which life certainly would not be possible.

Although far from a proven certainty, parts of Livingston's theory have received confirmation from surprisingly orthodox institutions and have created a stir among major research groups. Livingston published her finding on HCG in 1974 in the *Transactions* of the New York Academy of Sciences (Livingston and Livingston, 1974). Two years later, Herman Cohen and Alice Strampp of the Princeton Laboratories confirmed the "bacterial synthesis of a substance similar to human chorionic gonadotrophin" (Cohen and Strampp, 1976).

In 1978 another research group, headed by Hernan F. Acevedo, Ph.D., of the William H. Singer Memorial Research Institute, Allegheny General Hospital, Pittsburgh, confirmed the fact that *Progenitor cryptocides* produced the human growth hormone. Acevedo believed that a number of different bacterial strains isolated from the tissues of cancer patients also produced the hormone (Kellen, 1982a, 1982b).

A research group at Rockefeller University, headed by Samuel Koide, M.D., Ph.D., has also studied the microbe, and confirmed the fact that it produces a gonadotrophic hormone which appears to be identical to that of the human. This group also began looking at the germ from the point of view of a new approach to birth control. Since the hormone is apparently present in normal sperm, it might be possible to use it to prevent pregnancy (Koide, 1979).

Within a few years in the late 1970s Livingston appeared to have gained the respect of at least some established researchers, and the attention of many more. While none of these scientists became an open convert to the bacterial theory of cancer, Livingston was doubtlessly correct when she stated that the discovery concerning the HCG hormone "immediately gave credence and stature to the entire microbial theory'' (Livingston-Wheeler. 1977a:7).

An indication of Livingston's new stature can be gleaned by this comment from Acevedo's 1978 paper:

> The impact of these findings in the fields of oncology, bacteriology, epidemiology, genetics and molecular biology is so great that a detailed description will be beyond the scope of this communication. . . . It is apparent that this phenomenon exposes the need for a new approach to the analysis as well as to our current concepts of cancer (Acevedo, 1978).

Livingston believed she had such a new approach, and for several decades applied it in the treatment of patients. She had also discovered a natural substance present in many foods, abscisic acid, which, she said, neutralizes the HCG and thus should have an anticancer effect. Although difficult and expensive to purify for laboratory experiments, abscisic acid, similar to vitamin A, is plentiful in nature (see Table 6). Animal experiments have showed it to be a powerful anticancer agent (Livingston-Wheeler, 1977b).

In 1969 Virginia Livingston and her husband, Dr. A. F. Livingston, opened the Livingston Medical Clinic in San Diego and began immunization treatment of cancer patients. "My studies had led me to the conclusion that cancer is an immune deficiency disease based on infection by a definite etiological agent, the *Progenitor cryptocides*. On the basis of treating an immune deficiency in man, we began to accept cancer patients" (Livingston, 1972).

The treatment included a vaccine to fight the *Progenitor cryptocides*, antibiotics, antisera, immune stimulants such as BCG,* and a health-food diet. In addition, like many unorthodox practitioners, Livingston urged her patients to adopt a new, more relaxed way of life:

> It is ideally hoped that your whole foods will be grown in a naturally fertilized and composted home garden. Relaxation, plenty of rest, exercise and fresh air are as much a part of your new life as the food you will eat. They are all contributing towards your recovery. Most important is proper attitude. Negative emotion and its by-products waste much precious energy. A positive

---

*Bacillus Calmette-Guérin, the antituberculosis vaccine used as an immune stimulator in both orthodox and unorthodox clinics.

TABLE 6
Foods Containing Abscisic Acid

Fruits
Mangoes
Grapes
Avocados
Pears
Oranges, with the white underpeel and
  pulps
Apples, whole with the seeds
Strawberries

Fruit Blossoms and Leaves as Tea
Peach Flowers
Strawberry Leaves
Cherry Flowers
Apple Blossoms

Vegetables
Pea Shoots
Lima Beans
Potatoes
Peas, Dwarf
Yams
Sweet Potatoes
Asparagus
Tomatoes
Onions
Spinach

Root Vegetables*
All Root Vegetables—especially
  Carrots

Seeds and Nuts
Seeds and Nuts of all kinds

Leafy Vegetables
Mature Greens

*All seeds, nuts, fruits, root storage vegetables, and fresh vegetables with their mature greens
seem to contain abscisic acid.
(Information from Livingston-Wheeler, *Food Alive*)

attitude taken with this change in life style will allow your new way of life to
become a happy and rewarding experience (Livingston-Wheeler, 1977b).

In 1972 the Livingstons received as a patient a fellow physician, Owen
Webster Wheeler. Suffering from malignant lymphoma of the neck "the
size of a tennis ball," Wheeler made the "momentous decision" to be treated
by immunization alone, without conventional therapies. The deadly lymphoma, Livingston says, was completely gone in six months, and Wheeler
remained cancer-free and in good health for a number of years.

After the death of Dr. Afton Munk Livingston, Virginia Livingston and Owen Wheeler were married, and the clinic was renamed the Livingston-Wheeler Medical Clinic. In time, Wheeler's cancer came back and he died of its complications in December, 1987 at the age of 79 (Land, 1989).

With the medical discoveries concerning the HCG hormone and abscisic acid, the treatment at the clinic now routinely includes a heavy emphasis on the ingestion of food containing the vitamin A–like substance.

The treatment, however, is not cheap. Ten days of outpatient treatment costs between $3,500 and $4,000. The treatment also includes the services of a clinical psychologist who conducts group stress-reduction sessions among the patients twice a week. The patient leaves with a one-month supply of autologous vaccine. There is a monthly maintenance cost of $200–300 for the vaccine, but the amount of vaccine required tends to taper off over the years. Medicare will not pay for this treatment but private insurance companies often do pay, depending on the policy (Land, 1989).

Like many innovative practitioners, Livingston does not believe that the average American diet is adequate to maintain optimum health:

> In a society commercially oriented toward the profit system, mass production of cheap food, preservatives to prolong shelf life, exploitation of taste over quality, convenience, attractive packaging, the trusting and unsuspecting individual can become lost in a jungle of incomprehension, leading to poor health and general deterioration. . . . (Livingston-Wheeler, 1977b).

The great hope of Livingston and her followers, however, is to produce a really effective, universal anticancer vaccine. This may seem like a wild dream, but for years they have been hard at work on this project. In the late 1970s, she sent a colleague, John Majnarich of the BioMed Research Laboratories in Seattle, to Japan to learn firsthand the techniques of a Japanese immunologist, Dr. Chisato Maruyama. Livingston and her colleagues hoped to use this new technique with the *Progenitor cryptocides* to produce a vaccine which would be an effective form of cancer prevention and possibly a cure (Livingston-Wheeler, 1979).

At the same time, Alexander-Jackson, on the East Coast, prepared an autogenous vaccine for patients—that is, a vaccine derived from samples of their own microbes. About a dozen physicians commissioned Alexander-Jackson to grow these microbes from patients' urine; a medical laboratory then prepared the vaccines. She claimed that these vaccines were useful in the treatment of cancer if the patient was in the early stages of the disease, if radiation and chemotherapy had not destroyed the immune system, and if the patient had a proper diet and received other nontoxic forms of therapy.

Although Sloan-Kettering claimed to be unable to find the *Progenitor cryptocides* microbe when Alexander-Jackson worked there temporarily as a visiting scientist in 1973, she remained adamant that the microbes are real, have been correctly described, and can form the basis for an effective treat ment.

"Will there be a shot against cancer? Someday...probably yes!" This optimistic appraisal of the chances for a cancer vaccine came not from Livingston or one of her colleagues but from an American Cancer Society press release (New York City Division, February 2, 1976). It would be ironic indeed if such a shot came not from a beneficiary of ACS funds, but from scientists long considered deluded and incompetent by the cancer establishment.

1996 Update: Dr. Livington died on June 30, 1990. The 84-year-old physician was on a European tour with her daughter when she fell ill. She had recently spoken at the Office of Technology Assessment meeting of March 9. She succumbed to heart failure in the Greek islands before she could be moved to Paris for further treatment. Her clinic in San Diego remains open.

« 14 »

The Fiercest Battle: Burzynski and Antineoplastons

"The body itself has a treatment for cancer." S. R. Burzynski.

The Raid

On July 17, 1985, a cancer patient named Ron Wolin was lying on a couch in his doctor's waiting room in Houston, Texas. Suddenly there was a disturbance in the offices beyond the door. When Ron's companion, Avis Lang, put down her embroidery and went to investigate, she found agents of the U.S. Food and Drug Administration (FDA), accompanied by an armed U.S. marshall, on a "search and seizure" mission.

FDA Compliance Officer Kenneth P. Ewing, brandishing a search warrant, was helping his men load eleven four-drawer filing cabinets onto a large truck. The New York couple watched with amazement as the confidential medical records of over a thousand cancer patients were marched out the back door of the clinic to the waiting van.

Relying on the word of unnamed "confidential informants," FDA agents that day seized 200,000 medical documents. They looked through "every drawer, every trash can, every filing cabinet, every treatment room, everything," in the words of one of the doctor's attorneys (Lang, 1986). They went through the doctor's personal correspondence and even rifled his briefcase.

What physician presented such a danger to the Republic that Federal agents had to lay hands on every scrap of paper in his office? His name is

Stanislaw R. Burzynski, M.D., Ph.D., and by 1985 he had become a thorn in the side of the cancer establishment. The FDA has often been accused of overbearing tactics (Garrison, 1970). But not since G-men had burned the books of Dr. Wilhelm Reich in the fifties and cracked down on laetrilists in the seventies had they acted with such two-fisted methods against a cancer maverick.

The FDA raid followed the American Cancer Society's inclusion of Burzynski on its "Unproven Methods of Cancer Management" list. It came amidst a flurry of quack-busting: on the same day Lawrence Burton's unorthodox IAT clinic in the Bahamas was ordered shut (see chapter 13). The ostensible reason for the raid was to uncover the alleged distribution of Burzynski's unique drugs outside the state of Texas; the home addresses of persons to whom the drug had been distributed; patient treatment, accounts, and billing records; and insurance claims and receipt of insurance payments (Ewing, 1985).

This seizure created an intolerable situation for some patients. Struggling under the almost unbearable burden of malignancy, they suddenly found they had to confront their government as well. Cancer is a disease that can affect every aspect of a person's life, including the most intimate. Burzynski had asked them probing questions and gotten unguarded replies. Few patients worried that their answers might find their way into the hands of strangers. Yet now a middle-level government bureaucrat had access to a lot of embarrassing stuff. Later, when Ewing was asked if he had notified patients he was "looking through some of the most personal information in their lives," he answered in the negative (Lang, 1986:11).

Burzynski was allowed to copy only a small fraction of these records at the time of the raid. Subsequently, the FDA allowed him to copy his own files—on condition that he install his own photocopying machine at their office. But first he had to give the FDA a day or two's notice to find the records in question. Then a member of the doctor's staff had to travel sixteen miles across town and photocopy what was needed. This arrangement precluded optimum treatment in an emergency. Sometimes records such as lab results, necessary for proper treatment, would not reproduce clearly. In such cases, said the FDA, Burzynski and his patient would have to do without.

At other times the FDA misplaced or lost a particular set of records, as happened to a man named William Cody. Like several other patients, he demanded his medical files back after the raid. Ewing, he said, informed him that "those records were no longer my property. . . ." Cody finally got through to Ewing's superior, the FDA regional director in Dallas, who informed him that he could, in fact, have his records returned; all he had to do was apply to the FDA in Houston. When he did so, Ewing told him they could not be found (ibid.).

"I was outraged," said Cody. "I told him it was a matter of life and death and I felt by not giving me my records they were killing me."

Later, when matters came before a federal judge and Burzynski's attorney produced Cody as a witness, his records mysteriously reappeared. But, according to Dr. Burzynski, the files they handed him were incomplete and copies of some of the crucial tests were illegible (ibid.).

Over five years later, the 200,000 documents remain in the hands of the FDA. Burzynski has not been charged with any crimes. But the FDA will not give them back and the courts have so far refused to make them do so.

"Dr. B."

Listening to the two sides in this controversy is a peculiar experience. To the government, Stanislaw Burzynski is a clever opportunist, exploiting a mysterious and ineffective cancer "cure" of his own imagining. His treatment is bizarre, expensive, useless, and also possibly dangerous.

To Burzynski's patients and supporters he is "Dr. B.," a gentle physician who has saved or prolonged hundreds of lives with his innovative approach. His clinic's motto—*"Primum Non Nocere"*—is from Hippocrates: "Above all, do no harm." They are convinced Stanislaw Burzynski has made a major contribution to cancer therapy. In addition, he really cares about their well-being in an old-fashioned way rarely seen in today's oncology clinics. The government's attempt to destroy him and his treatment, they say, is one of the greatest crimes in the history of modern medicine.

Stanislaw R. Burzynski was born in Poland in 1943. One grandfather was a blacksmith in the Lvov district. The other owned a cement factory. Burzynski's father taught classical Greek and Latin, at first in the gymnasia (high schools) of Lublin and then, after the war, at the university. He attempted to teach his son these subjects as well as German and the violin, but "Stash" (as he is known to his friends) had little interest in languages. From the age of thirteen he showed a precocious ability in chemistry at the Zamoyski Gymnasium. In 1960 he was one of those who received a national medal in the chemistry "Olympiads," a high honor.

By the time he reached the medical academy, Stash had developed a passionate interest in biochemistry. He was given the run of the laboratory, a situation that created resentment among some of the other students. His first published papers on amino acids and peptides were done while still a medical student.

Stash graduated from the Medical Academy of Lublin in 1967—first in his class of 250. In the following year he received another doctorate, a Ph.D. in biochemistry. He was one of the youngest people in the history of the country to receive both advanced degrees.

His dissertation project turned out to be the beginning of his lifelong quest. It started quite serendipitously. His assignment was to study the blood of patients with various illnesses. He was to run these blood samples through two standard tests called paper and thin-layer chromatography, to find the association between the occurrence of particular amino acids or peptides and disease. Amino acids are the building blocks of proteins while peptides are small chains of amino acids.

When Burzynski ran these samples, he got the expected peaks but also noted three unidentified stripes on the filter paper. These were faint purple in color and not in the position of any of the clearly defined amino acids with which he was familiar. He inquired of his chemistry professor and found out that these stripes had actually been seen for many years, but no one had bothered to investigate them.

In Poland students must defend their Ph.D. theses in a public forum. Announcements of the time and place are even placed in the local newspapers. Burzynski was afraid that one of his examiners would ask him the identity of these three pale lines. He could see himself confessing his ignorance in front of the whole town. To ward off this embarrassment, he decided to analyze them further.

Using the laborious technology of the time, he repeatedly ran blood samples through paper chromatography. He collected many samples of the three purple stripes, then washed (eluted) them off the filter paper with a solvent. After concentrating the residues, he subjected each to high-voltage electrophoresis. This jolt of electricity broke each line into several better-defined ones. He did this over and over again, until out of the three original lines he had gotten 39 separate samples. Upon analysis, these turned out to be peptide fractions—clusters of medium-sized amino acid combinations. This was enough to get him through his exam without public humiliation.

Upon graduation Burzynski began to run into problems. Always independent-minded, he refused to join the Communist party, the prerequisite for academic advancement. In addition, his status as boy wonder of the Chemistry Department began to catch up with him. Although he was gentle and good-natured, his precocious success earned him a fair amount of jealousy. As a result, Stash Burzynski suddenly found himself in the Polish army—one of only two doctors from the academy drafted that year.

A Polish doctor's army service, he says, entailed an indefinite term, in which he would be unable to do any research. For two years he suffered through this. Finally, with the help of influential scientists, Burzynski was allowed to emigrate.

In 1970 he came to the United States and stayed with an uncle in the Bronx. At first he thought he might stay for a year, define his intriguing substances, and then return to Poland. Very soon, however, he landed a position as a researcher and assistant professor at Baylor College of Medicine in Houston, working in the anesthesiology department under Dr. George Ungar.

He struck a bargain with Ungar. He would work half-time on his boss's projects if he could have the rest of his time free. It was a mutually beneficial arrangement, and Stash was able to move quickly and silently to a further definition of his own mysterious peptides. Ungar was himself a controversial figure who believed that another set of peptides could hold the key to memory retention in rats. The implications for human memory were vast, and so Burzynski got his first taste of American scientific politics.

Burzynski had been working with blood—his own. In 1970 he switched to urine—also his own—as a peptide source. Urine is surprisingly similar to blood in its composition, but is even more complex. (By coincidence, it was a Pole, S. Bondzynski, who first discovered peptides in urine in 1897.) In Houston he was able to make use of sophisticated instruments unavailable in Poland. This included column chromotography and high-powered (3,000-volt) separation equipment. In 1974 he got a National Cancer Institute grant (approved in 1972) and used it to buy a free-flow electrophoresis machine, the first one at Baylor.

With this equipment, Burzynski worked quickly. He was able to break down the original 39 fractions into 119 medium-sized peptides (10 to 15 amino acids each) and to examine their biological activity. This was the exploratory phase of the work. There were startling results, which were published by Burzynski, Ungar, and E. Lubanski in a 1974 article (*Physiol. Chem. Phys.* 6:457). According to a standard review article on urinary peptides by two Du Pont scientists:

> When tested for an *in vitro* effect on intestinal smooth muscle and heart tissue, 90 out of 119 peptide fractions were found to be active; some produced only smooth muscle contraction of rat tissue, some caused positive and some caused negative inotropic effects [i.e., influenced muscular contractility], and one caused arrhythmia of frog heart muscle (Lou and Hamilton, 1979: 253).

The Baylor team also investigated the effect of these peptides on DNA and RNA, on protein synthesis and mitosis (cell division), and in laboratory cultures of human leukemia, osteogenic sarcoma, and HeLa cells.

Even when he was in Poland, Burzynski had suspected that some of these peptide fractions might have activity against cancer. The blood of one prostate cancer patient had proved almost entirely lacking in one of the three faint peptide streaks. The young doctor intuitively felt that these amino acid combinations might play some essential role in protecting the body from cancer.

Writing about Burzynski's early work, the Du Pont scientists remarked: "They found that some peptides could produce up to 97 percent inhibition of DNA synthesis and mitosis in the neoplastic cells of their tissue cultures" (ibid.).

The active peptide fractions consisted of two groups. One was strongly acidic; the other, broad-based and slightly acidic or neutral. The strongly acidic group had a very powerful effect on a limited number of tumor cell lines, especially osteogenic sarcoma, a kind of bone cancer. But the other kind stopped the growth of many different kinds of cancer cells. With many backward glances, Burzynski finally decided to focus his attention on this broad-based peptide band. And it was this admittedly ill-defined substance that Burzynski now dubbed Antineoplaston A. A new name was needed because these particular urinary peptides had never been described before. The name was derived from the Greek—*neoplasm* being a medical term for "new growth," or cancer. All subsequent forms of antineoplastons were ultimately derived from this substance.

One of the scientists who had helped Burzynski get out of Poland was Marian Mazur, a Warsaw professor who was a leading Polish expert on cybernetics. This is the influential "theory of messages" that forms the basis of today's computer languages (Wiener, 1954). This man became Burzynski's scientific mentor. From talking to Mazur, Stash began to formulate a cybernetic theory of the peptides' role that has formed the philosophical basis of all his subsequent work.

Many scientists tended to look on peptides as a kind of intercellular debris. Burzynski believed, however, that there was a biochemical communications system in man that complemented the white blood cells of the immune system. These small molecules could perform essential functions in the human body, such as regulating the interaction of normal cells (Ashraf et al., 1988).

"Instead of looking at peptides as such-and-such substances," Burzynski says, "I looked on them as words, pieces of information" (Lang, 1987a). In such terms, peptides could be seen as short, direct commands, e.g., STOP CANCER.

The second half of the twentieth century, says Stash, has been marked by the transition from energy- to information-processing. Medicine had to catch up with advances in the other sciences, particularly information theory. Cancer, according to this provocative view, was "a disease of information processing." Initially Burzynski's interest wasn't in cancer per se. "I picked up on cancer first," he says, "because cancer seemed to be the most intriguing" (ibid.). Cancer was a riot of misinformation—a lack of good instructions—working its havoc on the human body. Communication was the key to its eventual control.

The peptide discoveries were greeted with excitement in the scientific community and the press. Burzynski presented a paper at the 1976 Anaheim meeting of the Federation of Associations for Experimental Biology (FASEB), one of the largest scientific gatherings in the world. The work, done in conjunction with the vice president of the Department of Experimental Therapeutics at M. D. Anderson Tumor Institute, was publicized by FASEB's public relations department. Out of 3,700 papers, in fact, it became the lead Associated Press (AP) story on the gathering:

> A chemical with the power to change cancer cells back to normal cells has been extracted from human urine. . . . [It] apparently detects cells that are getting out of line and feeds them new information that returns them to normal.
>
> If the naturally occurring substance can be made artificially, Dr. S. R. Burzynski of Houston said Wednesday, it could be valuable in cancer therapy (*Houston Chronicle*, April 15, 1976).

The original broad-spectrum Antineoplaston A was eventually broken down (subfractionated) into A1, A2, A3, A4, and A5. In the early 1980s Burzynski made the breakthrough anticipated in the AP dispatch. Through a laborious process he managed first to analyze and then to synthesize one of the peptides in the original fraction. It could now be manufactured in the laboratory from off-the-shelf amino acids. This novel compound turned out to be a dipeptide (two amino acids), with glutamine arranged in a sixfold ring structure. Its chemical name was 3-phenylacetylamino-2, 6-piperidinedione. Burzynski dubbed it A10.

In the body, A10 broke down into two other substances, which were excreted in the urine. These were named AS2–1 and AS2–5. These three substances were soon being synthesized and manufactured in his Houston laboratory. Contrary to later charges, the composition of Burzynski's materials was not kept a secret. The doctor was eager for other scientists to learn his manufacturing methods. His procedures were the same as those of every other peptide chemist, but his discoveries were protected by the first of eighteen patents he obtained around the world on these unique substances.

These were productive and exciting years. He married a fellow emigré, Barbara Szopa, M.D., and for several years they settled down to a pleasant life. While at Baylor he authored or coauthored sixteen papers, five on peptides. He began to develop a private medical practice. He became a member in good standing of the American Association for Cancer Research (AACR) and the American Medical Association (AMA), and picked up enough awards and honors to fill two office walls. He combined these scientific accomplishments with a strong adherence to the Catholic church, especially its Polish-speaking pontiff.

After FASEB, the next logical step was to give antineoplastons to animals. There were two reasons for this: first, to test for toxicity, and second, to see if they had some effect on either the prevention or the treatment of cancer.

In every experiment they proved remarkably nontoxic, so much so that it was difficult to establish an "LD50," the median lethal dose at which 50 percent of the test animals died.

Results in the animal treatment experiments were spotty. Human antineoplastons did *not* generally cure animal tumors. Burzynski soon explained why. Since only Old World monkeys shared a precursor of antineoplastons with man (James et al., 1971) each species of animal seemed to produce its own specific kinds of antineoplastons.

Antineoplastons could be used preventatively in animals, however. For example, in tests performed by Dr. Craig Whitefield at the University of Arkansas in Fayetteville, chickens were injected with the virus that causes Rous sarcoma. Half of the birds were also given antineoplastons. Initially, "all the birds who did not receive antineoplastons got massive tumors and died," says Burzynski, "but *none* of the birds who received antineoplastons developed tumors." Eventually, however, even the antineoplaston-treated birds succumbed to their cancer.

Stories to this effect appeared in mass-circulation magazines such as *Family Circle* (February 1977) and *Prevention* (October 1977).

After the AP story appeared in the Houston papers, Burzynski came to the attention of the Baylor Cancer Research Center. In their eyes Burzynski was an important find, a scientist doing work of national importance in their own backyard. In 1976 he received $30,000 from the university to continue his research and a "Welcome Aboard" speech from the chief of the Baylor Cancer Research Center.

Burzynski was asked to become a member of the center. It looked like a promotion. There was one condition, however: he had to give up his budding private practice. Others might have grabbed at the chance and been happily absorbed into the cancer mainstream. There were, after all, ample rewards for doing so. But Burzynski hesitated. Perhaps it was his earlier brush with the Polish bureaucracy, but he hadn't come to America to become another cog in the wheel. Deep in his marrow, he feared institutionalization.

"Most medical breakthroughs," he later suggested with a sly touch of irony, "have happened because there was some lack of suppression by the supervisors of people doing some innovative work." Look at insulin, he said—discovered by a graduate student while the laboratory head was on vacation. In the backwaters of Baylor's anesthesiology department, "as far remote from cancer research as you can imagine," Stash Burzynski had received the precious gift of obscurity (Lang, 1987a).

In addition, his private practice gave him financial independence. "If I should join them," he said, "I would do exactly what they were telling me to do, even though I would have a separate lab" (ibid.). When he refused their offer, these well-established cancer researchers turned against him and began to make life difficult.

The year before, George Ungar had been ousted from Baylor in a power struggle. The school brought a 70-year-old anesthesiologist out of retirement and made him the head of the department. This man didn't like Stash, whom he regarded as his predecessor's protegé. Just before Christmas 1976, Stash was informed that his laboratory space was to be cut in half. NCI had to intervene to save him. The following year his NCI grant was approved but the funding was delayed. He knew he might have to wait up to four years to get the money to function—meanwhile, his laboratory expenses and staff salaries continued to mount up. He simply could not stay at Baylor without a grant.

Burzynski now stood at a crossroads. If he wanted to move forward with antineoplastons, he realized, he would have to leave the university. But this was wrenching because academic life was in his blood. He and his father before him had grown up in that seductive, cloistered atmosphere which, once experienced, is so difficult to give up. Leaving Baylor would mean turning his back on a secure, petit-bourgeois existence. It meant embracing unknown challenges to his livelihood, his reputation—and who knew what else?

In the midst of this personal crisis, an odd thing happened. Like a providential angel, his old mentor from Poland, Professor Marian Mazur, showed up unannounced in Texas. He had come to give a series of lectures at Rice University. Mazur listened to Stash's story and advised him to proceed with clinical testing. Burzynski raised all the difficulties this path entailed, but Mazur interrupted him: "If you are right about these peptides," he said, "everyone will eventually have to acknowledge it."

Burzynski's private practice had brought him into contact with living, and dying, cancer patients. It was torture to watch them waste away and know that he had a substance that might help them. Scientific curiosity gnawed at him. And financial considerations could not help but play their part. It escaped no one's notice that an effective treatment, locked in by patents, could be worth a fortune.

And so Burzynski made the most momentous decision of his life: to proceed with the testing of antineoplastons in people.

Although he received an impressive certificate for meritorious service from Dr. Michael DeBakey, the famous president of Baylor College of Medicine, his chairman's last words were not auspicious: "Just wait, Burzynski. They're going to kick your ass."

Texas prides itself on its maverick tradition. Looking for a place to try his novel compounds, Burzynski made contact with a self-described "old-fashioned country doctor," named William Mask. Mask was head of the Jack County General Hospital in Jacksboro, Texas. If Burzynski was looking for fellow mavericks, he found them a-plenty in Jacksboro, a town whose Wild West roots are celebrated in James Michener's novel *Texas*. "They hated bureaucrats," Burzynski adds, with a smile, "and were happy to cooperate."

The first clinical trials were among the most exciting moments in Burzynski's life. The compound had an effect—and sometimes a dramatic effect—on human cancer. Dr. Mask later testified at a court hearing in 1985:

> There's not any doubt in my mind. I'm convinced in my 40 years of experience in seeing cancer, this (treatment) is the best (*Houston Post*, October 11, 1985).

He also cited the case of a Wichita Falls man cured of bladder cancer in a second Jacksboro trial. Mast told the judge that he would recommend antineoplaston treatments in place of traditional chemotherapy and radiation, which "kill the good cells as well as the bad cells" (*Houston Chronicle*, Oct. 11, 1985).

Using these first results, Burzynski was able to convince previously skeptical doctors on the institutional review board of Houston's Twelve Oaks Hospital to allow him to begin treatments there as well. Twelve Oaks was a modern, 380-bed hospital near downtown Houston. In 1977 he reported on a clinical trial in which Antineoplaston A was given to 21 advanced cancer patients at Twelve Oaks. "Chronic intravenous administration of antineoplaston A to these patients showed pronounced antitumor effect without any significant toxicity," he wrote in a scientific journal (Burzynski et al., 1977). The medical language obscured a startling fact: antineoplastons were having an effect on cancers unresponsive to conventional forms of therapy.

Yet immediately after this, Twelve Oaks withdrew permission to treat patients with antineoplastons. According to Burzynski, he was told he would have to obtain approval from either Baylor College of Medicine or M. D. Anderson before he could proceed. Neither Baylor nor M. D. Anderson has any official regulatory power, of course, but they were powerhouses in Houston's massive medical complex. (From then on, although Burzynski retained admitting privileges at Twelve Oaks, he could no longer administer antineoplastons there.)

Burzynski's response was to open his own clinic nearby and start giving cancer patients antineoplastons. For the time being, the drugs were manufactured in a 2,500-square-foot garage space next door, while the doctor and his brother, engineer Tad Burzynski, scouted for a larger site.

To those familiar with the drug approval process it may seem strange—and suspect—that Burzynski did not first apply for Investigational New Drug (IND) status from the Food and Drug Administration (FDA) before administering his substances to patients.

The "normal" process is for a new substance to be discovered at a major medical center and then turned over to a drug company for development. If the company decides it is economically feasible, it will then battle its IND application through the FDA. This whole process takes on average ten years, generates truckloads of data, and costs on average over $100 million. Even then it is often unsuccessful.

But no drug company showed an interest in these nontoxic compounds. And so Burzynski decided to develop them himself. He would have liked to have gotten FDA approval. But in 1977 his capital amounted to exactly $5,000! Thus he was caught in a classic catch-22 situation. If he tested antineoplastons in humans, the FDA was sure to come down on him eventually. But if he didn't so test them, he could never win FDA approval, since antineoplastons, being species-specific, are not generally effective in animal treatment experiments.

His decision was thus to start treating patients, build up good records, let patient fees finance the future development of the drugs, and deal with the FDA later. When the battle heated up, some of his emotional motivation showed as well:

> I'm going to fight no matter what they do, because I believe I'm doing the right thing. I believe that this is our obligation to the people. If you find

something that's valuable, you must continue and I believe that we've found something that may be able to save lives (quoted in Null, 1979).

Texas at that time was what is called an unincorporated state. That meant that the rules of the FDA concerning new drugs were not yet incorporated into Texas law. (That happened only later, in 1985, possibly in response to Burzynski's notoriety.) According to his personal lawyer at the time, Ernest Caldwell, Burzynski had the freedom to use innovative medicines of his own. choosing as long as he was not involved in interstate commerce.

In 1978 Burzynski received his first site visit from the FDA. In light of FDA's later hostility, it was surprisingly friendly. They inspected his small manufacturing plant and gave him a good deal of constructive criticism.

"And in fact, there was a lot to criticize," said Burzynski. His manufacturing processes were still amateurish. The inspectors were cooperative, however, and gave excellent advice on how to improve his processes. "It was exactly as I thought the government should act in such a situation," he remarked.

His local colleagues were less tolerant toward this Polish emigré who was suddenly garnering all the headlines. In 1978 Burzynski became the focus of an investigation by the Board of Ethics of the Harris County Medical Society. The charge was using unapproved medications of his own devising. They repeatedly called him in for interviews and instructed him not to give any interviews to the press. For nearly two years he complied with their gag order.

This was only the beginning of his troubles, however. He was deeply in debt because he had to turn to bank loans to keep the operation alive; he was refused research money from the American Cancer Society; his former sponsor, the National Cancer Institute, now postponed his funding; and the May 1978 meeting of the AACR actually refused his abstract—something that rarely happens. (The chairman of the approval committee was a Sloan-Kettering chemotherapist.) In a mere two years, this rising star of cancer research had tumbled to the bottom of the heap!

The ethics board's news blockade was finally broken by Gary Null, a New York health crusader, in a 1979 article in *Penthouse* entitled "The Suppression of Cancer Cures."*

---

*Because of the intense interest of publisher Bob Guccione in the cancer problem, *Penthouse* for the last decade has been an unexpected outlet for favorable articles on unconventional approaches.

On October 22, 1981, Burzynski achieved national television attention when "The War on Cancer: Cure, Profit or Politics?" aired on ABC's "20/20." According to commentator Geraldo Rivera:

> The deeper we looked into the story, the more we realized that Stanislaw Burzynski is really not a maverick at all. His work is very much in the scientific mainstream, that burgeoning field of cancer research that's pinpointing the body's own natural materials, its own proteins, to control irregular cell growth. . . . Burzynski has simply decided to do things his way ("20/20," 1981).

After this publicity, hundreds of cancer patients began flocking to the Houston clinic to receive antineoplaston therapy. The spotlight of public attention seemed to freeze the Board of Ethics in its tracks. In any case, Burzynski never heard from them again after April 1980.

Instead, the baton was passed to various national agencies. In 1982 the Canadian Bureau of Human Prescription Drugs (Health and Welfare) requested information from their American colleagues on the effectiveness of antineoplastons. The U.S. National Cancer Institute reported it had no data but agreed to test three varieties of the drug—A2, A5, and the synthetic version, A10—in its standard animal assay.

Burzynski cooperated but was dubious. There were several test-tube and preventative models in which the drug had showed effectiveness, but the standard NCI pre-screen, P388 mouse leukemia, was not one of them. In June 1984 Burzynski sent samples of A10 to NCI. But he warned:

> Because of narrow specificity of antineoplaston A10, personally I do not believe the compound will display significant activity in the pre-screen P388. I decided, however, to submit antineoplaston A10 for such screening to satisfy scientific curiosity and to expand our knowledge of the compound (Burzynski, 1984).

As he had predicted, these compounds were not effective against mouse leukemia. Burzynski reasonably suggested that NCI try the antineoplastons in cell-culture assays that were similar to "human solid tumors, especially adenocarcinoma of the breast. . . ."

Burzynski was hardly alone in voicing doubts about the P388 mouse model. Ironically, it was Dr. John Venditti himself, chief of NCI's Drug Evaluation Branch, who in 1983 had coauthored an article in which he argued the limitations of this very mouse system.* Scientists at NCI had found, for instance, that of seventy-nine drugs which had previously been judged negative in the P388, fourteen showed "significant activity" when retested in cell culture assays:

> These initial screening results suggest that either the cell culture assay is more sensitive than the pre-screen or that it is detecting a different class of agents (Shoemaker et al. 1983).

Yet when a particular "different class of agents," antineoplastons, failed to have any effect in the P388 pre-screen, this fact took its place in government literature as the most damning piece of evidence against Burzynski's new method (NCI Statement on Antineoplastons, 1987).

In the early eighties, articles about antineoplastons also appeared in the Canadian print media, such as Maclean's and the *Windsor Press*. "20/20" was also widely seen north of the border. One of those who viewed that program was a Sault Ste. Marie oncologist named David Walde. Intrigued, he sent for Burzynski's literature, but did not feel his questions were adequately answered. In April 1982 he decided that he would go to Houston to investigate for himself.

Like most medical visitors, he arrived in a highly skeptical frame of mind:

> I had no idea what to expect upon my arrival there, and would not have been surprised to have found a backdoor operation directed to the exploitation of patients for financial gain, without the benefits of any therapeutic activity of the program. I also thought that documentation of the clinical cases would be poor and incomplete, making evaluation difficult, if not impossible (Walde, 1982).

What he found instead "was beyond my wildest expectations, and I had to rapidly backtrack on all my preconceived concepts of the situation. . . ." (ibid.).

---

*Leonard Kunst, M.D., and Harold Ladas, Ph.D., have made an interesting observation about this mouse leukemia standard: "The result of this selective research is an effective treatment against leukemia and little or no progress against the solid tumors which comprise by far the majority of all cancers. The choice of criterion . . . (the leukemic mouse standard) determined the area of success" (Kunst and Ladas, 1987).

Walde first visited the new antineoplaston production plant that Tac Burzynski was busy assembling in a block-long building in nearby Stafford The manufacturing guidelines were those suggested by FDA and the entir operation—with its highly sophisticated, computerized control panels, it safety codes, and its sterile precautions—was the same as one might find i any modern pharmaceutical plant.

> It was beyond my conception that an individual, without massive cash-flow funding from either commercial or government sources, would be able to single-handedly put together this sophisticated production capability. My impression was that the entire program, both research and production, was built on the financial backs of patients, supplemented by large personal bank loans by Dr. "B." (ibid.)

Walde's conclusion was that urinary peptides were an extremely promising area of cancer research. He also suggested that Burzynski submit his data for IND clearance in Canada. Once this was obtained, further studies should be coordinated with the Investigatory Drug Subcommittee of NCI Canada. And finally, that there should be "no sensationalism through the public media . . . as this could disrupt any investigatory program" (ibid.).

Burzynski agreed and proceeded to apply for an IND in Canada. The process moved swiftly forward, and for several months it looked as if Canada were going to be the first country to explicitly sanction the use of antineoplastons. But this was not to be.

In October 1982 the Ontario Deputy Minister of Health asked the Ontario Medical Association to appoint experts to review Burzynski's treatment. The Ontario Health Insurance Plan had stopped paying for antineoplastons, declaring them "experimental" treatment. Two Toronto doctors, Martin Blackstein, chief of oncology at Mount Sinai Hospital in Toronto, and Daniel Bergsagel, head of medicine at Princess Margaret Hospital, were sent to investigate.

On November 15, 1982, Drs. Blackstein and Bergsagel arrived in Houston. Burzynski first took them to the Stafford plant and then to his clinic to review records. In contrast to Walde's lengthy investigation, Blackstein and Bergsagel's review of the records lasted a total of two hours and fifteen minutes. Burzynski complained of "the hostility of Dr. Bergsagel" from the beginning of the visit "and his complete ignorance of pharmaceutical processing and testing . . ." (Burzynski, "Response," 1982).

When they returned to Canada, Blackstein and Bergsagel wrote up their conclusions. They had not a single positive thing to say about the treatment. In fact, their criticism was scathing:

1. The preparation of human urinary antineoplastons is not known and the structures of the synthetic compounds is [sic] secret.

2. We do not feel there is significant 'in vitro' activity of antineoplastons against tissue-cultured tumor cells, because such high concentrations are required before antitumor effects are observed.

3. There is no evidence that antineoplastons inhibit the growth of murine [i.e., mouse or rat] tumors.

4. After reviewing 20 case reports. . . . we were unable to identify a single case in which therapeutic benefit could be attributed to antineoplaston.

5. Dr. Burzynski has not filed a New Drug Application for the registration of Antineoplaston. . . .

6. We believe it is unethical to administer unproven agents such as antineoplastons to patients. . . . We also believe that it is immoral to charge patients for this unproven, experimental treatment . . . (Blackstein/Bergsagel, 1982).

A fuller treatment of the charges against Burzynski is given in section III below. But Burzynski himself was quick to refute these charges at the time and subsequent evidence has strengthened his assertions:

1. Far from being secretive, Burzynski said he attempted to explain his production techniques to the two doctors in great detail. They were shown the "70 different chemical and biological tests required for the production of antineoplastons" (Burzynski, "Response," 1982). However, Blackstein and Bergsagel evinced little interest, he said, in his lengthy production techniques.

When the author visited the plant in October 1988, the doctor spent the better part of an afternoon proudly explaining the minutiae of production technology, answering every question posed. Others have reported similar experiences. In addition, his processes are covered by five U.S. and over a dozen foreign patents, all of which reveal detailed manufacturing procedures. He has licensed Taiwanese, Filipino, Italian and Soviet companies to produce these products. These are hardly the signs of the secret formula usually associated with a stereotypical quack.

2. The doctors charge that the high doses needed to demonstrate an *in vitro* anticancer effect preclude its use as an effective drug in humans. This might be true of a toxic chemotherapeutic agent, but does not hold for compounds without serious side effects.

Relatively high doses of antineoplastons are required to achieve optimum effects in tissue cultures. But equivalently high levels of antineoplastons can and are routinely and safely maintained in patients' bloodstreams. This is possible because of the essentially nontoxic nature of the agents involved.

In regard to Burzynski's cell-line experiments, Blackstein and Berg-sagel claimed that "the growth of many mammalian cell lines can be inhib-ited by merely adding distilled water to the culture to lower the tonicity of the medium."

This remark is purely speculative. Burzynski follows the tissue-culture procedures recommended by the National Cancer Institute. In every such experiment, control tissue-culture flasks receive everything the experimental flasks receive *except the medicine under investigation*. Thus, if the drug is dissolved in distilled water, the control samples must receive the same amount of distilled water, only without antineoplastons.

If Blackstein and Bergsagel's objections were valid, *all* tissue-culture tests that follow NCI procedures would also be invalid. The reason such tests are acceptable is precisely because, like Burzynski's, they routinely utilize valid controls.

The two doctors also claimed that "a few of the fractions inhibited DNA synthesis to a modest degree (16–27 percent) and also inhibited the growth of HeLa cells in culture. . . . However, very large amounts of the fraction . . . [were] required to inhibit the mitosis of HeLa cell cultures by 77 percent."

In fact, antineoplastons inhibit up to 100 percent of the growth of cancer cells in culture. There is a dose-response curve: the more drug added, to the flask, the more inhibition. In the controls, on the other hand, there is uninhibited cell growth.

In one study, for example,

the exposure of HBL-500 cells to 0.125 mg/ml of Antineoplaston A5 reduced the colony number to approximately 60 percent of the control. At 0.25 mg/ml, only 14 percent of the cells were still able to form colonies and at 0.5 mg/ml no colonies were found (Lee and Burzynski, 1987).

Far from being a rare event, such tissue-culture assays are the routine way new batches of antineoplastons are tested at the Burzynski Research Institute. Every batch of the medicine isolated from urine has to show 80–100 percent inhibition before it is given to patients. This has been performed thousands of times by over a dozen different people around the world.

3. According to the two Canadians, "Dr. Burzynski speculates that the effect of antineoplastons is species specific." They hint that Burzynski may have had an ulterior motive for making this claim:

It should be noted that by introducing the concept that antineoplastons are specifies [sic] specific, that they are inactive in tissue culture, and only show antitumor activity after they are activated in the body, it becomes clear that the activity of these antineoplastons can only be tested by giving them to patients (Blackstein and Bergsagel, 1982).

But species specificity is a well-known phenomenon in nature. It is quite typical, in fact, for peptide hormones, such as insulin. The much-publicized drug interferon is species-specific. Independent studies of antineoplastons's precursors show that they differ in their amino acid composition from species to species (James et al., 1971). It is logical to suppose (although this is not yet proven) that antineoplastons do so as well.

In discussing the animal results, Blackstein and Bergsagel do not acknowledge or explain the frequent cases in which drugs fail the P388 prescreen only to be proven effective in more sensitive assays. This, for example, was the case with several now-accepted toxic chemotherapeutic agents, such as Vincristine, 6-Thioguanine, and hexamethylmelamine.

Furthermore, there is no mention in the two doctors' report of the preventative effect in animals, which is one of the drug's most prominent benefits.

4. Blackstein and Bergsagel claim that they reviewed "Dr. Burzynski's medical records on about 12 patients." They dismissed the significance of all of these, as well as those sent later by the Houston physician:

> The commonest problem we encountred [sic] was the fact that patients had received effective treatment before they were referred to Houston, and were responding slowly to this treatment. Dr. Burzynski started antineoplaston, and falsely credited the antineoplaston with the therapeutic response that was observed (Blackstein and Bergsagel, 1982).

In one case, for instance, the Canadian doctors were shown the X rays of a patient with metastatic lung nodules from a carcinoma of the colon. "The x-rays that we were shown demonstrated no significant change in the size of pulmonary nodules over a 4 to 5 month period," they concluded.

Yet months before, Burzynski had sent these chest X rays to a Houston radiologist, P. Amin, M.D., not associated with Burzynski's institute. Dr. Amin concluded:

> There is considerable improvement with almost complete resolution of the nodules in the right lung. . . . The nodule in the left suprahilar region which was seen on the previous radiographs has also completely regressed.

The other nodules show lack of definition but significant change in size . . . (Amin, P., M.D., Radiology Associates of Bellaire, June 24, 1982).

In two other cases, one of lung cancer and the other of soft-tissue sarcoma of the nose, the Canadian doctors complained:

> It is difficult to judge the response of a tumor on a CT scan if one is shown only a selected projection, because one must be sure that all of the projections are taken at the same level. We did not feel the selected projections had been obtained at the same level, and we did not think that either of these patients had shown a response to antineoplaston therapy (Blackstein and Bergsagel, 1982).

According to Burzynski, in both cases the projections were at the same level and showed a significant reduction in the size of the tumors. Again there was independent confirmation of this.

In the first case, according to Houston radiologist M. Calderon, M.D.:

> There is an interval change from April to June [1980] with an approximate 50 percent reduction in the size of the left hilar mass and no significant change in lymph node metastasis in the right hilum.
> From the examination of June 11, 1980 to June 22, 1980 we found slightly further reduction in the size of the left hilar region . . . (M. Calderon, M.D., Houston Imaging Center, August 8, 1980).

In the case of the soft-tissue sarcoma, Dr. Amin also confirmed Burzynski's contention:

> *CT/NASOPHARYNX & PARANASAL SINUSES:* In comparison with the previous examination of 7/6/82 there is further improvement with regression of the soft tissue involving the maxillary sinus and anterior and superior aspect of the right ethmoid cells. . . .
> *IMPRESSION:* There is further improvement. There is still approximately 30 percent soft tissue mass involving the right antrum and part of the ethmoid cells (Amin, P., M.D., Bellaire Tomography Center, August 31, 1982).

Burzynski says he was given time to show the visiting doctors records of only nine cases before they decided to leave. Six of these cases obtained complete remission and two obtained nearly complete remissions.

While the two doctors later wrote that patients had commonly received effective treatment before they were treated with antineoplastons, according to Burzynski only one of the initial nine was treated with radiation and chemotherapy and one additional patient received a very small dose of palliative radiotherapy.

> These patients were suffering from extensive and highly malignant cancers which usually do not respond to chemotherapy; such as, lung cancer, cancer of the liver, cancer of the cervix, colon cancer, mesothelioma, cancer of the larynx, sarcoma and stage IV malignant lymphoma. Each case was documented by biopsy, and the remission of each of them was confirmed by at least one other doctor not associated with our clinic (Burzynski, "Response," 1982).

Burzynski contends he urged Blackstein and Bergsagel to look at more cases, but they refused. He then suggested they take more cases with them to Canada. They refused. Finally he sent more to them in Toronto:

> Dr. Bergsagel and Dr. Blackstein were very anxious to leave the clinic as soon as possible. They did not want to look through any more cases, and they did not want to wait to take the copies of the additional case histories with them. Finally, we sent them sixteen additional case histories with most cases showing complete remission and not treated with radiation and chemotherapy (ibid.).

5. Concerning the FDA: At the time of the visit by the two doctors, Burzynski had not yet applied for an IND. But he had been in frequent touch with the FDA since 1978 and did apply for an IND in the following year (1983). The question of his IND was, strictly speaking, extraneous to the question the two doctors were in Houston to investigate—"to determine whether his treatment could be recognized as a promising approach to cancer therapy. . . ."

It was well known from the start that Burzynski had not yet gotten FDA approval to ship the drugs across state lines. In fact, if he *had* gotten an IND there probably would have been little likelihood or purpose for such a site visit.

6. The competing claims of consumer safety and freedom of choice raise many ethical dilemmas. One could just as well ask, however: Would it have been ethical for Burzynski to withhold his nontoxic treatment from dying patients, when no state or federal law at the time required him to do

so? When the regulatory barrier erected by FDA required an expenditure many thousand times what he possessed? When one million North Americans alone develop cancer every year and at least half of those, according to a 1985 Media General/Associated Press poll, want access to treatment with medicines not yet approved by the American FDA? (Chowka, 1987)

And what, after all, is an "unproven" method? Every method is unproven until it is proven, including all the highly toxic protocols that come out of the comprehensive cancer centers. And many drugs and procedures that have been considered proven in the past have turned out to be useless upon further examination, such as the Halsted operation or the indiscriminate use of radium. On the basis of historical precedent we can assume that in the future many of our present-day procedures will be considered useless, if not barbaric.

The two Toronto doctors found it "immoral to charge patients" for this therapy. Yet to avoid a double standard they would logically have had to condemn the entire fee-for-service medical system, which sometimes bankrupts people at their most vulnerable moments. Cancer is a multibillion-dollar business, and few oncologists work for free.

Not surprisingly, however, Blackstein and Bergsagel strongly recommended *against* insurance reimbursement for treatments at the Houston clinic. Their comments were widely circulated in the United States as well as Canada, and soon became the touchstone of opposition to Burzynski.

Shortly thereafter, in January 1983, the American Cancer Society launched a broadside attack. The condemnation of the peptide approach appeared in the January 1983 issue of *Ca,* a magazine the Society distributes free to nearly half a million medical readers (ACS, 1983). This statement, later incorporated into the *Unproven Methods* compendium, began with the usual litany: ACS "does not have evidence that treatment with antineoplastons results in objective benefit." It then repeated the usual charges.

Yet ACS also included data which undercut its own conclusions. For instance, it repeated that in the 1977 study, "twenty-one far-advanced cancer patients were treated with Antineoplaston A" and "some degree of clinical improvement was noted in 18 of the 21 patients (86 percent)." It also repeated the claim that there were "minimal or no side effects," and presented without criticism a chart showing complete remission in four cases, or 19 percent, and partial remission in another four.

"In contrast," wrote Robert G. Houston, "a study on Interleukin-2 in 25 patients with advanced cancer by Dr. Steven Rosenberg (1985) at the NCI produced an avalanche of attention because one patient (4 percent) had a complete remission" (Houston, 1987a:41). But Rosenberg was President

Reagan's surgeon and a powerhouse at NCI, which may have accounted for his technique's ready acceptance.

The blows now began to fall fast and thick. In April 1983 the FDA filed suit against Dr. Burzynski and his associates in an attempt "to force the permanent cessation of all their scientific and medical work on the development, manufacture and administration of antineoplastons" (Lang, 1986).

The judge, Gabrielle McDonald, ruled against the FDA, charging they had not brought in sufficient evidence to warrant such a sweeping measure. But on May 24, 1983, she did agree to an injunction against interstate shipment of antineoplastons until the FDA had received and approved a completed Investigational New Drug (IND) status. (An IND is the government's license to proceed with the testing of a drug.) Activity within the state of Texas was *specifically allowed,* however, by Judge McDonald's decree.

On May 6, 1983, as a result of the FDA action against him, Burzynski applied for an IND for Antineoplaston A10. At the end of the month, the FDA turned him down for the first of many times, putting the drug on "clinical hold," a state of suspended animation.

The reasons for the rejection were explained in a highly detailed letter from William J. Gyarfas, an official of the drug agency. The primary reason was the alleged lack of efficacy: Burzynski had failed "to furnish information indicating that Antineoplaston A10 . . . has activity against malignant cells of animal or human origin or against animal tumors . . ." (Gyarfas, 1983).

While the FDA official glossed over the positive data provided, his report noted all sorts of technical deficiencies. These would be tedious to repeat in full, but a few will give the flavor. FDA demanded:

- Statements from the "Quality Assurance Unit specifying the dates when inspections were made and the dates when the findings were reported to management and to the study director."
- Information on the "Institutional Review Board (IRB) as required by 21 CFR 56.103."
- Data "demonstrating the stability of antineoplaston [sic] A10 in the feed.
- Was the concentration of the drug in the feed adjusted weekly to account for the increase in weight of the animals?"
- A "table comparing the weekly food consumption for each dose group (male and female), animal weights, and weekly calculated drug dosage" (ibid.).

And so on for five pages, single-spaced. FDA also refused to accept Barbara Burzynski, M.D., as chairperson of the Institute's Quality Assurance Unit because she also chaired the Department of Pharmacy "in addition to being the spouse of the study director. . . ." The relevance of that last charge was not explained (Palmer, 1984).

These were the sorts of details that had made the American drug approval process a nightmare for even the biggest research institutions. By the late nineteen-eighties, in fact, the FDA drug bottleneck had become a national scandal.

AIDS patients in particular were taking the lead in demanding reform. On October 11, 1988, for instance, they attacked the headquarters of the FDA outside Washington, "where they lay on the ground with hand-painted tombstones at their heads, reading 'I Died for the Sins of the FDA,' 'I Got the Placebo' (*Wall Street Journal*, October 13, 1988).

Bitter opposition has also come from establishment sources. In his book *Understanding Cancer*, John Laszlo, M.D., senior vice president for research at the American Cancer Society, issued an eloquent plea for more open research:

> The FDA has changed its requirements for approving new anticancer drugs in a way that is likely to block further progress very significantly. . . . These problems are well known by cancer researchers as well as by the pharmaceutical industry; yet despite promises by recent Presidents to simplify government paperwork and bureaucracy, the cost of developing new drugs is constantly rising, partly because of these artificial barriers imposed by government (Laszlo, 1987:182).

The *Wall Street Journal* has been waging an editorial campaign for suspension of the 1962 Kefauver (efficacy) amendments. It is FDA's interpretation of these amendments that has provided the basis for its obstruction of innovative scientists, including, but certainly not limited to, Burzynski.

"If in fact the standard of approval is going to be 'definitive data,' " the *Journal* opined, "the FDA will definitively destroy a lot of raised hopes." It went on:

> In deciding over the years which drugs work and which don't, the FDA and most of the medical research community have set common sense on the shelf and put their faith in the arcane discipline of statistics. . . . The rigid worship of "definitive data" is why AIDS victims have virtually laid siege to the federal medical establishment ("Relief From Suffering" (editorial), September 19, 1988. See also June 15, July 14, and October 13, 1988).

For these establishment critics, FDA is bureaucracy gone wild. But if the FDA regulations are onerous for the ACS, imagine the burden they put on mavericks like Stash Burzynski.

In addition to the FDA, the ACS, and the NCI, even the Post Office got into the act. By the time of the raid, the U.S. Postal Service had developed a new, high profile in the war against quackery. In September 1985, for example, it cosponsored a national conference on health fraud. The conclave was called to publicize efforts by Representative Claude Pepper (D.-Fla.), the FDA, and the Pharmaceutical Advertising Council to push new antiquackery legislation (Caplan, 1987).

But while the Pepper bill was soon withdrawn amid a storm of controversy, the Postal Service kept up its pressure. In 1986 it sent chilling letters to Burzynski's patients informing them that "an investigation is being conducted into the activities of Dr. S. R. Burzynski and particularly regarding alleged improper insurance billing practices." Patients were informed they could expect to be contacted by a postal inspector in the near future "and it will be very helpful if you will have your records readily available regarding treatment by Dr. Burzynski" (letter of D. K. Beaty, September 12, 1986).

Had any patient filed a complaint about mail fraud? No. Nor was there any basis to these innuendos. After a few months, nothing further was heard about this investigation. One factor may have been that many patients angrily registered their refusal to cooperate.*

Despite such harrassment, Burzynski was not about to fold his clinic or leave the country. He maintained a serene confidence that his work on antineoplastons would eventually be vindicated, and that the American establishment would wake up to the facts.

He has doggedly attempted to comply with the government's requirements, repeatedly trying to fix his IND application to FDA's satisfaction.

On June 13, August 19, and October 12, 1983, for instance, he amended his Notice to comply with their requests. But each time FDA concluded that "it is still not reasonably safe to initiate your clinical investigation." This become a ritual: FDA asked for more data, Burzynski provided it, then FDA came back with yet more detailed questions and complaints. At least Burzynski was in technical compliance with Judge McDonald's order to apply

---

*To many, there was irony in the idea of the Post Office even entering the controversy over cancer therapies. The U.S. Postal Service is notoriously unable to keep its own "appointed rounds." A cover story in the *New York Times Magazine* revealed that bulk mail was delayed in 94 percent of the Eastern post offices, while first class mail and magazines were "discarded in trash bins" in 75 percent. Writer John B. Judis titled his story on the agency "Mission: Impossible" (September 26, 1988). Yet this same ailing Postal Service felt itself qualified to hound the discoverers of new cancer treatments.

for an IND. Thus, for the time being, he could legally keep his clinic open in Texas.

From time to time, in Kafkaesque fashion, the FDA would slip in some hint of eventual redemption. In 1983, for example, an FDA official conceded:

> The best assessment that can be made is that the disease remained stable in some of these patients, some of whom were also receiving other medications (Palmer, 1983).

In August 1988, Burzynski received a letter from the FDA which actually seemed to concede anticancer activity in a set of Japanese mouse studies. But by and large the line of the FDA and other establishment organizations has been consistent:

Burzynski is a menace. Burzynski has got to go.

The Case Against Burzynski

Since the Blackstein-Bergsagel visit, an elaborate case has been developed against Stanislaw Burzynski and antineoplastons. Many of the charges against him date from that Canadian visit. Others have been elaborated by the FDA and other opponents. It might be useful to try to reduce them to their essence and deal with them in turn. To Burzynski's opponents, then, there are five main objections: antineoplaston therapy is (1) ineffective, (2) bizarre, (3) unsafe, and (4) expensive. In addition, Dr. Burzynski himself is (5) unqualified to do clinical research.

1. "It just doesn't work."

The major charge against Burzynski is that antineoplastons are ineffective against cancer. And before FDA will allow clinical testing of a new anticancer drug, it requires proof that the product "has activity against malignant cells of animal or human origin or against animal tumors." The resistance to Burzynski is predicated on the idea that antineoplaston treatment is without proven effectiveness in such systems (Gyarfas, 1983).

Burzynski's work on cell lines was widely hailed in the mid-seventies. The peptides were "active against every type of human neoplasm we tested," he wrote, "including myeloblastic leukemia, osteosarcoma, fibrosarcoma, chondrosarcoma, cancer of the uterine cervix, colon cancer, breast cancer, lung cancer and lymphoma." In fact, "all antineoplastons inhibited up to

100 percent of the growth of neoplastic cells with less inhibitory effect on normal cells . . ." (Burzynski, 1986).

As we've seen, proving effectiveness to FDA's satisfaction primarily means passing an animal test called the P388 anticancer pre-screen. Burzynski correctly predicted his drugs would not have any effectiveness in this limited system. But despite the fact that many other useful drugs have also failed that particular test, the authorities tried to make that the end of the story.

It was primarily because of this failure that FDA refused Burzynski permission even to test antineoplastons for safety (Phase I studies). Over and over again it has harped on the failure in P388:

> Unless the drug has some antineoplastic activity in experimental systems there is no rationale for its administration to patients with malignant disease even though you propose only Phase I trials at this time (Gyarfas, 1983).

But there are other ways to evaluate a drug's efficacy besides P388. One of these is to test it against human cancer cells growing in a special kind of "nude" mouse. These animals are born without thymuses, and thus cannot mount host-vs.-graft reactions against transplanted human cancer tissue. In 1988, when Japanese researchers used antineoplastons in nude mice with breast cancer, the results were highly positive (Nishida et al., 1988; Shintomi, 1988).

In one case, 1.25 percent A10 in the regular mouse diet was able "to inhibit the growth curve of [human breast cancer cells] significantly after 35 days of treatment." There was a "61.345 percent inhibition in the antineoplaston A10 treated group." In addition, there was a "significant decrease in the number of mitoses [i.e., cell divisions] in the antineoplaston A10 treated group" (Nishida et al., 1988).

The second Japanese study more or less repeated the first, but with the A10 being given by injection. Once again, the tumor volume was dramatically less in the treated group than in the controls. "Histology of the tumor in the treated group," wrote the researchers, "showed necrosis but no lymphocyte infiltration" (Shintomi, 1988). This seemed to uphold Burzynski's original contention that antineoplastons are not dependent on the white blood cells for their action (Burzynski, 1986).

At this, there was flicker of interest from the FDA. John F. Palmer, M.D., the FDA official in charge of Burzynski's application, wrote the Texas doctor:

> The study . . . may provide a rational basis for concluding that the agent has antitumor activity (Palmer, 1988).

But did this mean Burzynski could begin testing? Hardly. Instead Palmer demanded a "detailed clinical protocol" of Burzynski's proposed study, including "a dissolution-time profile for antineoplaston A10 capsules . . . as a function of pH and . . . in the selected dissolution medium. An appropriate dissolution specification, with methodology, should be provided for the capsules." And so on: two more pages of questions, single-spaced.

"Until the required information is received . . . in triplicate," Palmer warned, "the studies . . . which you proposed in humans may not legally be conducted under this IND" (Palmer, 1988).

In October 1988 Burzynski supplied the additional information—over 6,000 pages worth—and began waiting for a reply. His IND application, stacked on the floor, was now over six feet tall.

Another way to evaluate drugs is to look for a preventative effect. Here antineoplastons shine, for they appear to be remarkably effective in *preventing* cancer formation. In one experiment, scientists administered a well-known carcinogen, benzo(a)pyrene (BP) to the A/HeJ strain of mice. This is of more than passing interest, since BP is an almost ubiquitous environmental pollutant, found in tobacco smoke, charcoal-grilled steaks, and hundreds of other products.

Two doses of pure BP, 3 milligrams each, were administered two weeks apart. Predictably, this caused an average of 6.86 tumors within 157 days in the control animals. Antineoplaston A10 was also given to another group of test animals—1 percent in their feed for one week prior to, and then throughout, the period of BP administration. The results were dramatic: a *70 percent reduction* in the total number of tumors in the test group (Kampalath et al., 1987).

A good rationale stands behind these exciting results: the physical structure of A10 makes it possible for it to intercalate (insinuate itself) into the double-helix strand of human DNA. Since carcinogens also do this, A10 may act by pre-emptively taking up the carcinogen's "parking spot" on the DNA strand. When the carcinogen comes along, it finds its usual spot already taken and, circulating around and around, is finally flushed out of the body. The mechanism is not original: some conventional anticancer drugs, such as Adriamycin, act in exactly this manner, but they bind with so many other normal cells that they are highly toxic (Lehner et al. 1986).

Another much-used experimental model is the "spontaneous" breast cancer in C_3H+ mice. These mice are doomed from birth: they all carry the breast cancer–causing murine mammary tumor virus (MTV). By their ninth or tenth month, 95 percent of the virgin female rodents already have developed breast tumors.

At the Medical College of Georgia in Augusta, Dr. Tom Muldoon and his colleagues demonstrated that A10 could significantly delay the appearance of these inborn tumors. Inclusion of A10 as a 1 percent dietary supplement from the age of three months "dramatically increased the disease-free interval," Muldoon wrote. At the age of 10–11 months, in fact, "none of the animals had developed tumors and the incidence reached 95 percent only at 21 months of age" (Muldoon et al., 1987). Thus antineoplastons had a dramatic effect in *delaying the appearance* of cancer in this widely used animal model.

In work presented at the 15th International Congress of Chemotherapy in July 1987, Muldoon also showed that A10 could have a marked effect on another carcinogen-induced cancer in virgin Sprague-Dawley rats. "A10 did not cause tumor regression," he and his colleagues reported, "but did eliminate production of additional new tumors." The researchers called it "remarkably effective" (Muldoon, 1988).

Animals were first divided into three groups. In the control, the carcinogen (the steroidlike compound DMBA) was given, but no A10. In this group, tumors began to form at fifty days after the "carcinogenic insult," and the appearance of new tumors increased in linear fashion for at least 140 days.

In the second group, A10 was given midway in the disease process— i.e., at 70 days. In this group it "blocked further tumor occurrence." Those tumors that had already formed, remained. But A10 functioned in this case as a "antitumorigenic, rather than tumoricidal" agent.

When A10, at one percent of dietary intake, was given ten days before administration of the carcinogen, the results were even more dramatic. It almost completely blocked the appearance of cancer in these animals. Whereas the mean number of tumors per rat in the untreated group reached four after 140 days, in the prophylactically treated animals it remained well under one per rat (ibid.).

In the summer of 1988, Naofumi Eriguchi and his colleagues extended these findings to yet another kind of cancer: urethane-induced lung tumors. They reported in the *Journal of the Japan Society for Cancer Therapy* that "Antineoplaston A10 reduced tumor number per mouse from 19.4 to 9.05," i.e., a 53.4 percent reduction in tumors. In addition, there were "no apparent side effect[s]" and it was "relatively non-toxic to the mice" (Eriguchi et al., 1988).

THE FIERCEST BATTLE

The Japanese researchers concluded that "we found antineoplaston A10 has a chemopreventive effect" (ibid.).

One might think that a new class of nontoxic agents that might prevent or delay the appearance of cancer would generate a great deal of favorable attention from the U.S. government. For instance, they could be tested as a preventative anticancer pill in populations highly prone to cancer, such as smokers or asbestos workers. Yet the government, found nothing of particular interest here, and focused instead on the alleged flaws in Burzynski's paperwork.

Human studies

There is also considerable and growing evidence that antineoplastons are effective in treating human cancer patients. Unlike some other unconventional practitioners, Burzynski is both willing and able to publish his findings and subject them to the scrutiny of his peers. He wants his compounds tested in many independent clinics, as quickly as possible. In fact, he is pursuing a strategy of spreading the clinical testing of antineoplastons around the world. It is the FDA that has hampered this development by refusing to allow Burzynski to ship antineoplastons to foreign medical schools where doctors have wanted to begin clinical testing (Hile, 1986).

In reviewing the evidence of antineoplastons' activity in humans, it would be possible to compile quite a few testimonials to the drugs' efficacy. Scientists generally discount such personal statements, however, because patients themselves can be subjective about the causes of their own improvement.

There are no controlled double-blind studies of antineoplastons' effectiveness. Burzynski is ready to assist qualified medical centers to conduct such studies as soon as he receives the IND he needs to ship the compounds out of Texas.

For a brief survey of some of the evidence, therefore, let us restrict ourselves to three published papers that give the results of over a decade of work with these peptides.

Varied tumors treated with A2. In an initial Twelve Oaks study, Burzynski treated fifteen patients with advanced neoplastic disease, including cancers of the breast, bladder, lung, kidney, esophagus, colon, and liver, as well as mesothelioma and glioma. These fifteen patients had all been given Antineoplaston A2 intravenously through a catheter between December 1979 and May 1980. The treatment had lasted from 53 to 358 days.

315

Since this was a Phase I safety study, particular attention was paid to questions of toxicity.

"Only minimal adverse effects were noticed sometime during the treatment," he said. Three patients experienced chills followed by fever at some point during the therapy. One patient experienced generalized muscle aches on the second day of treatment. These were infrequent and relatively minor problems, especially when compared to the harsh effects often associated with cytotoxic chemotherapy.

Burzynski also noted some of the therapeutic effects of the A2 treatment: nine of the fifteen patients showed objective response to the treatment. Six of these had *complete remission:* an adenocarcinoma of the lung, stage III (stage IV, according to current classification); a mesothelioma (asbestos-related cancer); a metastatic carcinoma of the liver with unknown primary site; and three cases of transitional cell carcinoma of the bladder.

In an additional case of adenocarcinoma of the breast, stage IV, the patient obtained complete remission of liver metastases and stabilization of bone metastases. Two other patients obtained partial remissions. Five patients had stable disease. One patient's disease increased.

Five years later he and a colleague, Dr. Eva Kubove, followed up on these fifteen patients and found:

> Three of the patients who obtained complete remission were cancer-free after five years.
> Three patients survived over four years from the beginning of the study. One died after four years and nine months. The other two were lost to follow-up after four years.
> Three patients survived over two years from the beginning of the study. "These patients discontinued the treatment with Antineoplaston A2 too early," they wrote, and subsequently died (Burzynski and Kubove, 1987).
> One patient was simply lost to follow-up.
> Five patients died within two years of the beginning of the study (ibid.).

Bladder cancers treated with various antineoplastons. In a workshop at the 15th International Congress of Chemotherapy, July 19–24, 1987, Burzynski reported on the treatment of bladder cancer with antineoplastons. There are approximately 46,000 new cases of this disease in the United States each year. It is the fifth most common cancer in men. Surgery and radiation are the principal treatments, although in recent years combination chemotherapy (CISCA, M-VAC, and CMV) has also been used. According to the American Cancer Society, the five-year survival is 88 percent in an early stage, but drops to 41 percent when it is more advanced. There are still over 10,000 deaths a year from this type of malignancy (ACS, 1988).

Burzynski reported on the treatment of nineteen bladder cancer patients, grades II to IV, without distant metastases, who were treated and followed up to ten years. "At the end of the study," he wrote, "68 percent of the patients were diagnosed with complete remission, 11 percent with partial remission, 5 percent with stable disease, and 16 percent with increasing disease. . . . [T]herapy with antineoplastons is associated with [a] high percentage of objective responses and minimal adverse reactions" (Burzynski, February 1988a).

These findings were made in the course of Phase I safety trials. Burzynski believes that Phase II clinical trials should give a much higher response rate.

Brain tumors treated with various antineoplastons. When they enter the clinic, all of Burzynski's patients are enrolled in one of forty-one different protocols. In 1988 he reported on the results with his first cohort of brain cancer patients. There are over 15,000 cases of primary brain cancer each year in the United States, with 9,000 deaths. It is a particularly tragic type of illness, because it often entails disastrous effects on the seat of intelligence and emotions.

In his article in the June 1988 *Advances in Experimental and Clinical Chemotherapy*, Burzynski reported on the results of a Phase I trial in twenty patients. "Fifty-five percent of patients responded objectively to the treatment," he indicated, "25 percent had increased disease, and 20 percent had stable disease with symptomatic improvement." Especially good results were observed in the treatment of astrocytoma, glioblastoma multiforme, and metastatic lung cancer.

He cited the case of a woman with an astrocytoma, Grade II to III. In adults this type of brain tumor often grows rapidly and invades extensively. In December 1985 her doctors predicted that she could not live for more than two months. On January 8, 1986, however, she began treatment with AS2-1. After five months she no longer had any signs or symptoms of her disease by physical examination. Two years later she still did not have any symptoms, felt well, and was living a normal life. She continued to take a maintenance dose of antineoplaston capsules.*

Two things are clear from this report. First, these results, if confirmed, would be among the best currently being achieved in such advanced cases;

*This woman, incidentally, filed a lawsuit against her insurance company when it refused to pay for the treatment. This was taken to court in Lander, Wyoming, and the judge ruled in her favor. He concluded that the patient's treatment was "usual and customary based on her condition" and that the patient's cancer was in remission.

second, antineoplastons are not a "magic bullet," a sure-fire cancer cure, nor does Burzynski present them as such. Those who have remissions sometimes relapse, although Burzynski attributes some of these to the patients' failure to take the medicine in the prescribed way.

2. "It's bizarre."

Antineoplastons were originally derived from human urine. Today most of it is synthesized from off-the-shelf chemicals in the laboratory, but some is still collected. Where does one get 20,000 gallons of urine (the capacity of the laboratory's huge underground tanks)? One contracts for it.

In the past, Burzynski's contractor obtained urine from Texas penitentiaries, Houston sports stadiums, even Gilley's well-known bar. Due to political pressure, these sources literally dried up and the price went higher than Texas crude. Today the main sources are Houston city parks, where special separators have been installed underneath the urinals, for ultimate use in the clinic. (A city map on Burzynski's wall locates the urine depositories with colored markers.)

There may be a humorous aspect to the trials and tribulations of a urine collector. Essentially, however, this is a serious business: because of the urine blockade, many patients cannot receive the natural forms of antineoplastons that in the past have demonstrated the greatest effectiveness against their particular form of cancer, such as A2 for bladder tumors.

Urine occupies a curious cultural niche. Try to tell people about Burzynski's treatment and they are usually sympathetic—until you mention the source. Then noses wrinkle up. Scientists know that urine is an important medical tool. But in our collective mind it is dirty stuff, a four-letter word.

At first Burzynski worked with blood serum, and in fact the two are roughly equivalent as sources of peptides. Yet urine, as he discovered, "is not really waste material, but probably the most complex chemical mixture in the human body; it therefore can deliver virtually any information about the body." It is "a concentrated filtrate of blood plasma" (Lang, 1987a).

Many rumors have been spread about the alleged contamination of Burzynski's urine supply. A visit to the Stafford, Texas, laboratory would put those concerns to rest. The urine is put through an elaborate purification process. The first is a set of millipore filters that weed out all particles greater than 0.2 microns in diameter. This does away with not just cigarette butts but all microbes and viruses as well. The residue is then heated, treated with chemicals, and finally freeze-dried. All that is left is a sterile, white powder, repeatedly tested for purity and potency.

By the time it reaches the drug stage, it has been so processed and purified that it has no more relationship to the original source than do approved urine-derived drugs such as urokinase or Premarin.

History

The use of urine in medicine originated in antiquity. The Greek physicians Serapion of Alexandria (third century B.C.) and Xenokrates (second century A.D.) spoke of its use, and they were almost certainly drawing on much more ancient Egyptian traditions.

The medieval physician Johannes Actuarius wrote:

> He who masters the two sciences of the pulse and the urine will possess almost all that is necessary for diagnosis and prognosis. Conversely, he who knows only one of these two sciences will be prone to a thousand errors, for in the study of diseases, the science of urines is as valuable as that of the pulse (quoted in Frank et al., 1983).

During the seventeenth century there was practically a cult of urine analysis. The *matula,* or urine flask, became a symbol of the medical profession. Later the use of urine in any form became a sign of quackery. Nowadays one can find small texts in out-of-the-way health food stores advocating the therapeutic ingestion of urine. One group, the Water of Life Institute, is even promoting such treatment for AIDS (see *Seven Days,* November 23, 1988).

Urine made a scientific comeback when biochemists learned to respect it as a source of interesting chemicals. Urea was among the first organic substances to be isolated (Rouelle, 1773) and synthesized (Wohler, 1828).

"The investigation of urinary peptides and amino acids in normal human urine has been pursued for the past half-century," two Du Pont researchers wrote in a 65-page review article. "Because of the great number of amino acids in urine and the complexity of some of the amino-acid-containing constituents, good separation techniques are a prerequisite . . ." (Lou and Hamilton, 1979).

Modern techniques were pioneered in 1951 with column chromatography. In 1958 the ion-exchange chromatographic technique became automated. Gel filtration was introduced in 1959 and thin-layer chromatography (TLC) a few years later. These, plus electrophoresis, were the standard techniques Burzynski used to reveal the presence of peptide fractions. From a urinary point of view, then, Burzynski was well within the mainstream.

Because of the immense number of naturally occurring peptides and the complexity of extraction techniques, even many doctors do not understand how these compounds are isolated from urine. For odd reasons, understanding about urinary peptides has spread slowly. Today, however, many naturally derived peptides are making their way into medicine, including vasopressin, enkephalins, plasma kinins, and angiotensins. There are forty such factors already known and more on the way.

These developments have put Burzynski in eminent company, and there is a growing openness to his concepts among biochemists. But some medical people still regard urinary products—and peptides themselves—with suspicion. Thus, Burzynski's enemies can strike a receptive note when they link him to antineoplastons' humble origins.

3. "They're unsafe."

Every scientific study of antineoplastons has emphasized their safety and nontoxicity. They are natural products and appear to be well tolerated by the body even in high doses, without any of the serious side effects routinely associated with cytotoxic chemotherapy.

Burzynski reports adverse reactions in a scrupulous way. In the aforementioned brain cancer study, for instance, he recorded what might otherwise be considered inconsequential effects. For example, about half the patients reported minor and transient rashes, headaches, flushing or dizziness—but generally of only one or two day's duration during treatment that lasted from 42 to 872 days.

It is ironic, therefore, that government authorities have tried to depict antineoplastons as particularly dangerous. Unable to claim that the drugs are themselves toxic, they have fallen back on indicting one particular route of administration: subclavian catheterization. This is the surgical insertion of a small plastic tube beneath the collar bone to facilitate delivery of a drug into the bloodstream. It has been routinely used in cancer chemotherapy since the 1970s.

Burzynski himself does not insert the subclavian catheters. That is done by surgeons in the Houston area, particularly Dr. Younan Nowzaradan. No problems with these procedures have come to Dr. B.'s attention.

"Two of Dr. Burzynski's patients in Canada are reported to have contracted septicemia from the catheter used to administer antineoplaston," the FDA states in a form letter, "and one of them is reported to have died from the septicemia," or blood poisoning (Wetherell to Bentsen, 1984).

The FDA claim is vague: ". . . are reported. . . ." By whom? To whom? Dr. Burzynski has never received a report of any of his patients dying from septicemia. Yet this charge is repeated in every argument over antineoplastons. This widely repeated accusation seems to be derived, ultimately, from the Blackstein-Bergsagel report:

> "The administration of antineoplastons into subclavian catheters for prolonged periods by *unsupervised* patients is not safe, and we know of two Ontario patients who developed septicemia . . . after returning from Texas; one of the patients died as a result of the septicemia" (Blackstein-Bergsagel, 1982, emphasis in original).

The two Canadians do not specify the names of the patients, nor do they provide proof that the alleged septicemia was the *result* of the catheterization. Yet FDA scientists feel comfortable repeating these unsubstantiated rumors.

Let us assume for the sake of argument, however, that these critics are right: that two patients contracted septicemia and one of them died. The sad fact is that such things happen in all cancer clinics—*even under doctors' supervision*. Cancer patients often have weak immune systems, which are further compromised by cytotoxic drugs and radiation. Many patients also pick up iatrogenic (doctor-caused) infections in the hospital. The death rate for septicemia in 1986 was fairly high: 7.1 per every 100,000 in the general population—more than for emphysema, for example (Hoffman, 1987).

Burzynski is frank about the dangers. "One of the risks of having a catheter, for any purpose," he points out, "is septicemia." But isn't FDA applying a double standard when it warns of the use of catheters for antineoplastons but approves of their use for conventional chemotherapy?

Blackstein and Bergsagel seem particularly upset about the *self-help*—"unsupervised"—aspect of antineoplastons. (If patients can give themselves the treatment, the need for medical specialists is greatly decreased.) But this would seem to be one of the great advantages of nontoxic therapy. It not only increases the patients' own participation in their cure, but promises to lower the rapidly escalating cost of high-tech medicine. After all, many diabetes patients give themselves frequent injections of insulin without getting infected. Why can't cancer patients perform a similar task?

Perhaps there are cases in which Burzynski's patients should be receiving their drugs from licensed local physicians. But in those cases it is the FDA's own intransigence that has denied patients the right to receive medically supervised antineoplaston therapy outside the Lone Star State.

At the same time, Dr. B.'s critics drop broad hints that people are harmed in other ways as a result of antineoplaston therapy.

In a September 1985 form letter about Burzynski circulated to Congressional representatives the FDA added, ominously, "People have died as the result of taking untested drugs" (Cannon, 1985).

Despite appearances, they are *not* talking about the risks of antineo-plastons here but of untested drugs in general. FDA's reasoning seems to be as follows: unproven drugs kill people; antineoplastons are unproven drugs; ergo, antineoplastons kill people. The fact that antineoplastons have repeat-edly been shown to be safe does not break into this illogical syllogism. This statement also obscures the fact that people have *really* died while using FDA-approved drugs. In 1982, for example, more than a dozen people were killed by the newly approved anti-arthritis drug Oraflex before FDA and the manufacturer, Eli Lilly, woke up and took it off the market (Gieringer, 1986).

The truth is that all drugs carry some risk. Cytotoxic anticancer drugs, given in high doses, carry a large risk of side effects, such as hair loss, ulcers, deafness, and even death. In many animal toxicity studies and over 1,400 human cases, no one has demonstrated anything more than minor, transitory symptoms from antineoplastons.

If FDA would allow scientists to proceed with carefully controlled clinical studies of large numbers of patients as part of an approved IND, the entire safety question could quickly be laid to rest. This it will not do, thus keeping alive a controversy it then attempts to exploit.

4. "They're expensive!"

The FDA decries "the financial hardship that results from spending money for unproven cancer remedies that raise false hopes . . ." (Wether-ell, 1984).

Leaving aside the moot question of "false hopes," it is certainly true that antineoplaston therapy is expensive. These costs are no secret but are spelled out in the Burzynski Research Institute's patient brochure. The drug itself costs from $315 to $685 per day. The monthly cost of outpatient ther-apy is between $3,000 and $5,000. This does not include the cost of room and board in Houston, transportation, etc.

These costs go toward several things: the manufacture of antineoplas-tons; the expense of research and development and of preparation of the IND; legal expenses; and finally, staff salaries, including that of Dr. Bur-zynski.

The Institute employs over one hundred people, including thirteen at the doctoral level. No one can tour the Stafford laboratory without realizing the enormous expense involved in developing and manufacturing these drugs.

These are experimental medicines, produced under adverse conditions unknown to the large and well-connected pharmaceutical companies. There is no way that this can be done cheaply.

Compare the consumer's costs for some recent medicines produced by orthodox drug companies working with the FDA's approval. One drug, Factor VIII (Armour), which speeds blood clotting, costs $25,000 a year. AZT (Burroughs Wellcome), for AIDS, runs $8,000 a year. Genentech's TPA, a clot-dissolving agent, costs $2,200 *per injection!*

"The drug companies evidently feel that they can get away with whatever the market will bear," said Representative Henry A. Waxman (D.-Calif.), who heads the House Subcommittee on Health and the Environment (*New York Times,* February 9, 1988). The FDA does not generally complain about these outrageous costs. It only discovers the "financial hardship" of modern medicine in the case of unconventional therapies.

The cost of antineoplaston therapy often becomes a personal hardship when insurance companies refuse to reimburse for it. But this, too, can be laid at the feet of the government. At the October 1985 hearing, FDA employee Kenneth P. Ewing admitted that he not only warned companies who called him about Burzynski but actively *initiated contact* with Blue Cross of Texas, telling them that antineoplastons were an "unproven remedy" that had not shown efficacy in treating animal tumors (*Houston Chronicle,* October 4, 1985).

Burzynski lost hundreds of thousands of dollars in billings as a result of FDA's opposition. Today about half of the insurance claims are honored, but some companies, such as Aetna Life Insurance, have become particularly bitter opponents. In fact, Aetna has gone so far as to file a civil Racketeer Influenced and Corrupt Organizations ("Rico") suit against Burzynski. Aetna's consultant on this is a Washington attorney named Grace Powers Monaco, who has become a prominent opponent of "questionable" cancer therapies (Monaco, 1988). (Insurance companies have always had a large stake in the cancer field. Morgan Brainard, president of Aetna, was even one of the founders of the American Cancer Society. Ross, 1987).

If their insurance plans will not pay, then the cost of antineoplaston therapy must be personally absorbed by the patient. This can be considerable, running into tens of thousands of dollars. In this respect, it is no different from any other treatment for chronic illness in America, which can bankrupt an uncovered victim.

Nevertheless, there are many stories of Burzynski's exceptional generosity. At the 1985 hearing in U.S. District Court, Richard A. Sharpe testified that he owed Dr. Burzynski $70,000, which he probably would never be able to repay. Billy Brown is another who had been treated free of charge since Prudential Insurance Company refused repayment.* William Cody has been treated gratis for years. Despite many offers, the Burzynski Research Institute has never employed a collection agency (Lang, 1986). How many of Burzynski's medical critics can make the same statement?

"Why do you continue to treat [Mr. Cody], Doctor?" Burzynski was asked at the 12-day hearing.

"Because we care for his life," was his simple reply (ibid.).

The question of cost inevitably raises the question of freedom of choice, since presumably an informed consumer has the right to spend her money however she wishes.

It is startling to realize that FDA objects to the cost of the treatment even when fully informed adults, acting as careful medical consumers, willingly spend their money in exchange for these medical services. The patient can feel she has made the best investment in her entire life, but FDA is still against it.

"The FDA obtained the injunction against Dr. Burzynski," one of its officials wrote Senator Lloyd Bentsen, ". . . to protect cancer victims, including those who would willingly undertake the risk and expense of antineoplaston therapy" (Wetherell, 1984).

The FDA's working premise seems to be that the patient is a fool. When it comes to cancer, we and our most trusted advisers cannot think for ourselves. Stung by the revelations that alternative cancer patient are more educated and intelligent than the average, FDA responds:

> Even the best educated and most rational of us are likely to have a vulnerable spot. . . . [W]e may want to believe in a secret chemical that cures cancer. And our wish to believe in miracles may conquer our common sense at times" (FDA Commissioner Young in *FDA Consumer*, Dec. 1985–Jan. 1986).

In fact, it is often the orthodox who exploit the hope of "miracles" for cancer—such as interferon, monoclonal antibodies, or interleukin-2. Burzynski is always moderate in his claims.

Yet over and over, Burzynski's opponents repeat that antineoplastons' "promoters" claim it is "a cancer cure" (Cannon, 1985). They trot out the same stale and unproven argument that "false hope" in unconventional therapy may divert patients from the conventional path.

*On February 20, 1989 Brown won a major victory against Prudential in his court battle. A jury ordered the giant company to pay him $500,000 in punitive damages in addition to medical and legal costs (Johnson, 1989).

> Dr. Burzynski does harm by misleading patients and giving them false hope. Furthermore, some patients may be diverted from standard curative therapy by the lure of a false siren (Blackstein and Bergsagel, 1982).

They hold to this even when that conventional path offers *no* hope to the 500,000 Americans who die of the disease each year.

Needless to say, it is the establishment itself that is bent on deciding for us what is common sense and what is a delusion. Odysseus-like, its ears plugged with wax, the FDA intends to shepherd gullible cancer patients past the "false siren" of antineoplaston therapy!

It must give these public saviors pause that despite their easy access to the major media and their control of widely disseminated house organs, most of their intended beneficiaries are not convinced. Fifty-two percent of the public, in a Media General–Associated Press poll, said they would seek "a medical treatment that promised a cure" even when the treatment was rejected by the established medical community (*New York Daily News*, November 11, 1985).

"People are very angry at the medical profession," responded Helene Brown, a director of the American Cancer Society. In a remark which sounded odd coming from a long-time quack-baiter, she added ". . . .there are portions of the medical system who are not willing to allow patients to participate in their own treatments" (ibid.).

Hence the FDA's recourse to police power, the settlement of scientific questions by main force.

FDA's position on Burzynski, however, is in no way the unequivocal law of the land. Although there has been no definitive Supreme Court ruling on medical freedom of choice, there are a number of court decisions that favor this right. Most important is the Second Circuit U.S. Court of Appeals verdict in the case of *Schneider v. Revici* (1987). This was a malpractice case defended by Sam Abady of the New York law firm Abady and Jaffe. In a landmark decision, the court opined:

> We see no reason why a patient should not be allowed to make an informed decision to go outside currently approved medical methods in search of an unconventional treatment. While a patient should be encouraged to exercise care for his own safety, we believe that an informed decision to avoid surgery and conventional chemotherapy is within the patient's right 'to determine what shall be done with his own body' (817 *Federal Reporter*, 2d Series:987–996, 1987).

FDA's behavior not only flies in the face of this court decision but against a whole tendency of democratic opinion that has sought to establish the rights of patients, including access to alternatives (Annas, 1978).

Medical freedoms, like the rights of privacy in general, were not explicitly spelled out in the Constitution. (One organization, the Coalition for Alternatives in Nutrition and Healthcare, Inc., or CANAH, has proposed a 27th Amendment to the Constitution to do just that. Davis, 1988.)

Two hundred years ago, Benjamin Rush, M.D., a signer of the Declaration of Independence, warned about the consequences of that omission:

> The Constitution of this Republic should make special provisions for medical freedom as well as religious freedom. To restrict the art of healing to one class of men and deny equal privileges to others will constitute the Bastille of medical science. All such laws are un-American and despotic (cited in Burk, 1974).

Justices Benjamin Cardozo and Louis Brandeis spoke favorably about a patient's right to choose.

The consequences of experimental "treatments," where the patients' rights were trampled in the dust, were amply demonstrated by the Nazis. For that reason, the Nuremberg Code, adopted after World War II, held that the patient "should be so situated as to be able to exercise free power of choice, without the intervention of any element of force, fraud, deceit, duress, over-reaching or other ulterior form of constraint or coercion" (World Medical Association, 1981).

The Declaration of Helsinki, adopted by the 18th World Medical Assembly in Helsinki, Finland, in 1964 and approved by the U.S. Congress, also affirmed that:

> In the treatment of the sick person, the doctor must be free to use a new therapeutic measure, if in his judgment it offers hope of saving life, reestablishing health, or alleviating suffering (ibid.).

By its paternalistic attitude, the cancer establishment deprives the patients of their right to choose, and the doctor of a chance to make a vital contribution to medicine through the accumulation of essential clinical knowledge.

5. "Burzynski is unqualified."

The most surprising charge is the government's challenge to Burzynski's qualifications to do the clinical research on antineoplastons. After he submitted his first IND proposal, FDA wrote:

> Please submit information concerning your training and experience in oncology which would qualify you to undertake clinical evaluations of the safety and effectiveness of drugs for the treatment of malignant disease (Gyarfas, 1983).

What sorts of qualifications does one need to test new drugs? Burzynski has both an M.D. and a Ph.D.; has worked for seven years at a prestigious medical center; has come up with new concepts and findings hailed by his peers; has lectured and published all over the world; and has created, from scratch, both a thriving medical clinic and a pharmaceutical company. Yet, oddly, none of this seems to impress the FDA.

This problem is not unique to Burzynski, but afflicts all would-be medical innovators in the United States. It has become clear that the kinds of qualifications FDA requires have more to do with economics than with medicine: A revealing article in the *New York Times* explained that many biotechnology innovators are actually being forced to turn their companies over to "high-powered outsiders hired from the giant drug companies to run the show." In some cases they must sell the budding firm to one of these companies in order to get even a small share in the fruits of their own discoveries. Why do this? Because FDA regulations are so constructed that only big drug company executives have the requisite skills and connections to work their way through the regulatory maze. "Approval from the FDA can mean the difference between profits and bankruptcy," says the *Times* ("Staying Alive in Biotech," November 6, 1988).

Given this Byzantine environment, it is amazing how far Burzynski has gotten with sheer persistence. Succeeding, however, takes more than determination. It requires a protracted struggle by the people most directly affected by the outcome of this war—the cancer patients themselves.

To The Patients' Defense

Many alternative cancer therapies have come and gone. Most of these have been defeated or driven underground, not primarily for scientific reasons but because they failed to mobilize public opinion and correctly translate that into organizations with sustained political power. In other words, they failed to build democratic movements for the attainment of cancer patients' rights.

Today, despite a concerted effort by the FDA, ACS, NCI, Postal Service, Aetna, the Texas Health Department, and Texas State Board of Medical Examiners, Burzynski holds on. Part of the reason is the vigorous support he has received from his patients, their families, and their friends. Central to this have been the efforts of two determined individuals, Ron Wolin and Avis Lang, founders of the Patient Rights Legal Action Fund.

Ron and Avis feel they have good reason to be grateful. Ron was diagnosed with lymphocytic lymphoma in September 1983. His doctors at Lenox Hill Hospital in New York recommended conventional chemotherapy, but held out insufficient hope. "I was sweating bullets," Ron says, "but I knew I would not undergo toxic chemotherapy." He didn't know what to do, however, and so he procrastinated.

By July 1984 he had reached stage IV. There were enlarged nodes all over his body; one, under his arm, was the size of a grapefruit. This athletic fifty-year-old (who had once ridden his bicycle across the country) could no longer walk up the steps of the subway station without pausing and gasping for breath. Tumors were beginning to encroach on his ureters; his bone marrow was all but destroyed (Lang, 1989). He was sinking fast when he found out about Burzynski from Michael Schachter, M.D., a Rockland County physician.

"The most I got from Dr. Burzynski was guarded optimism," Ron says. "He promised no miracles but I was impressed by his scientific attitude." On August 3, 1984, he began outpatient treatment. For the next eleven months he and Avis lived in a small furnished apartment in southwest Houston. He received not just daily antineoplaston therapy but nine blood transfusions and several canisters of oxygen "during one especially terrifying period" (Lang, 1989). In fact, at one point he was near death.

Although Ron Wolin died of complications of his cancer on March 4, 1990, for five and a half years after his initial diagnosis, most of his tumors and other symptoms were gone. "I'm doing sixty sit-ups a day," he wrote, "and my overall health is better than at any time in the past five years. I owe it all to Dr. Burzynski and his antineoplaston therapy" (Wolin, 1988).

Ron had spent the previous twenty years in New York as an organizer in the antiwar movement and other campaigns for social change, and even as he lay on the couch on the fateful day of the FDA raid, the wheels were turning. "Though his body was weak," wrote Avis, "his organizer's mind was as perceptive as ever" (Lang, 1989). As a university lecturer in art history, Avis had also been an activist in feminist cultural circles. Even before returning to New York, Ron and Avis had started a grassroots organization called the Patient Rights Legal Action Fund (PRLAF). The overall goal of PRLAF was to raise public consciousness about cancer patients' rights and how they were being trampled in the U.S.A.

PRLAF's first campaign was to assure Dr. Burzynski's patients uninterrupted access to the medicine and treatment that they believed was sustaining their lives.

This meant bringing the FDA into federal court for violations of a constellation of basic democratic rights, including the breach of privacy and confidentiality represented by the FDA's seizure of the patient records (Lang, 1987b).

Whatever happened to the sanctity of the doctor-patient relationship? they asked. The world was horrified when Nixon's "plumbers" stole medical files. Yet it looked on complacently when the FDA, in broad daylight, seized the records of over a thousand individuals.

For several years PRLAF joined Burzynski in waging a protracted court battle to get the patient records and the medical and insurance files returned to their original storage location in Dr. Burzynski's office; they also sought to win a ruling that cancer patients have a right to seek the medical treatment of their choice, without fear of interference from governmental bodies.

They saw it as "a struggle to protect ourselves from the excesses of a federal bureaucracy whose only possible legitimate mandate is to protect the citizenry from harm" (ibid.).

The campaign raised consciousness among patients, their families, and supporters as well as certain members of Congress and other elected officials. The clinic has remained open, and patients have continued to receive antineoplaston therapy—major, though indirect, effects of the legal action.

The case itself was dismissed, however, and the pre-1985 records remain in the hands of the FDA. After losing the battle in the lower courts, PRLAF took the question to a three-judge panel in the U.S. Court of Appeals, Fifth Circuit. Judge Alvin B. Rubin sided with the FDA against the patients:

> "This court . . . must not allow sympathy for the plight of persons suffering from cancer to cause us to interfere hastily with the mission of FDA . . ." (United States v. Burzynski, et al. and Kuharzyk, et. al., 798 F. 2nd, 5th Circuit).

A costly attempt to bring the case to the Supreme Court also failed when the Justices refused to hear the case.

Yet PRLAF has persisted in organizing hundreds of cancer patients and their supporters. This is never an easy task, given the difficulty of people trying to fight their illness and their government at the same time.

In September 1988 the Texas State Board of Medical Examiners scheduled a hearing in Austin on the question of whether to revoke Burzynski's medical license. The Board routinely examines charges brought by dissatisfied patients. In this case no patients had complained, and so their own Director of Hearings brought the charges himself. The Board in effect would serve as both prosecutor and judge in the case of Stanislaw Burzynski.

The charges were based on supposed violations of a technical and administrative nature—things that had nothing to do with the quality of care provided by Burzynski. The New York law firm of Abady and Jaffe, which specializes in the defense of unconventional physicians, represented the Houston doctor. To PRLAF, this hearing was not only an outrage but a direct threat to hundreds of lives.

As soon as the Texas Board's summons came to light, PRLAF swung into action. They began a nationwide emergency campaign "to mount the public and political pressure it will take" to get the Board to "drop their spurious, unwarranted charges against Dr. Burzynski and to stop jeopardizing the lives of his cancer patients" (PRLAF, September 18, 1988).

Supporters of PRLAF were asked to send mailgrams and letters to Dr. G. V. Brindley, Executive Director of the Board, urging him to drop the charges and warning him that the actions he was contemplating were "tantamount to genocide." Copies of the letters were also to be sent to the governor of Texas, to congressional representatives, and to George Bush and Lloyd Bentsen, two Texans running at that moment for national office.

These hundreds of letters were eloquent documents of support from Burzynski's patients and their families and friends. More than just testimonials, however, they were moving cries for elemental justice.

For instance, one man wrote:

> As a patient who is having excellent results from the Burzynski treatment (X-rays of my lung cancer show considerable tumor shrinkage within the first two months), and having observed the dramatic improvement in many other patients, I am also aware that interruption of treatment in all cases is dangerous and life-threatening in the extreme. . . . Are you prepared to take that responsibility?

A researcher in Texas communicated his fears:

I am writing to you out of great concern for the future of the Burzynski Research Institute in Houston. As a patient, I feel that any interruption of the treatment I began last December for malignant lymphoma would be very harmful to me.

The mother of Paul, a seven-year-old with a brain tumor, wrote from a small town in Michigan about her son's positive response to the treatment. She pointed out that her entire community was aware of the boy's progress "and has been rejoicing with us at Paul's improvement." Then she added:

Please do not do anything that would put our son's life in jeopardy. He needs this treatment. Dr. Burzynski is a fine man. I trust him with my son's life. I would get down on my knees and beg you to allow Dr. Burzynski to continue treating my son if that would help you to decide in our favor. I would do that for Paul's life.

But perhaps the most touching letter came from a Midwestern teenager:

I am 13 years old and I have a 7 year old brother. We love our father very much. Thanks to Dr. Burzynski's treatment, my father's tumor has stopped growing. All of the doctors in my home state of Missouri said there was no cure for my father's disease. Dr. Burzynski gave him a chance for life again. Please don't take that away from us.

At the rambling Board meeting on September 23, 1988, such voices were not heard. Instead the Board quibbled over procedural matters and then decided—by a split vote—to postpone making a decision.

Had the hundreds of letters had some effect? PRLAF said yes.

Although the Board and the Governor of Texas will never admit it, every letter, mailgram, or phone call they get helps stay the hands of the Texas authorities in their crude and inhumane attempts to railroad Dr. Burzynski . . . (PRLAF, October 8, 1988).

Although the delay represented a victory of sorts, the Damoclean sword of license revocation still hangs over Burzynski's head, and will until he either gets complete FDA approval for his work or public pressure results in a breakthrough for the patients' right to choose.

Conclusions

Despite all the opposition, Stash Burzynski remains remarkably confident of ultimate victory. In October 1988 he resubmitted his IND application, answering the latest FDA objections. On November 28, 1988, Dr. Palmer responded with a dozen more requests and recommendations (Burzynski, 1989).

It has been said that the last stage of establishment opposition is "we knew it all along." If so, then Burzynski may be nearing victory. In late 1988 he appeared on a Midwest talk show opposite George Sledge, M.D., an oncologist at Indiana University School of Medicine. Burzynski presented an outline of his work. While denying Dr. B. credit, Sledge responded:

> The basic concept is a very reasonable one. . . . It is an approach that is being widely used and widely investigated in standard medical research at this time. It's an approach that's been around for many years. It's an approach for which undoubtedly there will be Nobel Prizes awarded sometime within the next few years ("A.M. Indiana," October 18, 1988).

But perhaps the most significant development has been the growing interest in antineoplastons in other countries. Burzynski was even invited to speak as an honored guest in Poland in the summer of 1989—nearly two decades after he left as a disaffected emigré with twenty dollars in his pocket.

Production of antineoplastons is scheduled to begin in Switzerland, Taiwan, the Philippines and the Soviet Union. He has signed a licensing agreement with a major Italian pharmaceutical company. The mainland Chinese, and especially the Japanese, are experimenting with his substances. Their involvement is not just humanitarian. A special section of the *Wall Street Journal* called "The Final Frontier" (subtitled "Japan Assaults the Last Bastion: America's Lead in Innovation") gives a practical reason for this interest (November 14, 1988).

"Japanese business is trying to buy the world's best science and scientists," according to the president of Japan's National Institute for Research Advancement.

"Grabbing the nascent idea and commercializing it, ahead of the U.S. and Europe, is a large part of Japan's strategy for the 1990s and beyond," said the *Journal* (ibid.).

Of particular interest to students of antineoplastons is an 892-page book entitled *Japanese Technology*. This "guided tour of the Japanese science establishment's vision of the future" reveals that Japan's long-term goals include the following:

> *By the year 2002*—prevent the spread of cancer in the human body.
> *By the year 2005*—correct the abnormal division of cancer cells and return them to normal cells (cited in ibid.).

If the latter goal sounds familiar, it should, for it is an exact description of the rationale behind Burzynski's therapy. America, through its FDA, may reject and revile innovative concepts such as antineoplastons. But others are not so shortsighted, and America may no longer dominate cancer research worldwide.

They still can try, however. In January 1986 Dr. Hideaki Tsuda, chief of clinical investigation of anticancer drugs at Japan's Kurume University School of Medicine, formally requested of the FDA the right to import 1350 bottles of A10 "for investigational purpose upon human patients" (Tsuda, 1986).

According to the Japanese doctors, "this drug may be legally used and imported . . . for investigational use and treatment of cancer" (ibid.).

But the FDA turned down this request, claiming that since the drug was unproven it could not be exported! (Hile, 1986) Since it was precisely such a test as the Japanese researchers were proposing that might have settled the issue, it once again appeared that the FDA was trying to prevent a resolution of the controversy.

In November 1988, nearly three years later, the FDA announced it was sending two investigators to Kurume. Ordinarily such a site visit might be the sign of impending approval. But given the history of the question, Burzynski's supporters were afraid that FDA was looking for a way to discourage Japanese interest in antineoplastons. In December 1988 the Japanese researchers received approval from their own Ethics Committee to begin clinical trials on humans using antineoplastons, according to Burzynski's office (Burzynski Research Institute, 1989). The antineoplastons will be purchased from a Swiss pharmaceutical manufacturer (Burzynski, 1989).

This skirmish over antineoplastons can best be understood as part of what the *Wall Street Journal* calls "the biggest economic battle of the future . . . America vs. Japan" (November 14, 1988). The Japanese are already challenging the United States in pharmaceutical production. Antineoplastons thus might become an object of worldwide competition.

Burzynski has continued to pursue his foreign connections. In November 1988 he signed a licensing agreement with a group of major investors from Taipei to manufacture antineoplastons. The Chinese plan to open a clinic on Taiwan and to follow that with a clinic in the Philippines and the exportation of antineoplastons to the countries of southeast Asia (BRI, 1988b).

In March 1989 Burzynski's institute announced that it had signed a letter of intent with Sigma-Tau, Italy's largest pharmaceutical company, authorizing them to conduct laboratory, preclinical, and clinical studies on A10 and AS2-1. The countries involved in this agreement are Italy, Spain, France, the United Kingdom (European territories only), Ireland, Holland, Luxembourg, Belgium, West Germany, Switzerland, Austria, and Denmark.

BRI will share the data from these studies and try to use them to gain approval for the drugs in the U.S., Canada, or Mexico (BRI, 1989).

The fact that Stash Burzynski is by birth a foreigner turns out to be an asset, for he does not suffer from a narrow or parochial outlook. He has kept his international point of view and connections. From a global perspective, he feels, the future looks bright.

"We are at the end of the war," Burzynski says, with infectious optimism. "But at the end of the war," he adds, "comes the fiercest battle."

Postscript

In an unexpected turnabout, on March 16, 1989, the Food and Drug Administration finally approved Dr. Burzynski's IND application for one kind of antineoplaston in one type of cancer.

Dr. Palmer's letter was short and to the point:

We have concluded our review of your application . . . and have concluded that it is reasonably safe to proceed with your proposed study. Consequently, the 'clinical hold' on this application is removed (Palmer, 1989).

Palmer cautioned that the IND applied only to a proposed Phase II study of the effect of A10 capsules on fifteen patients with advanced breast cancer to be conducted at an independent institute in the Midwest. He also warned that investigators were not allowed to charge for the drug in the study and had to report any fatal or life-threatening experiences encountered with the treatment (ibid).

While Burzynski's supporters were celebrating with vodka and caviar, some seasoned observers suspected a trap.

Burzynski has never published the results of his ongoing protocol for A10 in breast cancer. What if it does not work well on this tiny group of patients with this type of disease? Would that perhaps throw into question the whole peptide approach? As the ACS vice president for research has noted about analogous cases:

> Some drugs may be effective in only one or two types of cancer out of more than one hundred, so although the drug may be found inactive in several types of cancer, it still might have important anticancer activity if only the right tumor is chosen (Laszlo, 1987:195).

Burzynski intends to follow up this IND with others, for different forms of antineoplastons in varied kinds of cancer, to yield a broader picture of the drugs' effects (BRI, 1989).

Many other possibilities should be considered. Burzynski still faces two serious challenges to his career. The first is the suit by the Aetna Life Insurance company, for which Burzynski Research Institute employees are currently giving depositions. The second is the still-pending activity of the Texas State Board of Medical Examiners.

Burzynski had hoped that a federal IND would clear away the challenge to his medical license. Instead it may work against him. The Board may choose to interpret the IND to mean that Stash can treat only metastatic breast cancer—and that only with A10 capsules—in the state of Texas as well. At the same time the FDA could refuse to license him to treat even that kind of cancer, since it is the Midwestern oncologist—and not Burzynski himself—who was authorized to treat patients under the IND. Thus the discoverer of antineoplastons may find himself unqualified to use them anywhere in the United States. The combined action of the state of Texas and the Food and Drug Administration could turn out to be a pincer movement to immobilize him, while the massive Aetna lawsuit would bankrupt him and put him out of business.

No doubt Burzynski's staff and attorneys will exert themselves to prevent this, but the only things that can stop it are the threat of foreign competition and, especially, patient action.

What about the IND itself? Without an effective patients' rights movement, even a successful double-blind test will not result in automatic acceptance. The case of hydrazine sulfate proves that. Nor can one necessarily count on open and aboveboard dealings when it comes to unorthodox treatments for cancer. How much was known about the Midwest clinic that Burzynski had chosen to conduct the study? Could this be another laetrile-type coverup in the making?

It is, of course, too soon to know if any of these nightmare scenarios are accurate. In any case, without taking away from the credit due the Burzynski Research Institute for obtaining this IND, it is necessary to probe behind the press releases to understand the reasons for this change.

The FDA is a pressure-sensitive institution. Despite appearances, ultimately even FDA feels the heat of public disapproval or condemnation. And in 1989 FDA faced unprecedented opposition. What other agency is currently facing sixties-style sit-ins? Who has generated more acrimony, especially on the emotional issue of AIDS policy?

The fact is, FDA's control over the new-drugs approval process is slipping. It is not inconceivable that it will be forced to give up its right to enforce the efficacy requirements in the future. Commissioner Young has already liberalized the three-stage drug-approval process (Young, 1989). There is a developing national consensus that FDA should loosen its control.

Such pressure is coming from many quarters and is symbolized by what the *New York Times* called the "odd alliance" between militant AIDS advocates and conservatives such as the Competitive Enterprise Institute (November 24, 1988).

The blue-ribbon Lasagna Commission, appointed by Armand Hammer and sanctioned by President Bush, gave an impetus to this alliance. While making ritualistic knee-bends in FDA's direction that affirmed the beleaguered agency's control of both "safety and efficacy," its obvious intention was to lessen the FDA's almost dictatorial power over new drug development (Chabner, 1989). In fact, according to one eyewitness account, an NCI official suggested that "his preference would be that the FDA didn't exist" (Dumoff, 1989).

Antineoplastons are rarely mentioned in such august proceedings. But by allowing a small IND study of an ACS-certified "unproven method," the FDA has taken some of the pressure off itself on the contentious cancer front.

It has to be emphasized that antineoplastons, being drugs, present less of a challenge to the status quo than radical life-style approaches such as the Gerson diet, metabolic therapy, or macrobiotics. These may involve drugs but are more like paradigmatic challenges to an established way of thinking. Antineoplastons are unorthodox in being essentially nontoxic—a not inconsiderable distinction—but in other ways are not unlike the kind of thing FDA is used to dealing with: in the case of A10, a pure, synthesized substance of known chemical composition with a good scientific rationale for its action.

Finally, it should be noted that at the very moment of this approval, the FDA itself was under congressional investigation for allegations of bribery and favoritism in the approval of drugs.

"We gather that the size of that scandal is growing," said Representative John D. Dingell, the powerful Michigan Democrat who chaired the Oversight and Investigations Subcommittee of the House Energy and Commerce Committee. "When we started out on it, it looked like a small, isolated matter. As we have gotten more deeply into it, it looks like there is a rather startlingly large number of individuals and companies involved" (*Baltimore Sun,* March 4, 1989).

According to the Reuters news agency, a criminal investigation is being conducted by a federal grand jury in Baltimore. It anticipated that several FDA employees and six drug companies would be indicted (ibid.). This may not have directly affected FDA's decision, but it certainly reinforces the impression of an agency under siege.

In any case, Dr. Burzynski has gotten his foot in the door. Antineoplastons still represent a powerful challenge to toxic chemotherapy. It remains to be seen if the FDA, or anyone else, will be able to slam that door shut again.

1996 Update: The focus of the cancer alternative controversy has increasingly become centered on Dr. Burzynski and his treatment. Whatever happens, this promises to be an extremely bitter and hard-fought battle. It may well be that the fate of alternative cancer medicine hangs in the balance.

The U.S. Attorneys in Houston, after failing in three attempts to get a Grand Jury to indict him, succeeded in November, 1995. Dr. Burzynski was finally indicted on 75 counts of mail fraud, contempt, and violations of FDA laws. He faces up to 300 years in federal prison. The trial is scheduled to begin in the fall of 1996.

The case itself hinges on the government's contention that Burzynski broke the law when he allowed out-of-state patients to take antineoplastons back home with them. Burzynski claims that he has always acted in accordance with Judge McDonald's 1983 consent decree. The government also claims that he has defrauded insurance companies.

It appears that Dr. Burzynski's 200 patients will be allowed to continue receiving antineoplastons. But it is less likely the judge will allow the Texas doctor to enroll any new patients into his program. This would destroy the financial base Burzynski will need to wage an adequate defense.

Burzynski has been besieged on multiple fronts over the last few years. There was a damaging attack in the June 3, 1992 *Journal of the*

American Medical Association by Saul Green, Ph.D, entitled, "Antineo-plastons—An Unproved Cancer Therapy." The article failed to mention that members of Emprise, Inc. of which Dr. Green was scientific director, served as consultants to Aetna in its RICO suit against Dr. Burzynski.

There have also been almost constant attempts by Texas authorities to remove Burzynski's medical license. This case has see-sawed back and forth in the courts. At present, against unbelievable odds, he is still practicing.

Various insurance companies have sued him, attempting to recover money paid out to cancer patients for this treatment. However, the Aetna suit was thrown out in March 1992 by US District Court Judge Kenneth Hoyt.

In an unanticipated event, in October, 1991 the National Cancer Institute sent a site visit team to look at Burzynski's cases. Dr. Nicholas Patronas and other scientists concluded that Burzynski's treatment had indeed significantly shrunk tumors in six cases of brain tumors. NCI then announced that it would sponsor clinical trials on antineoplastons at Memorial Sloan-Kettering, using $750,000 provided by the Office of Alternative Medicine. In 1995, however, unsatisfied with the pace of these trials, NCI, Sloan-Kettering and the FDA decided among themselves to significantly alter the protocols, allowing in patients far more advanced than agreed to. They did this imperiously, without consulting either Dr. B. or OAM. When Dr. Burzynski strenuously objected, the trials were cancelled.

All in all, there has been a tremendous amount of sympathy for Burzynski—among the patients he allegedly exploits, from the general public, and even in the mainstream media and in Washington.

Congressman Joe Barton (R-TX) has held a series of hearings of the Investigations Subcommittee, in which he raked FDA over the coals for its handling of the Burzynski case. (It did not go unnoticed that Burzynski's indictment came down within days of FDA Commissioner Kessler's humiliating appearance before the subcommittee.)

Typical of favorable media coverage was an April 4, 1996 report by CBS Anchor Dan Rather on the TV news program "48 Hours." It showed patients, some of whom were in complete remission, organizing, lobbying and raising money for Burzynski's defense. One patient, uncontradicted, referred to the FDA as "the monster." It seems that for now Burzynski is winning the battle for the hearts and minds of the American people. It remains to be seen whether such support will help keep him out of federal prison.

PART THREE

Prevention

« 15 »

Preventing Prevention

Can cancer be prevented? This question has split the cancer field as profoundly as the debate over unorthodox methods of treatment, and perhaps more profoundly, for an effective program of prevention would render all methods of therapy—orthodox and unorthodox—obsolete.

The traditional establishment answer to this question has been that only a few types of cancer can be prevented. According to a long-standing American Cancer Society statement:

> Some cancers, not all [can be prevented]. Most lung cancers are caused by cigarette smoking, and most skin cancers by frequent overexposure to direct sunlight. These cancers can be prevented by avoiding their causes. Certain cancers caused by occupational–environmental factors can be prevented by eliminating or reducing contact with carcinogenic agents (ACS, 1988).

In a 1962 poll of 1,400 physicians a researcher associated with the American Cancer Society reported in *JAMA*, the journal of the American Medical Association, that

> the idea of preventing cancer seemed vague and doubtful to the [physician] audience as a whole. Added to this discouragement is the fact that not one

idea, lead or theory on cancer prevention was suggested by the entire professional audience (McGrady, Sr., 1964:394).

Today the situation is somewhat better, and many doctors urge their patients to stop smoking.

The ACS now devotes four and a half pages of its influential *Facts and Figures* booklet to prevention. Some of what it includes under this rubric is in fact early detection. Much space is given to tobacco use. In addition, it provides what it calls a "common sense approach" to nutrition and cancer, which centers around noncontroversial advice to "avoid obesity" and "keep alcohol consumption moderate" (ACS, 1989).

One can of course argue with the details of ACS's go-slow program. The main point is that prevention has become such a popular issue that even the Cancer Society has been forced to deal with it.

In fact, in many ways the establishment's yielding on the diet-cancer link is one of the most important developments of the decade. Although some dietary approaches (such as macrobiotics) continue to be listed on the unproven methods list, the Society itself now advocates some special foods, such as the cruciferous family of vegetables (cabbage, broccoli, brussel sprouts, kohlrabi, and cauliflower) to prevent cancer. This is a far cry from the days when anticancer diets were considered the very hallmark of quackery.

But beyond these largely verbal measures, little is done to stop the incidence of cancer before it occurs.

For many years it was a small, but growing, number of mavericks who maintained that cancer was a preventable disease. The pages of health magazines were filled with their claims. Often they urged a return to a more simple, organic diet as a way to prevent what has been called the "disease of civilization."

Others, working in the laboratory or compiling statistics on cancer's victims (epidemiology), proposed evidence that showed a link between chemicals encountered at home or at work and the rising rate of cancer.

What are these chemical factors, or carcinogens?

Scientists pinpointed at least two dozen that are known to cause cancer in laboratory animals and almost certainly contribute to cancer in man. These include tobacco and particularly its smoke, which can cause not only lung cancer but tumors of the mouth, throat, and bladder; smoked foods, which have been implicated as a cause of stomach cancer; alcohol, suspected of being a cocarcinogen, potentiating other cancer-causing substances; various drugs, including those used to treat cancer itself; female hormones; food colorings; pesticides; and nitrosamines, formed by a combination of nitrites or nitrates and amines in the body (Fraumeni, 1975).

Industrial chemicals that cause cancer may afflict workers on the job, people who live in the vicinity of factories, or even consumers of products containing such chemicals. These carcinogens include asbestos, benzene, cadmium, arsenic, nickel, vinyl chloride, and the dye chemical beta-naphthylamine. All radioactive substances are potentially carcinogenic. As everyone is now aware, the list of suspected carcinogens grows steadily, almost with every passing day.

An effective strategy for dealing with cancer might be to reduce or eliminate exposure to these chemicals and environmental pollutants. Some physicians, familiar with the poor record of conventional treatments, believe this is the *only* effective way to fight cancer.

Minnesota pediatrician Ronald J. Glasser has warned: "We are not doomed to die of cancer—unless we persist in dooming ourselves . . . unless we take steps right now to defend ourselves, the incidence [of cancer] will continue to rise in the decades to come" (Glasser, 1979:172).

Giulio J. D'Angio, M.D., former chairman of the Department of Radiation Therapy of Memorial Sloan-Kettering Cancer Center, expressed a similar sentiment after many years of treating cancer with radiation:

> It is natural for physicians to focus on treatment. A far better focus is prevention. The recent identification of environmental oncogenic [cancer-causing] factors, some of them prenatal, some of them found even in the household, and their elimination are obvious and totally effective ways of curing cancer, before it develops (D'Angio, 1975).

The elimination of these cancer-causing substances might at first sight appear to be a simple and rational way to reduce the incidence of cancer. It may be rational, but it is certainly not simple. Critics charge that the main obstacle is the power of industry to hinder such changes:

> Today, more than ever before, the price of health is vigilance, and this vigilance means that we must recognize not only the poisons in our environment but also the efforts on the part of industry to resist, in the name of profit, the removal of these carcinogens and mutagens, as well as government tolerance of these efforts (Glasser, 1979:173).

In a classic study of environmental carcinogens, *The Politics of Cancer*, Samuel S. Epstein, M.D., professor of occupational and environmental medicine at the School of Public Health, University of Illinois, attempts to dissect the eight-part strategy that industry uses to prevent the prevention of cancer (Epstein, 1978):*

(1) *Minimizing the risk:* Industry will try to downplay the importance of a particular compound, and chemicals in general, in the causation of cancer. For example, Exxon Corporation and the industry trade group Manufacturing Chemists Association claimed that although benzene may cause leukemia, this was no longer an environmental problem. Scientific reports showed, however, that chemical workers continued to be exposed to dangerous levels of this substance (ibid.:132–33).

(2) *Diversionary tactics:* Industry spokesmen will attempt to drag a red herring across the scene to divert attention. For example, they will demand a degree of precision about the effects of a putative carcinogen on humans that they know is impossible to achieve. Or they will call for more research into a known hazard. This has been a favorite tactic of the tobacco lobby.

(3) *Propagandizing the public:* With tremendous resources at its disposal, industry has been able to confuse the public about the risk of cancer-causing substances. In fact, historian David F. Nobile has called this "the corporate ideology of the 1980s" (Nobile, 1979). Mobil Oil, he reports, spent $3.2 million on "grass-roots lobbying" in 1978; Monsanto spent $5 million a year on television spots, newspaper ads, and pamphlets for school children; and Union Carbide formed a communications department to "engage in public policy dialogue on issues that affect our business" (ibid.; Epstein, 1978:394).**

In the late 1970s, as Nobile explains, there was a shift in corporate strategy:

> In the past when regulators identified a chemical as carcinogenic, that charge alone was enough to alarm the public. . . . Today, corporations like Union Carbide have begun to shift the very nature of the debate. They now readily concede that their products are carcinogenic, but blandly insist that the acknowledged risk of cancer be put in "perspective," that it be compared with other risks and traded off against product benefits. Life, after all, is risky (Nobile, 1979).†

*Much of the information that follows is derived from Epstein's excellent book.
**William S. Sneath, Union Carbide president, was a member of MSKCC's board of overseers.
†Similarly, when critics charged that the American Cancer Society-National Cancer Institute breast screening program would *cause* as many deaths through radiation-induced breast cancer as it would save through early detection, ACS vice president Arthur I. Holleb, M.D.,

As tough antismoking laws have proliferated around the country, the tobacco industry has fought back with a nationwide campaign to organize opposition to such legislation. They spent $20 million in California in 1988 in an unsuccessful attempt at defeating a 25-cent-a-pack increase in the cigarette price. They also flew high-powered Washington lobbyists into small towns, such as St. Charles, Missouri, to stop antismoking ordinances from passing (*New York Times,* December 14, 1988).

In May 1987, RJR Nabisco and the Tobacco Institute coordinated an effort to overturn an antismoking ordinance in the town of Rancho Mirage, California. RJR Nabisco threatened to move its golf tournament out of town, and the Tobacco Institute organized the prosmoking forces, including restaurant owners.

"It was close to a mob mentality," said Mayor Jeffrey Bleaman, who supported tough legislation. "There was screaming and booing. In my wildest dreams I would never have imagined something like that." And the ordinance was, in fact, seriously weakened after the incident (ibid.).

(4) *Blaming the victim:* Industry will sometimes claim that cancer is not really caused by chemicals, but is the fault of the person who gets the cancer. Thus industry spokesmen have postulated a "hyper-susceptible worker" who is genetically predisposed to contract the disease. This has been a favorite concept with the asbestos industry, said Epstein (1978:94).

(5) *Controlling information:* While independent scientists have gathered quite a bit of information on carcinogens, most of the public's and Congress's information about chemicals and their effects must necessarily come from the manufacturers.

This situation leaves the door open for distorted presentations or even outright fraud. The *Congressional Record* of July 30, 1969, cites numerous instances of data manipulation with such drugs as MER/29, for which executives of Richardson-Merrell Company were convicted of criminal charges; Dornwall, for which Wallace and Tiernan Company were found guilty of submitting false data; and Flexin, about which McNeil Laboratories failed to submit toxicity data on drug-related liver damage, including eleven deaths, in their reports to the FDA (cited in ibid.:303–04).

"Prescriptions for Profit," a recent television documentary, detailed

---

replied in identical fashion: "From the moment of birth we face innumerable risks that not only threaten our existence, but also carry the potential of temporary or even permanent infirmity. To avoid most risks one would have to take to the bed—a considerable circulatory risk in itself—and shun normal activities" (Holleb, 1976). Thus, women should ignore the risk of breast cancer and take their mammograms. Despite this, an NCI panel ruled against the routine use of mammography in women under fifty (see chapter 2).

numerous instances of drug company duplicity in the marketing of Oroflex and other painkillers. Data was often withheld or downplayed in the presentations made to doctors (Frontline, 1989).

(6) *Influencing policy:* Even if a substance is proven carcinogenic, it is a long way from being regulated, controlled, or banned. It took more than half a dozen years of consumer lobbying to gain passage of the Toxin Substances Control Act of 1976. But not only did the Manufacturing Chemists Association manage to tone down that once-promising legislation, through daily conferences with congressional representatives and their staffs, but little has been done since then to enforce the control of toxic substances.

(7) *Exhausting the agencies:* The regulatory agencies often show little inclination to control industry. But if they ever do, industry is able to overwhelm the would-be regulators with legal paperwork. One or two major cases, such as Shell's protracted defense of its cancer-causing pesticides aldrin and dieldrin, can totally exhaust the resources of a government agency.

Even when Shell finally lost its aldrin/dieldrin case, it used the *identical* arguments and tactics in the almost identical chlordane/heptachlor pesticide case. Industry has insisted that every case must be argued separately, on its own merits, instead of on the basis of commonly agreed-upon cancer principles. Thus, a would-be regulator of industry is in the same plight as Sisyphus, in Greek mythology, whose punishment in Hades was to roll a giant rock to the top of a hill, only to have it constantly fall back to the bottom again.

(8) *The flight of the multinationals:* If all else should fail, the giant corporations can pick up their operations and move to regions or countries more receptive to "dirty" industries. With the passage of the Occupational Safety and Health Act of 1970, such runaways within the United States have become more difficult. But the manufacturers of asbestos, benzidine dye, pesticides, plastics, and copper have moved their carcinogenic processes out of the country.

It should hardly shock anyone that industry will use a wide variety of tactics to protect its investments. What is more surprising is the degree to which leaders of the cancer field have also helped to obscure the need for prevention.

Memorial Sloan-Kettering Cancer Center, which has often been the pace-setter for other institutions, has done surprisingly little in the field of prevention. Some research was conducted on the link between tobacco and cancer in the 1950s and 1960s, but this almost entirely came to a halt when

Dr. Ernst Wynder left the Center in 1969.* Some other work on chemical carcinogenesis was carried out at the Walker Laboratory of Sloan-Kettering. But this work was of a rather abstract nature and never entered the public debates on the cause of cancer.

The tone for Sloan-Kettering was set by its leaders, and these men were fully in accord with industry's view that cancer was not caused, to any appreciable degree, by products of industry.

In the mid-1960s, for instance, Frank Horsfall, the director of Sloan-Kettering, was asked by a reporter if he thought that certain occupations were dangerous with respect to cancer. This was more than a decade after scientists had proven that bladder cancer could be caused by the chemical beta-naphthylamine. Many other industrial causes of cancer were either then known or strongly suspected. Horsfall's answer was a very qualified yes:

> A farmer, for instance, who works in the sun all day, with the ultraviolet rays beating on his skin. This, plus the dirt that gets in the crevices of the skin, may lead to skin cancer (*U.S. News and World Report*, April 19, 1965).

Granting that "certain petroleum products and such things" could contain "incitants," Horsfall cautioned his audience:

> These should not be emphasized, because the frequency with which they lead to cancer is very low indeed, and industry has been particularly effective in detecting and getting rid of them. Industrial hazards of this kind are of progressively smaller importance (ibid.).

After Horsfall's death, Leo Wade, M.D., became acting director of the Institute. Wade had a long career in industry before coming to Sloan-Kettering as first vice president. He was medical director of Standard Oil of New Jersey from 1951 to 1961, and was a member of the American Petroleum Institute, the Manufacturing Chemists Association, and the National Association of Manufacturers—organizations that have generally been unfriendly to stringent government health regulations.**

*Wynder became president and medical director of the American Health Foundation. He remained a consulting epidemiologist at MSKCC.

**Wade's publications at Standard Oil included the articles "Why People Don't Work" and "Medical Public Relations for the Physician in Industry" (Wade, 1958, 1953). Biographical information on Wade from MSKCC press release, May 16, 1961, and obituary, in the *New York Times,* January 6, 1975.

In 1964 Wade granted that some workers show an increased incidence of certain types of cancer. Nevertheless, he remained unconvinced that particular chemicals could actually *cause* that cancer:

> Although some assume a true cause-and-effect relationship to have been established, I believe the relationship more properly considered as one of association. The common causes of cancer in man are still unknown (Wade, 1964).

The Sloan-Kettering leader considered the provisions of the Workmen's Compensation Act, which reimbursed workers for occupationally induced cancer, "a 'gold mine' for those willing to exploit medical ignorance" (ibid.). Efforts to control chemicals suspected of causing cancer were "both futile and suspect" (Wade, 1962). Far from being a problem created by industry "cancer is now widely believed to consist of a heritable, and therefore genetic" problem (Sloan-Kettering, 1969).

The ascension of Robert Good to the directorship of Sloan-Kettering in the early 1970s seemed to augur a new, more liberal approach to this question. The 1972 *Annual Report* (prepared in 1973) promised "the development and use of better laboratory techniques for determining which chemicals in our environment cause cancer" (MSKCC, 1972:9). Even had he wanted to, however, Good could not change the composition of the body he reported to, the MSKCC board of overseers, which is made up predominantly of bankers and industrialists (see Appendix A). Nor could he alter the long-established relationships between scientists at Sloan-Kettering and big business.

In 1974, in the midst of the furor over the potential danger of pesticides, Memorial Sloan-Kettering pathologist Stephen Sternberg headed the Shell Chemical Company Ad Hoc Committee of Pathologists which claimed that aldrin and dieldrin were *not* carcinogenic (Epstein, 1978:261). Sternberg is now head of the American Council on Science and Health, which is funded by big business and, with the exception of tobacco, generally takes pro-industry positions on questions of environmental pollution.

Few steps have been taken to make preventive medicine a major focus at the Center. One long-anticipated move was the establishment in July 1976 of an Epidemiology and Preventive Medicine Service within the Department of Medicine. The first major study this group undertook was an investigation of cancer in petroleum workers, which was funded by the American Petroleum Institute, a trade association of the largest oil companies (MSKCC *Center News*, September 1975 and September 1978).

At Sloan-Kettering Institute, only a small percentage of the overall research effort was ever directed toward prevention. Of approximately one hundred laboratories listed in the 1976 *Annual Report*, for instance, only one—Chemical Oncogenesis—was exclusively occupied with the question of cancer prevention. In a few other laboratories, researchers worked on questions of prevention, but often on a part-time basis. The 1987–88 "Sloan-Kettering Institute: Research and Educational Programs" revealed no projects directed toward the question of industrial pollution.

In the past, this situation was partially the result of a lack of funding for such studies from the National Cancer Institute, the American Cancer Society, and private donors; today it is mainly the result of the pro-big business attitudes and policies at MSKCC itself. (The link between the directors of MSKCC and cancer-causing industry is further explored in chapter 17 and in Appendix A.)

The American Cancer Society

In the public's mind, the American Cancer Society (ACS) is associated with the first really large-scale cancer prevention project ever attempted in the United States: the campaign against cigarette smoking. In the 1950s and the 1960s, the Society carried out a massive and expensive study on the relationship between smoking and health. About one million people were questioned by ACS volunteers, and the Society kept track of more than 90 percent of these people for a dozen years.

This ACS study provided much of the basis for the Surgeon General's report of 1964 that condemned smoking as a cause of lung cancer. It linked the number of cigarettes smoked to the dramatic increase in lung cancer in certain populations. Follow-up studies in this country, England, and Japan have confirmed the basic validity of the ACS work.

Historically ACS has tended to rely on education and to downplay legislation or other activist measures. For example, an official in the 1970s said that the Society "had used [its] resources to uncover the health risks of smoking. Now it was up to the government to take a stand and respond accordingly" (cited in Epstein, 1978).

The Society was one of the first health groups to ask President John F. Kennedy to take action against tobacco in 1961. But when a consumer activist petitioned the Federal Communications Commission for equal time against tobacco ads in 1971, "the Society refused to support him, let alone defend the subsequent FCC ruling in his favor" (ibid.).

Epstein called the Society's efforts against tobacco "weak and diffuse" (Epstein, 1978:424); he himself helped form a Cancer Prevention

Committee within the Illinois Division of the Society, to try to swing the ACS toward a more activist stand.

Obviously stung by this sort of criticism, in 1978 the Society initiated a National Commission on Smoking and Public Policy, which recommended the following strictures: prohibition of smoking in most public places, as well as in the working environment and in schools; phasing out the government tobacco price-support system; a Food and Drug Administration study of potentially harmful cigarette additives; reduction of insurance rates for nonsmokers; basing the cigarette tax on tar and nicotine content; adoption of quit-smoking programs by all hospitals and clinics; banning all advertising of high tar and nicotine cigarettes and curtailing use of models in ads; holding the tobacco industry accountable to the FDA or the Consumer Product Safety Commission for the safety of its products; and an HEW interagency council to coordinate antismoking activities of different departments (ACS, 1978:15).

On balance, however, it must be granted that the ACS's record on tobacco is generally very good. They initiated the "Great American Smokeout," in which people are encouraged to quit smoking for a day (ACS, 1978:14). That program is now over a dozen years old. They distribute "I Quit Kits," and run effective groups to help people stop. Together with the American Heart and Lung Association, ACS forms the Tri-Agency Tobacco-Free Young America Project. In recent years, ACS has focussed much of its attention on convincing young people to stop, or never start, smoking (ACS, 1986).

All of this is positive and represents a more activist course than the Society pursued in the past. And a determined stance is absolutely necessary in the light of the alarming increase in lung cancer: in the thirty years between 1953–55 and 1983–85, for example, the death rate for men went up 161 percent and for women an astonishing 396 percent! (ACS, 1988:29). The $55-billion-a-year cigarette industry is vigorously attempting to stop any legislation which is aimed at stopping this plague. It wields enormous resources but is facing a mass movement of opposition. Over the last twenty-five years, ACS has helped spearhead that movement.

That said, it is necessary to raise serious questions about ACS's overall stance on environmental carcinogens. Although tobacco is an important—in fact crucial—issue, there are other pollutants and other sources of cancer, even lung cancer.

And here ACS has not done nearly as well.

While the fight against tobacco is important, it sometimes seems as if the ACS uses this fight as a smoke screen to hide its inaction in the overall field of environmental and occupational cancer. The Society's Board of Directors has contained many business leaders and bankers. Science writer Peter Barry Chowka contended that many of the known carcinogens "are by-products of profitable industries in which its [ACS's] directors have financial interests" (Chowka, 1978b).*

During the public debate on the banning of saccharin, the American Cancer Society took the side of the manufacturers and the Calorie Control Council (a soft-drink lobbying group) to argue that this known animal carcinogen should be allowed in foods and drinks because it is of great medical benefit and safe. In effect, the Society came out against the Delaney Amendment, which states that no substance known to cause cancer in animals may be added to the food or water supply. Although many experts question the value of saccharin even for diabetics, ACS official R. Lee Clark declared that "banning saccharin may cause great harm to many citizens while protecting a theoretical few" (*New York Times*, April 6, 1977).

"The ACS has done the American people a really great disservice," declared Nobel Prize-winner David Baltimore, an ACS-fund recipient whose picture had appeared on page one of the Society's 1975 *Annual Report*. He added, "ACS has been playing into the Calorie Control Council's hands" (Chowka, 1978b). The Council's members utilized 75 percent of the nation's saccharin supply.

A key member of the Calorie Control Council was the Coca-Cola Company, which manufactured the saccharin-sweetened diet soda Tab. In its 1976 *Annual Report,* the ACS acknowledged that "a generous grant from Coca-Cola supported transportation" for a large delegation of the Society's executives and volunteers who visited the Soviet Union in that year. In addition, a vice president of Pepsico, another prominent Calorie Control Council member was on the ACS Commission on Smoking and Public Policy (ibid.).

For an organization that claims to devote "considerable effort to studying the link between the environment and cancer," the ACS has taken a number of other questionable positions. For example, the synthetic hormone DES (diethylstilbestrol) is a known carcinogen.** For years, it was given to live-

*Dan Greenberg has called the ACS House of Delegates "a Who's Who of the American establishment." In the seventies it included eighteen officers or directors of banks, seven members of investment firms, thirteen business or industrial executives, with the remainder drawn from communications, advertising, media, manufacturing, insurance, and pharmaceuticals (cited in Chowka, 1978b).

**"When DES was first synthesized in 1938, it was also found to be carcinogenic, inducing breast cancer in male mice. Subsequent studies showed that DES was approximately ten times more potent as a carcinogen than natural estrogens. . . . Administration of female sex hormones has been shown to induce cancer of the uterus, cervix, vagina, breast, and ovary in women, and of the breast in men" (Epstein, 1978:219–20).

stock to fatten them up, on the assumption that the hormone itself does not enter the food supply. In 1971 doctors discovered a link between DES and cancer of the female reproductive system. In 1972, residues of the hormone were discovered in beef, and public-interest groups demanded an immediate ban on the food additive. However, the American Cancer Society refused to take any position on the matter, and thereby deprived the consumer advocates of what could have been their most powerful support (Epstein, 1978:232).

Similarly, when the Food and Drug Administration suggested a patient package insert for Premarin and other hormone-containing drugs, indicating that these may increase a woman's risk of cancer, the ACS opposed the move on the grounds that this would "interfere with the practice of medicine" and "discourage patients" from taking such drugs (ibid.:236).*

In 1987 Dr. Epstein issued a blistering attack, "Are We Losing the War Against Cancer?" which Representative Henry Waxman (D.-Calif.) inserted into the Congressional Record (Epstein, 1987).

After reviewing the runaway growth in polluting substances, as well as the government's failure to regulate these, he zeroed in on the cancer establishment. This establishment "continues to mislead the public and Congress into believing that 'we are winning the war against cancer.' " It periodically "beats the drum to announce the latest 'cancer cure' and dramatic 'breakthrough,' " such as interferon or interleukin-2. It emphasizes the lifestyle aspects of cancer, such as smoking and diet, and all but ignores the industrial sources.

Epstein, in fact, points out that in 1982 Congressman David Obey (D.-Wisc.) discovered that NCI had "pressured the International Agency for Research on Cancer (IACR), funded in part by NCI, to downplay the carcinogenicity of benzene . . ." (ibid.).

But the particular target of Samuel Epstein's wrath is the American Cancer Society. As indicated, Epstein had previously tried to work from within the ACS to change its priorities. "Following nearly a decade of fruitless discussion with the ACS," he wrote, "at a February 7, 1987 press conference, a national coalition of major public-interest and labor groups headed by the Center for Science in the Public Interest . . . and supported by some 24 independent scientists [including Epstein] charged that the ACS is 'doing virtually nothing to help reduce the public exposure to cancer-causing chemicals" (ibid.).

*The wording is from a suit filed in the U.S. District Court in Delaware against the FDA by the Pharmaceutical Manufacturers Association, the drug industry's lobbying group, and the American College of Obstetricians and Gynecologists in September 1977. The ACS supported these groups in their protest.

The ACS, he charged, not only "fails to make its voice heard in Congress and the regulatory area," but more specifically:

> It has failed to support critical legislation that seeks to reduce or eliminate environmental exposure to carcinogens. It refused to join a coalition of major organizations, including the March of Dimes, the American Heart Association, and the American Lung Association, to support the Clean Air Act.
>
> ACS statements are "expressly or implicitly hostile to regulation" of polluting industries.
>
> Its approach to cancer prevention is a "blame the victim" philosophy. For instance, it blames the higher incidence of cancer among blacks primarily on diet and smoking, rather than on the fact that "blacks work in the dirtiest, most hazardous jobs and live in the most polluted communities" (ibid.).

A few days after the press conference, Epstein says, ACS announced a "new set of policies," passing resolutions for improved regulation of asbestos and benzene. "However," the University of Illinois scientist commented, "there has been no evidence of any real change of heart in the ACS since then" (ibid.).

In the *Congressional Record* and in interviews Epstein has courageously called for an economic boycott of the $300-million-a-year American Cancer Society. Such a boycott is "long overdue," he told reporters (*Chicago Sun-Times,* November 29, 1987).

It is difficult to summarize the ACS's overall stand on cancer prevention. On the one hand, it has done more than any other organization to establish the link between tobacco and cancer, and to help people stop smoking. It has given support to some researchers in the environmental field (see chapter 16), yet the overwhelming share of research funding has gone to efforts to improve the three orthodox treatment methods. It speaks about cancer prevention, yet at critical junctures has taken public positions that have hindered the effort to control carcinogens.

As an institution dependent on small donations for its continued existence, the ACS, in the words of Lane W. Adams, a former executive vice president, must watch out for "disturbing signs of skepticism about the effectiveness of the struggle against cancer" (ACS, 1978:3). It therefore must acknowledge the widespread and growing conviction that environmental factors are responsible for a good deal of the cancer in the United States, and that prevention may well be "the only cure." On the other hand, ACS's ties to a treatment-oriented medical profession and to big business dampens its enthusiasm for really strong measures to enforce prevention. The ACS

sounds like the sophisticated corporate spokesman who grants a link between cancer and the environment with one hand—only to take it away with
the other. According to one ACS *Annual Report:*

> We are steadily extending our knowledge of cancer-causing agents. How-
> ever, some misunderstanding has grown up around the probable extent of "en-
> vironmental" cancer—an unexamined assumption that a very high percentage
> of human cancer is caused by dangerous chemicals in our air, food, water and
> work places. . . .
>   While the evidence is mounting that substances we eat, breathe or contact
> are contributing causes of most cancer, only a minority of these are industrial
> "chemicals" or by-products (ACS, 1978:6).*

Ten years later ACS was only slightly more positive. While granting
that "most cancer cases in the United States are believed to be environmentally related," it was quick to downplay the role of toxic chemicals encountered at work, school or home:

> Occupational hazards, although associated with only a small percentage
> of cancers, are under close surveillance. Virtually every suspected major chemical
> and other substance in the workplace presumed to be a health risk is under
> investigation. Each study can require years and hundreds of thousands of dol-
> lars to complete (ACS, 1988:27).

With such an attitude, it is unlikely that the American Cancer Society
will play a very active role in the struggle against man-made carcinogens.

The National Cancer Institute/National Cancer Program

The policy of the National Cancer Institute (NCI) toward prevention
resembles that of the American Cancer Society. This is more than a coincidence. ACS was instrumental in the founding of the government's cancer
institute in 1937 and in the passage of the National Cancer Act of 1971,

---

*"An informed consensus has gradually developed that most cancer is environmental
in origin and is therefore preventable" (Epstein, 1978:23). Studies by R. Doll, B. Armstrong,
and other epidemiologists have established that from 70 to 90 percent is environmental in origin
(ibid.: 514). The lack of research on occupational cancer has hindered the effort to determine
how much of this is due to chemicals. But Epstein estimates that "30 to 40 percent of cancers
in the general population" may be due to pollution just from the large petrochemical plants
(ibid.:27).

which quickly quadrupled NCI's budget. ACS and NCI personnel interlock on many committees (see chapter 17). Historically it has been the ACS that has influenced the larger, but more weak-willed, NCI. An "ACS-controlled clique . . . dominates NCI policy and funding decisions," according to journalist Ruth Rosenbaum. "They've [ACS] turned it into a dollar pump," a House Appropriations committeeman added graphically (Rosenbaum, 1977).

From the 1940s to the 1960s, NCI's involvement with environmental and occupational carcinogens centered around one man, William C. Hueper. A German-born physician, Hueper came to the United States in 1923 and established himself as an expert on environmental causes of cancer.

Hueper predicted correctly that dye workers at E. I. Du Pont de Nemours & Co. would soon start succumbing to bladder cancer. When the prediction came true (such occupational cancers were already known in Europe), Hueper was hired by the company to "solve the puzzle" of this disease. He received little cooperation from the company. When he made an unauthorized visit to a Du Pont factory, he discovered large, uncontrolled amounts of carcinogenic chemicals. He reported this to the top management of the giant chemical company.

"The result of that letter," Hueper recalls, "was that I was never permitted to see the dye works again" (Agran, 1977:176). Restricted to the laboratory, Hueper demonstrated that one of the chemicals used in the dye works (beta-naphthylamine) produced bladder cancer in dogs. Eventually, 339 out of 2,000 workers at Du Pont exposed to this chemical died of bladder malignancies (ibid.).

In 1942 Hueper published *Occupational Tumors and Allied Diseases,* now considered a classic of the epidemiological approach to cancer ("a definitive summary," Shimkin, 1977:230). In 1948 he was appointed chief of the Environmental Cancer Section of the National Cancer Institute.

Hueper's job was carrying out field studies to determine which chemicals were causing cancer among workers and the general population, and laboratory studies to determine the effect of chemicals on animals. This ambitious program was hampered by the fact that Hueper's total budget for 1948 was $90,000—out of a $14.5 million allocation to NCI. In fact, when Hueper retired from the Institute sixteen years later, his budget was *still* about $90,000, although NCI's allocation had jumped by 1,000 percent (Epstein, 1978:321).

Hueper was also concerned with the danger of radiation, and he attempted to warn the Colorado Medical Society of the peril faced by uranium miners. Hueper's director at NCI refused to allow Hueper to do so, reportedly telling the scientist, "You shall omit that from your presentation" (Agran, 1977). Hueper responded, "I did not join the Public Health Service [of which NCI was a branch] to be made a liar!'' (ibid.). Corroborating recent revelations about the suppression of information on radiation's dangers (see chapter 4), Hueper explained, "You see, the AEC [Atomic Energy Commission] was afraid that publication of that kind of information might interfere with the continued production of atomic bombs" (ibid.).

Similarly, when Hueper was asked to testify before Congressman Delaney's (D.-N.Y.) Select Committee Investigating the Use of Chemicals in Food and Cosmetics, his supervisors at NCI refused to allow him to use much of his data on additives and even suggested that he refuse to testify. He therefore testified as a private citizen and contributed to the passage of the Delaney Amendment, which bans carcinogens from the food supply (ibid.).

For the second time in his career, Hueper was restricted to his laboratory and not allowed to contact state health departments or industrial concerns. But he poured out a steady stream of articles and books, eventually totaling over 350, detailing the manner in which occupational and environmental factors cause cancer (ibid.).

Although of major theoretical importance, Hueper's discoveries did not have a significant impact on NCI policy or direction. With the passage of the National Cancer Act of 1971, NCI did not indicate any pressing interest in expanding work on the environmental causes of the disease (unless one defined putative cancer viruses as "environmental causes"—as NCI did). Instead the emphasis was put on finding a cure. Reviewing the war on cancer, British science writer Dr. Roger Lewin commented:

> The scientists have brought their own distortions . . . emphasizing the glamorous and exciting areas of research, such as virology and immunology, while ignoring to an unjustified extent topics such as epidemiology and environmental carcinogenesis (*New Scientist*, January 22, 1976:168).

NCI's record on tobacco is worse than that of the American Cancer Society. NCI's Smoking and Health Program, discontinued in 1977, was designed not to fight tobacco consumption but solely to devise a so-called safe cigarette. The Tobacco Working Group, which NCI established to oversee the program, included vice presidents and research directors of Liggett & Myers, the Brown and Williamson Tobacco Company, R. J. Reynolds Industries, Lorillard Research Center, and Philip Morris—all giant cigarette manufacturers.*

*Epstein presents evidence that it may be impossible to create a safe cigarette, since there are hundreds of potentially harmful chemicals in tobacco smoke. Carbon monoxide, the result of incomplete combustion, is itself a health hazard. The new flavor additives, which

A critical role in the direction of NCI's research is played by the National Cancer Advisory Board (NCAB), which reviews the Institute's budget twice a year, considers all grant applications over $50,000, and made recommendations on which ones were to be funded (NCI, 1986). To consider the validity of grant applications concerning the environmental causes of cancer, the NCAB established a Subcommittee on Environmental Carcinogenesis, first chaired by Dr. Philippe Shubik.

For an expert on environmental cancer, Dr. Shubik took a surprisingly lax stand on the control of chemicals. For example, he attacked the "cancer principles," which would have allowed regulatory agencies to treat all carcinogens the same. This action led to the refusal by an Environmental Protection Agency administrative law judge to ban the carcinogenic pesticides chlordane and heptachlor (Epstein, 1978).

In November 1975 Shubik was successful in getting NCI to abandon its "Memoranda of Alert," in which it warned the public about early findings in its animal testing program. This action came shortly after NCI had issued a memorandum of alert on a chemical used by General Foods to decaffeinate coffee. Shubik also testified against banning a proposed Procter and Gamble detergent that contained a potentially harmful chemical. So vehement was Shubik's defense of this detergent that Dr. Umberto Saffioti, associate director of NCI's Carcinogenesis Program, was compelled to ask: "Would you for the record identify what capacity you are here under?"

Shubik replied, "Procter and Gamble" (ibid.).

It turned out that Shubik, an NCAB official, was also a paid consultant to General Foods, Royal Crown Cola, Abbott Laboratories, Miles Laboratories, Colgate Palmolive, the Flavor and Extract Manufacturers Association, and the Calorie Control Council.

On most cases, however, Shubik spoke like a good environmentalist. "It is the universal opinion that cancer can be attributed to environmental factors, in the main," he has said. "Cancer is largely a preventable disease." He also expressed "general astonishment" that the National Cancer Program "does not appear to have accorded an adequate priority or sense of urgency to the field of environmental carcinogenesis" (*Science and Government Report,* April 1, 1975; *New Scientist,* January 22, 1976:168).*

make low-tar-and-nicotine cigarettes more appealing to smokers, may be carcinogenic. There is even evidence that people who smoke low-tar-and-nicotine cigarettes may have a higher incidence of lung cancer, since they inhale more deeply and smoke more than those who smoke unfiltered high nicotine cigarettes (Epstein, 1978:163–65).

*In 1978 Dr. Shubik came under congressional scrutiny for possible conflicts of interest in relation to millions of dollars in NCI grants to the Eppley Cancer Research Institute, of which he was the director (Epstein, 1978).

Shubik does not appear to be alone in his connections to industry. According to the *Cancer Letter:*

> Why [Congressman David R.] Obey [D.-Wisc.] has singled out Shubik as a target for conflict of interest charges is a mystery. Nearly every scientific member of the Board, the President's Cancer Panel, and the various advisory committees could be subject to such charges (cited in Rosenbaum, 1977).

For example, the chairman of the NCAB turned out, under congressional inquiry, to be a director of Pennwalt Corporation, a conglomerate with both pharmaceutical and chemical interests. NCAB member Frank Dixon was a consultant to Eli Lilly Co. (*Cancer Letter,* June 11, 1976). The business connections of former NCAB members Benno Schmidt and Laurance S. Rockefeller are dealt with elsewhere (see Appendix A).

The chairman of the President's Cancer Panel throughout most of the 1980s has been Armand Hammer, head of Occidental International Corporation. Among Occidental's subsidiaries is Hooker Chemical Company, implicated in the chemical pollution of the environment.

Hammer began his tenure by offering one million of his own dollars to the scientist "who achieves a cure for cancer similar to that discovered by Dr. Jonas Salk with the polio vaccine" (*Science,* December 18, 1981).

This headline-grabber was yet another variation on the thesis that cancer could be cured by an infusion of cash. "But the money is unlikely to speed up the discovery of an ultimate weapon against cancer," wrote Marjorie Sun in *Science,* "given the billions of federal dollars that have been pumped into the cancer program so far . . ." (ibid.).

At his first public meeting Hammer was heckled by members of a group called Citizens Concerned About Corporate Cancer. They charged that as head of Occidental, he was unfit to be a cancer panel member.

"Your chairmanship is a fraud," said one young man wearing a T-shirt emblazoned with *Love Canal: Another Product Brought to You by Hooker Chemical.* The protesters were eventually "escorted out of the room" (ibid.).

Under pressure from Congress and the public, NCI has claimed that a major portion of its work is relevant to environmental and occupational cancer. In 1976 Frank Rauscher, then National Cancer Institute director, told Congress that 20 percent of his agency's budget was devoted to the study of environmental carcinogens (Epstein, 1978:326 ff).

Rauscher's statement was based on the fact that the Division of Cancer Cause and Prevention commanded 18 percent of the Institute's budget. This division included most of the work on cancer viruses, which are, technically speaking, environmental factors. The virus program received approximately half of the division's yearly budget. However, the departments that studied the chemical causes of cancer and tabulated the results of epidemiological surveys, Carcinogenesis Program and Field Studies and Statistics, together received only 12 percent of the Institute's budget—a vast improvement since Hueper's day but less than what was needed, according to many critics (ibid.).

More important than the number of dollars spent was the dearth of results. Under Rauscher's directorship, NCI's chemical-testing program achieved little. Most of the testing of chemicals for carcinogenicity was farmed out to an industrial contractor, Tracor Jitco, Inc. In 1973 about 100 new chemicals were tested each year. By 1976, however, the program appeared to be grinding to a halt. Only 30 compounds were tested in that year. (There are 4 million compounds listed in the Chemical Abstract Service computer registry, and over 30,000 of them are in *common* use in the United States [ibid.].)

Only five scientists were employed at NCI to test chemical compounds for their carcinogenic potential, and only half a dozen reports were issued in the mid-seventies. Dissatisfaction increased, and in early 1976 Rauscher was directed by federal legislators to increase emphasis on prevention and was allocated the money to do so. He was specifically told to hire a staff of sixty new people for the Carcinogenesis Program and seventeen scientists for a newly created Epidemiology Branch (ibid.).

In April 1976, however, NCI was shaken by the resignation of Dr. Umberto Saffioti as associate director of the Carcinogenesis Program. In his letter of resignation, Saffioti complained of a lack of manpower for the program and a general lack of support for cancer prevention. Following his departure, the rest of the staff of the Carcinogenesis Program also resigned, leaving NCI with almost no cancer prevention program at all (ibid.:330).

"It had become clear," wrote Epstein, "that Rauscher was not only crippling any possibility for using the vast resources of the NCI to prevent cancer, but that he failed to understand why he should do so" (ibid.:331).

Rauscher's inaction on this politically sensitive issue had become a liability to the Ford administration, especially in an election year. On November 1, 1976, Rauscher resigned his NCI post and assumed a position as vice president for research at the American Cancer Society.*

In July 1977 Dr. Arthur Upton was appointed director of NCI by President Jimmy Carter. Many scientists, labor leaders, and public-interest groups supported his nomination because they considered Upton an expert on radia-

*Rauscher attributed his resignation to financial factors: his salary at ACS, $75,000, was more than double what it was in government (Epstein, 1978:331n). By 1987 his salary exceeded $104,000.

tion as a cause of cancer, and he seemed to express many of the same concerns as Rauscher's critics.

Upton's personal attitude toward the carcinogen program seemed far more supportive than Rauscher's. Nevertheless, he inherited a situation which may well have been beyond his capacity to change.

Just when his administration had succeeded in clearing up a backlog of 207 unwritten technical reports on possible carcinogens, Upton was hit with a barrage of government criticism in mid-1979. Investigations by the General Accounting Office (GAO), the government's financial watchdog, as well as by two Congressional committees, made the following charges about NCI's carcinogen-testing program:

As of June 1979, NCI was sitting on the results of 223 additional studies completed before 1977—this in addition to the 207 reports previously disclosed.

The Institute had been financially manipulated by its largest contractors, and given shoddy work at exhorbitant prices. For example, it had agreed to pay Litton Bionetics a total of $225 million for its management of the Frederick Cancer Research Center, at which much of the animal (bioassay) studies of carcinogens was conducted. Yet according to the House Appropriations Committee, Litton "has muddled along from catastrophe to catastrophe in the animal colony" (*Science*, June 22, 1979). For example, gaps underneath the doors permitted test animals which got loose to roam from room to room, spreading disease. Outbreaks of pinworm, salmonella infection, hepatitis, and other infections led to the slaughter of over 100,000 carefully bred animals, at a cost of almost $500,000 to the taxpayer.

The animal-testing facilities of another major contractor, Tracor Jitco, were similarly inadequate. A GAO investigator found "holes and cracks in the ceilings, walls and floor," inadequate air exchange, and other problems in their facilities. Yet NCI not only did nothing to penalize these companies but gave them a "handsome profit" on a cost-plus basis, a profit that a House investigation called "probably exorbitant" (ibid.).

The result of these deals was not only to shortchange the public, but virtually to cripple the already inadequate chemical testing program. One reason for this, said *Science,* was that the top leaders of the cancer war had no enthusiasm for government testing of environmental carcinogens:

Benno Schmidt, the chairman of the President's Cancer Panel, is on record as favoring chemical testing by industry, not NCI, and members of other NCI advisory groups have said the same thing. To some extent, the attitude persists even among NCI staff (ibid.).

Having industry supervise tests on its own chemicals is similar to appointing the wolf to guard the sheep. Because of NCI's neglect of the program,

> some important details of numerous studies on chemicals used in insecticides, drugs, food, and manufacturing remain in NCI files. And NCI, apparently, has little enthusiasm about ferreting them out (ibid.).

A spirit of rebelliousness seemed to be growing in Congress as officials felt increasing pressure to show real progress in the cancer struggle. During a break in one of the 1979 congressional appropriations hearings, Dr. Upton said that he felt as if he were being "marched up to the scaffold" by the questioners (ibid.). And the chairmen of these committees hinted that NCI's budget might suffer as a result of these scandals.

And, in fact, after hitting the billion-dollar mark in 1980, the NCI appropriation slipped back for three consecutive years (see Table 7). This had more to do with Reaganomics than with congressional dissatisfaction. In Reagan's second term this amount increased significantly. By 1988 NCI was receiving almost $1.5 billion annually. In fact, total appropriations in the fifty years since its founding (1938–1988) totaled $18,314,894,283 (NCI, 1987).

In 1983 NCI established its "Year 2000 Goals," an ambitious plan for reducing the cancer mortality rate in the United States by 50 percent by the year 2000. The plan is based around four main areas:

1. *Tobacco*—reduce the proportion of people who smoke from 36 percent in youths and 34 percent in adults to 15 percent in both groups;
2. *Diet*—reduce the average consumption of fat from 40 percent to 30 percent or less of total calories; increase the average consumption of fiber;
3. *Early diagnosis*—increase the percentage of women who have mammograms and Pap tests;
4. *Treatment*—increase the adoption of state-of-the-art treatments, including improved treatment of micrometastases (ibid.).

While few would argue with the smoking and dietary goals, it is questionable if the measures NCI intends to adopt will be strong enough to reach

TABLE 7
Appropriations of the NCI During
the "War on Cancer"
(1972–present)

1972	$ 378,794,000
1973	492,205,000
1974	551,191,500
1975	691,666,000
1976	761,727,000
1977	815,000,000
1978	872,388,000
1979	937,129,000
1980	1,000,000,000
1981	989,355,000
1982	986,617,000
1983	987,642,000
1984	1,081,581,000
1985	1,183,806,000
1986	1,264,159,000
1987	1,402,837,000
1988	1,469,327,000
Total	$15,865,424,500

Source: National Cancer Institute, "Fact Book,"
1987.

the stated goal in a dozen years. For instance, when it comes to smoking, in fiscal year 1987 NCI's main activities were:

- The Smoking, Tobacco and Cancer Program (STCP), which supports sixty large-scale prevention and cessation clinical trials targeted toward women, heavy smokers, minority and ethnic populations, adolescents, and smokeless-tobacco users;
- A major consensus conference of over 200 smoking-control researchers and experts to examine state-of-the-art tobacco-use prevention and cessation techniques. Recommendations of this conference were to guide future program plans of STCP;
- Several new programs by epidemiologists "clarifying the cancer risks associated with various smokeless tobaccos, including snuff, chewing tobacco and exposure to passive smoking" (NCI, 1987).

It is difficult to see how such weak, if well-intentioned, measures will make a serious dent in the tobacco industry, much less reduce consumption by one-half. One need only point out that cigarette smoking is not just an unhealthy practice but an actual addiction. Cigarette manufacturers spent $2.4 billion in 1986 on advertising—almost twice NCI's entire budget!—and tens of millions more opposing antismoking legislation (*New York Times,* December 24, 1988).

The situation in some ways is getting worse, not better. Lung cancer in 1986 overtook breast cancer as the leading cause of cancer death among women, as it has long been in men (*New York Times,* January 11, 1989).

Fifty million Americans still smoke, especially within the working class and minority communities. Children, especially girls, are smoking at younger ages. From 1980 to 1987 smoking among high school seniors levelled off after years of decline. Many children begin to smoke in the sixth grade (ibid.).

In the preface of a major report on smoking (released on the twenty-fifth anniversary of the first famous report on smoking), Surgeon General C. Everett Koop wrote:

> The critical message here is that progress in curtailing smoking must continue, and ideally accelerate, to enable us to turn smoking-related mortality around. Otherwise, the disease impact of smoking will remain high well into the 21st century (ibid.).

Koop also pointed out that while a smoke-free society is "an attainable long-term goal" for the United States, "the looming epidemic of smoking and smoking-related disease in developing countries does not encourage similar optimism" (ibid.)

It is this sort of bracing realism—and not NCI's wishful thinking—that is necessary if we, as a society, are going to confront an epidemic that is held responsible for the death (from cancer, heart disease, respiratory disease and ulcers) of 390,000 people a year in the United States alone (ibid.).

When the National Cancer Advisory Board (NCAB) held a series of public meetings around the country, this was the message they heard: "More aggressive programs at all levels of government are needed to combat cancer" (*New York Times,* February 9, 1989).

The Board projected that at current rates, 576,000 Americans will die of cancer in the year 2000, as against the 494,000 who died in 1988 (ibid.).

The Board's recommendations were that Congress reclassify tobacco as a drug and make it subject to regulation by the Food and Drug Administration, and that diagnostic tests for breast, cervical, and colon and rectal cancer be made available to all people at a "fair price" (ibid.).

Meanwhile the clock is ticking, and America's death rate pushes steadily upward. The new director of the National Cancer Institute, Dr. Samuel Broder, took over on January 10, 1989, and quickly affirmed his belief in the value of prevention.

"Each time a patient comes in and needs cancer therapy, you could say it was a failure of prevention," Broder said (*New York Times,* February 7, 1989). One can only hope that the new director will be able to turn around NCI's generally weak performance in the field of prevention and help lead the fight for a militant cleanup of the environment.

The Food and Drug Administration

Any analysis of the cancer-prevention problem must include a discussion of the Food and Drug Administration (FDA). This government agency has prime responsibility for keeping carcinogenic substances out of the public's food, beverages, cosmetics, and drugs. Critics contend, however, that the FDA is too close to the industries it is supposed to regulate, is a cumbersome bureaucracy incapable of decisive action, and is financially incapable of doing the job it has been assigned.

Long delays have often accompanied FDA action against a carcinogen in the food supply. The synthetic hormone DES (diethylstilbestrol) was shown to be carcinogenic at the time it was discovered in the late 1930s. The story of DES is one of the great medical tragedies of the twentieth century. It was the first synthetic hormone, first manufactured in 1938. Because it was easy to make and had many uses, it quickly became popular. By 1951 there were nineteen different manufacturers.

DES was widely used as a drug and also as a growth stimulant for poultry, hogs, and cattle because it makes animals grow fatter on less feed and come to market sooner. But problems soon came to light. Commercially raised minks became sterile after being fed the heads and necks of chickens which had received DES pellet implants as a growth stimulant. Scientific tests showed residues of DES in the muscle meat and especially the livers of animals which had received such pellets. In 1959, for example, some poultry were found to contain *1,000 times* the amount of DES necessary to cause breast cancer in mice (Epstein, 1978).

Rather than lead the fight to have DES removed from the food supply, the Food and Drug Administration often appeared to be the protector of the pharmaceutical industry that produced the synthetic hormone, and of the food industries that used it. When Representative James Delaney (D.-N.Y.) questioned the cancer-causing potential of DES in the *Congressional Record* in 1957, the FDA immediately issued a counterstatement denying that the hormone was carcinogenic (ibid.).

After passage of the Delaney Amendment, the FDA argued that the rule could not be applied retroactively: DES must stay because it had been introduced before passage in 1958 of Congressman Delaney's amendment to the 1938 Food, Drug, and Cosmetic Act.* For years, the FDA sought to annul the Delaney anticancer clause (ibid.).

After extensive lobbying by the industries involved, DES was explicitly exempted from the Delaney Amendment. Manufacturers simply promised to monitor their own poultry and livestock for DES levels. The FDA was still supposed to monitor meat for residues, but rarely did. Even if the agency found excess DES residues, the results of its inspections were kept secret. In 1970, at the request of Eli Lilly Co., the principal manufacturer of the hormone, the FDA allowed an across-the-board doubling of the DES that could be given to livestock. Even the rather feeble limitations of the "DES clause" were thus superseded (ibid.).

In the late forties a doctor named O. W. Smith proposed the use of the synthetic hormone in preventing "late pregnancy accidents" such as abortion, premature delivery, and intrauterine death of the fetus. The idea caught on even though it was unproven. "By the early 1950s its use was widespread in the United States," said R. B. Stewart in his excellent study, *Tragedies from Drug Therapy* (Stewart, 1985).

But other investigators failed to confirm Smith's contention. In fact, in 1953 Dr. W. J. Dieckmann criticized Smith's theory because it was based on clinical observations without adequate controls. He and his colleagues decided to test the therapy on over 2,000 women. The result was resounding proof that DES did none of the things for which it was being prescribed. Stewart comments:

> Physicians, just like everyone else, tend to be creatures of habit and once they begin treating a condition in a certain established way, habits are hard to change. After the published report describing the ineffectiveness in DES in pregnancy complications, use of DES decreased but was still widely used for this purpose into the 1960s (ibid.).

*The Delaney Amendment states that "no additive shall be claimed to be safe if it is found to induce cancer when ingested by man or animal, or if it is found after tests which are appropriate for the evaluation of safety of food additives to induce cancer in man or animal" (Public Law 85-929, September 6, 1958).

In 1971 doctors at Massachusetts General Hospital discovered that the daughters of women who had taken DES to prevent miscarriages were succumbing to vaginal cancer a dozen or more years later. This created a furor, and the U.S. Department of Agriculture began a series of tests for DES residue in animals. They found such residues as high as 37 parts per billion—a seemingly minute amount, but six times the amount needed to cause breast cancer in mice (Epstein, 1978).

The USDA is said to have attempted to squelch these findings, but news leaked out. DES, it was now realized, was highly dangerous in both its prime uses: as a livestock growth stimulant and as a drug for pregnant women.

Congressional hearings were held in November 1971, at which it was pointed out that twenty foreign countries had already banned DES and many Europeans would not eat American beef—specifically because of its DES content (ibid.). At the hearings, the commissioner of the FDA appeared on behalf of industry's position and spoke against the ban. Charles C. Edwards, the commissioner at the time, argued that the amount of DES found was insignificant and American industry would lose between $300 and $400 million a year if DES were banned.

The regulatory agencies opted for a seven-day waiting period between the last DES treatment and the slaughter of treated animals. How did they know that this waiting period was sufficient to rid the meat of DES residue? According to Epstein, the decision was apparently based on an FDA experiment involving *one cow* which received *one dose* of the hormone (ibid.).

As often happens, the FDA found itself pushed by the consumer movement on the one hand and powerful industries on the other. There was a temporary ban on the additive for the better part of 1973, during which industry switched to the more expensive synthetic hormones Ralgro and Zeranol.* A federal district judge ruled in January 1978 that industry had the right to use the additive as long as residues were kept at the lowest possible level at which the drug could be monitored.

Consumers, however, rebelled against the use of this chemical and its manufacturers.

In April 1971 Dr. Arthur Herbst and his colleagues published a paper in the *New England Journal of Medicine* that linked DES use in pregnancy to cancer of the vagina and cervix in offspring of DES-treated women. It is now considered a classic case of medical detective work.

How many women and their children were affected? According to one

---

*Ralgro and Zeranol are manufactured by Commercial Solvents. H. Virgil Sherrill, then a director of the company, is an overseer of Memorial Sloan-Kettering Cancer Center.

study, "perhaps 2 million pregnant women were given DES to prevent miscarriage" (Hecht, 1986). "DES daughters" were at increased risk of dysplasia, a condition of the cervix and vagina that sometimes may lead to cancer. "DES sons" have been reported to have increased risk of genital abnormalities, although further studies dispute this claim (Moira and Potts, 1987). And "DES mothers" turn out to have one and one-half times as great a risk of breast cancer, according to the report of a task force convened by the Department of Health and Human Services (ibid.).

The response of the various health agencies was slow and inadequate. In 1971 FDA ordered manufacturers to include a warning in the package insert that the drug was not to be used in pregnancy. But it did nothing to stop the manufacture of the drug. Ironically, it is still sold—for the *treatment* of advanced cancer of the breast and the prostate (PDR, 1988).

It wasn't until 1978 that the Department of Health, Education and Welfare (as it was then called) convened the first DES task force. The task force tended to downplay the damage caused by the drug (Hecht, 1986). A second task force, assembled in 1985, "concluded that there is now greater cause for concern than there was in 1978, although a causal relationship has not been established" (ibid.). At the present time the Mayo Clinic is following 4,000 DES-exposed daughters as well as 1,300 unexposed women, in a review of their cases. In the NCI-funded study, Mayo doctors send the women questionnaires in the mail.

The ACS seems disinterested in these women's plight. There is no reference to DES mothers or children in the 1988 *Facts and Figures*. In the section on the risk factors for uterine cancer they list "early age at first intercourse," "multiple sex partners," "history of infertility," and so forth. No DES.

There is only passing reference to DES in ACS vice president Laszlo's book. His single comment is singularly detached: "This was the first demonstration of the passage of a carcinogen across the placental barrier into the fetus, a very significant finding." DES was not one of modern medicine's great moments, and Laszlo seems eager to downplay the entire touchy topic of iatrogenic (doctor-caused) cancer. "Drugs," he opines, "are believed to account for fewer than two percent of all cancers" (Laszlo, 1987).

"The DES affair seemed to have little impact on the drafting of new drug regulation," said Dr. Stewart. "It did, however, send the women who had been exposed to DES to their attorneys" (Stewart, 1985).

Not content with government action, women who took DES to prevent miscarriages, and their daughters, organized DES-Action groups in New York, Washington, D.C., San Francisco, and other major cities. Many women lost lawsuits because of the difficulty of identifying the actual manufacturer of the drug. This is not surprising, as there were 142 manufacturers of the drug. In fact, a recent book lists almost eighty brand names for this product (Moira and Potts, 1987). The big breakthrough came in July 1979 when a twenty-five-year-old social worker was awarded nearly $500,000 in a damage suit against Eli Lilly Co. after undergoing a hysterectomy and a vaginectomy for cancer at the Albert Einstein Medical College Hospital. Her mother had taken DES to prevent miscarriage (*New York Times*, July 17, 1979).

The legal significance of this case was that Eli Lilly was sued not as the actual manufacturer but as one of the twelve companies that had gotten the drug approved by the FDA; Lilly's package insert was then used as the model for all the other companies as well (Stewart, 1985).

Twenty-seven Massachusetts women have also filed a class action suit against all the manufacturers of DES. This suit, known as *Payton vs. Abbott Laboratories,* made it much easier for DES-exposed women to obtain justice in the courts (ibid.).

The story of DES—and particularly of the Food and Drug Administration's involvement—is not unique. It resembles FDA behavior toward most food additives and potential carcinogens.* FDA laxity toward the nation's largest manufacturers stands in sharp contrast to its eagle-eyed stand toward small businessmen, scientific innovators, and nonconformists, as demonstrated in the previous chapters.

Conclusions

An increasing number of scientists now believe that much cancer is environmentally induced and can therefore be controlled. Cancer prevention not only spares the victim the agony of suffering from the disease, but is ultimately far cheaper than the enormous and ever-growing social cost of treating a major ailment after its occurrence.

In the case of cancer, prevention means regulating and controlling some of the largest and most lucrative industries in the country. Particular targets must include the petrochemical, food, drug, rubber, automotive, mining, and other giant companies. Perhaps most urgent is control of the nation's runaway nuclear weapons and power facilities.

Although prevention is certainly economical in the long run, it would probably cost a great deal in the short run, both in terms of lost profit op-

---

*See Epstein for numerous other examples. As a derivative of coal tar, the first known chemical carcinogen, Red Dye #2 should have been high on the FDA's suspect list. Instead the agency took years before it banned the chemical, and has refused to move against other, similar food dyes.

portunities and increased environmental controls. Industry has traditionally resisted such threats to its profits, shunning responsibility for its share of the cancer problem.

Large industry not only spends millions of dollars to argue against the need for stringent control of carcinogens, but appears to play a powerful role in shaping the direction of cancer research and management. The Board of Overseers of Memorial Sloan-Kettering Cancer Center is composed predominantly of men and women closely associated with the very industries under attack. The American Cancer Society is similarly tied to big business and to the treatment-oriented medical profession. A crucial position at the government's National Cancer Institute is occupied by the National Cancer Advisory Board, which has been dominated by big businessmen and investors such as Benno Schmidt and Laurance S. Rockefeller. The Food and Drug Administration, which has ultimate responsibility to keep carcinogens off the shelves of America's stores, appears to be biased in favor of industry and to consider the consumer's interest secondarily—if at all.

In short, the road toward prevention, although theoretically a bright and simple highway, is a tortuous path, filled with numerous roadblocks and dangerous pitfalls. The difficulty involved in establishing a substance as a cause of cancer and bringing that substance under control can be illustrated by the case of one such pollutant—asbestos.

« 16 »

Asbestos: The Harvest of Death

Not long ago, *asbestos* was a reassuring word. Literally meaning "unquenched" or "unceasing," the name refers to a family of minerals that share the unique and useful quality of being unharmed by heat or fire. For all practical purposes, asbestos will not burn.

Some 4,500 years ago, Finnish potters incorporated asbestos into their cooking utensils to insulate them against heat and fire. By the twentieth century, asbestos had become a big industry. Mined mainly in upper Québec, Canada, by the giant Johns-Manville Corporation, asbestos was manufactured into over a thousand different products, including such household items as aprons, floor tiles, mittens, potholders, stove linings and mats, and table padding. About 75 percent of asbestos was used in construction. In all, at least 25 million tons of it surround us in the United States alone.

Asbestos is remarkable in other ways. It is a rock that can be spun like a fabric. It is relatively inexpensive and abundant. It is truly a "magic mineral" as the asbestos manufacturers always claimed.

There is only one problem: Asbestos is also one of the most dangerous environmental pollutants ever discovered. Originally used to protect us from a major hazard—fire—it has now turned out to be a hazard of nightmarish proportions on its own.

Asbestos fibers are virtually indestructible. When released into the air, they take a long time to settle. People who work or live in the vicinity of loose asbestos breathe in the microscopic fibers. They often do not breathe them out, however, for 50 percent of the fibers are trapped by the membranes of the lungs and the linings of the lungs and other parts of the body. Once there, by mechanisms still not completely understood, the fibers irritate the delicate cells, creating "asbestos bodies"—harmful lesions visible only under the microscope.*

If exposure persists, scarring of the lungs take place. The condition is known as asbestosis. Eventually after many years, scar tissue replaces healthy lung tissue. The victim progresses from persistent coughing to difficulty in breathing. Finally he dies—from a lack of oxygen or from heart failure caused by the strain of pumping blood through the scarred lung tissue. It's a terrible death.

But asbestosis is only one of the dangers. The main problem is cancer. Lung cancer forms within and around the scar tissue. Another form of cancer attacks the linings of the lungs (mesothelial tissue). This is called mesothelioma. Once a rare disease, it has now become common among asbestos workers. Other kinds of cancer are also typical results of asbestos exposure.

It was once thought that only asbestos workers were in danger of these diseases. It is now known, however, that people who have worked near asbestos, and even people who have lived in proximity to it, are also in danger. Since these diseases take a long time to reveal themselves, often as long as thirty years, the millions of workers exposed during and after World War II are only now beginning to show up in the cancer clinics.

"The harvest time of the disease has now arrived," said Dr. Philip Polakoff, a specialist in occupational medicine in Berkeley, California (cited in Weinstein, 1978). It is a harvest of death for thousands.

Equally frightening is the fact that almost all of us have now been exposed to asbestos to some significant degree. A high percentage of all urban dwellers have asbestos bodies in their lungs at autopsy—even if they never worked near asbestos (Brodeur, 1974). Some government officials have now stated that 10 to 15 percent of *all* cancer deaths are due to asbestos alone.

Since the mid-1970s, government officials and scientists have begun to acknowledge the dangers of asbestos and to warn those who were exposed

---

*Asbestos bodies are inhaled asbestos fibers that have been altered by the reaction of the lung tissue and coated with a substance rich in iron. Scientists at Mt. Sinai Medical Center are beginning to understand how asbestos causes cancer. It was found that fibers can transport DNA into cells where this foreign genetic material may interfere with the cell's own genes. Or, possibly, the asbestos might activate an oncogene, a fragment of the genetic code that helps promote cancer when it is inappropriately switched on (*New York Times*, October 18, 1988).

to get medical checkups. These officials often add that science has only recently learned of this danger. This, however, is not true. The perils of asbestos have been known for many years. But few scientists spoke out on behalf of workers and the public, and those who did were not listened to by the institutions that stood to gain from asbestos's continued use.

In 1900 a London physician first identified a new disease, which he called asbestosis. The London doctor didn't even see fit to publish his findings in a scientific journal but simply passed his observations on to a government commission, where they lay buried for several decades (Kotelchuck, 1974).

The medical profession in the early part of this century may have been ignorant of this disease and the peril of asbestos. But the people most concerned with the production of asbestos were not unaware of its dangers. The records show that many workers quit their jobs in asbestos mining and manufacturing soon after being hired because they considered it dangerous. In 1918 U.S. and Canadian insurance companies stopped selling personal life insurance policies to asbestos workers—a clear indication that these companies were also well aware of the asbestos hazard. It is a fair assumption that the asbestos manufacturers also knew of the dangers (Brodeur, 1974).

In 1924 the medical profession rediscovered asbestosis when Dr. W. E. Cooke reported in the *British Medical Journal* the untimely death of an asbestos worker. This thirty-three-year-old woman had been an asbestos factory worker since the age of thirteen. On autopsy, Cooke found massive amounts of asbestos in her scarred lungs. Eleven more cases of asbestosis were reported in Great Britain in the 1920s. American doctors at the Mayo Clinic and Yale University also reported cases of asbestosis among U.S. workers. In fact, by 1935 twenty-eight cases of asbestosis had been reported in the leading medical journals of Great Britain and the United States (Kotelchuck, 1974).

The British government responded by making asbestosis a compensable disease under their workmen's compensation acts and instituted safety rules. American asbestos manufacturers began a campaign to *prevent* the same thing from happening in the United States. Internal documents show how the various giant manufacturers—especially Johns-Manville (J-M) and Raybestos-Manhattan—colluded to prevent the hazard of asbestos from being known. In the early 1930s,for example, the editor of *Asbestos*, a trade magazine, wrote to Sumner Simpson, the president of Raybestos, asking if the time might not be ripe for an article on "dust control" in American factories.

The Raybestos president forwarded the letter to a top Johns-Manville attorney with the comment, "I think the less said about asbestos, the better off we are," a statement that neatly summarized the strategy and thinking of the entire industry in those years. He added, however:

> At the same time we cannot lose track of the fact that there have been a number of articles on asbestos dust control and asbestosis in the British trade magazines. The magazine *Asbestos* is in business to publish articles affecting the trade and they have been very decent about not reprinting the English articles (Weinstein, 1978).

On the specific request of the Raybestos president himself, Johns-Manville's lawyer wrote back:

> I quite agree with you that our interests are best served by having asbestosis receive the minimum of publicity. Even if we should eventually decide to raise no objection to the publication of an article on asbestosis in the magazine in question, I think we should warn the editors to use American data on the subject rather than English (ibid.).

"American data" on the subject was far less extensive than that of the British and, as shall be shown, much of it was paid for by the manufacturers and biased in favor of industry's position that asbestos was harmless. In order to counter the anti-asbestos studies, Johns-Manville and Raybestos-Manhattan sponsored a study of asbestos workers carried out by doctors at Metropolitan Life Insurance Company and the Department of Public Health at McGill University, Montréal. Although the study appeared to be an objective, academic report, it was actually guided by the asbestos industry.

According to South Carolina Circuit Judge James Price, internal documents showed "written evidence that Raybestos-Manhattan and Johns-Manville exercised an editorial prerogative" over this Metropolitan Life study. In fact, Price granted a new trial to the family of a dead asbestos worker after seeing these documents (ibid.).

Specifically, minutes of a meeting between a Metropolitan Life doctor—Anthony J. Lanza—and a Johns-Manville attorney and other industry officials on November 28, 1933, revealed that the attendees felt that Lanza's study "would be helpful to us, if favorable, in the event we should ever be involved in litigation" (ibid.). Before Lanza finished his study, he dutifully sent it to industry officials for their comments before publication.

In a letter to Dr. Lanza in December 1934, the Johns-Manville attorney wrote:

> I am sure you understand fully that no one in our organization is suggesting for a moment that you alter by one jot or title [sic] any scientific facts or inevitable conclusions revealed or justified by your preliminary survey. All we ask is that all of the favorable aspects of the survey be included and that none of the unfavorable be unintentionally pictured in darker tones than the circumstances justify.
>
> I feel confident that we can depend upon you and Dr. McConnell to give us this "break" and mine and (others') suggestions are presented in this spirit (ibid.).

The Metropolitan Life study was conducted on Johns-Manville workers between 1929 and 1931 but was not published until 1935. ("The name of the game is not truth, of course, but delay," said David Kotelchuck, a student of the asbestos controversy [Kotelchuck, 1974].) A total of 126 workers in Canada and the United States were examined for signs of asbestosis. The authors did not conclude that there was any serious problem of asbestosis among J-M workers. In fact, they claimed that the workers appeared healthy and were not at all disabled.

So much for the conclusions. If one looks at the *actual data* in their report, however, it reveals that of the 126 workers examined, 67 definitely had asbestosis, 39 may have had it, and only 20 appeared free of the disease. Thus 84 percent seemed to show signs of lung scarring (the positives plus the doubtfuls), and only 16 percent were definitely clear at the moment they were examined.

In addition, out of 121 physical examinations, 96 workers—or 79 percent—complained of persistent coughing and shortness of breath, the classic signs of early asbestosis. In response to this finding the authors of the Metropolitan Life report state that "too much emphasis should not be placed on statements of subjective symptoms" (cited in ibid.).

This study was then quoted by the United States government as proof that asbestosis was *not* a serious health hazard. In fact, the U.S. Public Health Service published the Metropolitan Life study as an official government Public Health Report. "Few actions more clearly illustrate the interlock between industry and government," wrote Kotelchuck (ibid.).

The asbestos companies were quite concerned that the United States would follow the example of Britain and make asbestosis a compensable disease under the Workmen's Compensation Act. This had in fact been proposed in New Jersey. A Johns-Manville lawyer therefore wrote to Dr. Lanza:

As it is the policy of Johns-Manville to oppose any bill that attempted to include asbestosis as compensable, it would be very helpful to have an official report to show that there is a substantial difference between asbestosis and silicosis [a similar disease caused by inhalation of silica dust], and by the same token, it would be troublesome if an official report should appear from which the conclusion might be drawn that there is very little, if any, difference between the two diseases (Weinstein, 1978).

Dr. Lanza complied with these requests and never made any comparison between asbestosis and silicosis, which was recognized as a compensable disease. (Had asbestosis been recognized as compensable, the company might have been held liable for damages.) In fact, asbestosis did not become compensable in New Jersey until after World War II.*

But the problems of the asbestos workers were not over. In 1935 two doctors at the Medical College of South Carolina performed an autopsy on an asbestos worker and found lung cancer amid the scar tissue. By 1942 ten such reports had followed in the medical literature, and it became known— at least among specialists—that asbestos also caused lung cancer in workers.

With this revelation, the industry took a more aggressive policy. They commissioned a study in 1938 from scientists at Saranac Laboratory, an Adirondack tuberculosis sanatorium and research center with a long history of cooperating with industry. The asbestos manufacturers paid $15,000 to support the study, and the J-M attorney wrote to another industry official:

It would be a good thing to distribute the information among the medical fraternity[,] providing it is of the right type and would not injure our companies (Weinstein, 1978).

The Saranac study, conducted by Dr. Arthur Vorwald and John Karr, simply dismissed the asbestos-cancer link by commenting that the workers found to have lung cancer were not a random sample of asbestos workers. They also had asbestosis. Perhaps, the scientists argued, there was some special relationship between asbestosis victims and lung cancer. The only way the asbestos-lung cancer link could be definitely proven was by carrying out a cancer study among a large number of asbestos workers, irrespective of any other disease. But industry controlled the medical records of the

---

*Dr. Lanza rose from assistant medical director at Metropolitan Life to chairman of the Institute of Industrial Medicine at New York University Medical School. He was the author of well-known textbooks on lung diseases and remained a leading expert on asbestos until his death in the early 1960s (Kotelchuck, 1974).

asbestos workers, and it was not about to open these records to inquisitive scientists. Thus the entire matter lay dormant for many years. Kotelchuck remarked:

> Scientists did not protest the industry's denial of access to this information or insist in their scientific papers that epidemiological studies be carried out. True to their professional codes, they kept silent. So nothing happened—except 20 more years of growing profits for the asbestos industry (Kotelchuck, 1974).

And, it might be added, twenty more years of cancer for asbestos workers.

In 1956 the Québec Asbestos Mining Association (QABA) commissioned a study from the Industrial Hygiene Foundation (IHF—now the Industrial Health Foundation). Based in Pittsburgh, the IHF performs research for industry and is considered pro-management.

The IHF study examined 6,000 Québec asbestos miners' health records for evidence of lung cancer. They found none. However, they had ignored one of the cardinal principles of such studies: the twenty-year time lag between first exposure to an agent causing lung cancer and the clinical appearance of the disease. This is known as the twenty-year rule for lung cancer. According to Dr. Irving Selikoff:

> For lung cancer the percentage of all deaths that occurred at 10 years or less was trivial; it was not until 25 years after onset of employment that deaths [from lung cancer] became common [among shipyard workers] (Selikoff, 1978).

These facts were certainly known to the authors of the QAMA report, for they themselves cite studies, by Hueper and others, that contain explicit reference to the "twenty-year rule." But by studying a relatively young group of workers, two-thirds of whom were between twenty and forty-four years of age, the industry-sponsored scientists were able to make the report come out favorable to the companies.

By the early 1960s the asbestos health hazard had begun to receive increasing attention. A doctor in South Africa discovered a high incidence of mesothelioma among asbestos workers. This disease was once so rare that it was not even listed as a separate cause of death in the International Classification of Causes of Death. The best estimates, based on autopsy series, was that only one out of 10,000 people died of it.

But among asbestos workers it was soon found that 7 or 8 percent were dying of this cancer of the lining cells—somewhere around 1,000 times the number expected. At about the same time, Dr. Irving Selikoff and his coworkers at Mount Sinai Medical Center in New York broke through industry's monopoly of health data on asbestos workers by going directly to the unions involved.

Selikoff's findings were a bombshell. He, too, found that among young workers there was little change in their X rays. "In the New York area," he said, "when we examined somewhat over a thousand asbestos insulation workers, we found that of the 725 with *less* than twenty years from onset of exposure, most had normal X rays." After twenty years, however, extensive disease began to appear with appalling frequency (ibid.).

In 1943 there were 632 men in a New York pipefitters union. All of them were "followed" by Selikoff and his colleagues. By 1977, the outspoken physician told a medical meeting,

> instead of the 330 anticipated deaths (given their ages in 1943) there were 478 deaths. Why did some 150 people die who were not expected to die? Well, there should have been 56 deaths from cancer, and there were 210. Instead of 13 deaths from lung cancer there were 93. One out of every three asbestos workers dies of lung cancer. This is simply a disaster! (ibid.).

"Interestingly, too, instead of 15 deaths from cancer of the esophagus, colon, stomach and rectum there were 43—a modest increase," Selikoff added ironically. "Obviously, anyone who inhales dust also tends to ingest it."

Selikoff next followed up this New York study with a more extensive report on thousands of asbestos pipefitters across the country.

> On January 1, 1967 there were 17,800 men in the international union. By 1977, there were 2,270 deaths, instead of 1,661 expected. . . . Once again, instead of 320 deaths due to cancer there were 994 (ibid.).

Selikoff and his Mount Sinai colleagues were able to draw some lessons from these studies.

First, until this time it had been assumed that the main hazard of asbestos came from asbestosis. In fact, as late as 1968 government officials shrugged off suggestions of any other danger (Brodeur, 1974:23). But, said Selikoff, "the major excess [of deaths] was from cancer" (Selikoff, 1978).

So prevalent was cancer among asbestos workers, their family members, and even neighbors of asbestos plants that the Mount Sinai doctor remarked, ominously, "We're beginning to understand why one out of every four Americans—if things go as they are—will have cancer in his or her lifetime and why 20 percent of all deaths in this country are now due to cancer" (ibid.).

Second, not only workers are susceptible to the ravages of asbestos and other environmental hazards. *Consumers* of these products are also in danger, and with over one thousand products made of or with asbestos, that includes almost everyone. In fact, said Selikoff, sometimes consumers are at greater risk than workers, since in a factory carcinogens may be totally enclosed. There are *some* health regulations for production, but consumption is largely uncontrolled and unregulated.

Third, other chemicals may interact with asbestos to incite an even greater risk of disease. For example, asbestos workers who also smoke have an even greater risk of contracting lung cancer (Fraumeni, 1975:468). "They are sitting targets," said Selikoff.

Fourth, although even a brief exposure to asbestos can be hazardous or even fatal, in general the chance of contracting the disease is related to the length of time and the extent of exposure. The risk is obviously higher for those most heavily involved in the production of asbestos, who can inhale up to 8 billion fibers and fibrils (submicroscopic fibers) of asbestos a day, 50 percent of which are retained in the lungs.

Nor have workers generally been told when their health was threatened by asbestos exposure.

For example, Dr. Kenneth Wallace Smith, medical director of Johns-Manville until 1966, testified in a lawsuit that he could see early X-ray changes in a patient perhaps ten, twelve, or fifteen years before he developed any clinical signs of disability.

But Smith did not tell the J-M workers they were coming down with asbestosis or cancer. In a 1949 confidential report to management he urged:

> As long as the man feels well, is happy at home and at work and his physical condition remains good, he should be permitted to live and work in peace. . . . Should the man be told of his condition today, there is a very definite possibility that he would become mentally and physically ill, simply through the knowledge that he had asbestosis (cited in Weinstein, 1978).

Many experts believe, however, that "early detection of asbestosis is critical since it is irreversible when fully developed and gradually destroys

379

the lungs." If, on the other hand, the disease is monitored closely, the patient's life can be prolonged (ibid.).

Theoretically the government should be a watchdog and should prevent such abuses from occurring. In fact, however, government scientists have been among the most vocal advocates of industry's position. Lewis Cralley, a top official of the Public Health Service's Division of Occupational Health, carried out a study of health conditions in the asbestos industry. He "suppressed its findings for six years," said Kotelchuck, "until they were released by other . . . officials over his objections" (Kotelchuck, 1974).

Although the asbestos industry has largely blocked investigations of the asbestos peril, Cralley told reporter Paul Brodeur, "all I know is that the first real interest came from industry. They asked for our help back in 1964, and they have cooperated with us magnificently" (Brodeur, 1974).

During Cralley's tenure as head of Occupational Health, government investigators were not required to identify individual factories in their reports on hazards, forward interpretations of data to state agencies, or even make any recommendations to factory owners (ibid.). In fact, says Brodeur in his award-winning study *Expendable Americans,*

> in order not to embarrass management or make workers apprehensive, the government engineers who took air samples during the environmental surveys not only were forbidden to discuss the nature of their activities with any workers they encountered but were also instructed not to wear respirators, which would have afforded them some protection against the hazard of inhaling asbestos dust (ibid.).

Through scientists such as Cralley, industry was afforded an entrée into the inner circles of the medical establishment, including such prestigious universities as New York University, McGill Medical School, Wayne State, the University of Pittsburgh, and Carnegie-Mellon, and such groups as the American Public Health Association, the International Union Against Cancer, and the American Academy of Occupational Medicine. In fact, Dr. Lee B. Grant, medical director of Pittsburgh Plate Glass Company—a major asbestos user—eventually became president of the American College of Preventive Medicine (ibid.).

Over the years most cancer scientists have shown a lack of interest in the asbestos problem, just as they have failed to deal with environmental factors in general. For many years, in fact, Selikoff and his group were among the few asbestos researchers in the United States.

In the 1970s the American Cancer Society gave financial support to Selikoff's lab, and a page and a half of ACS's 1974 *Annual Report* was taken up with a description of its joint work with the Mount Sinai team. In that same year the Society gave Selikoff about $150,000, two-thirds of which went for research on asbestos (Garfinkel, 1979). While this seems to be a large sum, it represents only a fraction of 1 percent of what ACS garnered from the public that year ($108 million). By 1978 support for the Mount Sinai group had risen to $286,000 for all of Selikoff's projects, including asbestos research, while public donations to ACS had risen to almost $140 million (ibid.; ACS, 1978). This increase was a modest recognition of the growing public awareness of the asbestos problem.

The record of Memorial Sloan-Kettering Center is worse. The 386-page 1976 *Annual Report* of the Sloan-Kettering Institute, which detailed hundreds of research projects, contained no mention of studies on asbestos. A dozen years later there were still no research projects specifically concerned with asbestos.

This lack of interest in asbestos (as in other environmental and occupational causes of cancer) has had some unfortunate consequences for MSKCC employees, as well as for the public, which might benefit from such investigations. In 1976 the Center's administration began renovating two of the older buildings in the complex. Dust flew in the corridors of the hospital that summer and fall, but no one outside the administration knew that these clouds contained asbestos, which had accidentally been freed from old pipe coverings by workmen.

Jane McGill, head of the Employee Health Service, wrote in her 1976 annual report that there had been certain "environmental problems." One of these, she noted, was that "asbestos-containing pipe-covering had been removed by the contractors by dry technique and not according to OSHA [Occupational Safety and Health Administration] precautions."

"It was determined that one area was contaminated with asbestos fibers," she said (McGill, 1976). Later that year *Second Opinion,* the "underground" employees' newsletter at MSKCC, obtained a copy of this report and publicized it (Second Opinion, June 1977). No official announcement was made that for several months employees, visitors, and possibly patients had been exposed to asbestos-laden dust.

Apparently MSKCC did not have an expert sufficiently versed in the problems of asbestos to deal with the question, for Dr. Irving Selikoff and Dr. Arthur Rohl, both from Mount Sinai, and Dr. Robert Sawyer of Yale University were called in and asked to assess the extent of damages (McGill, 1976).

Although there is more public awareness of the asbestos peril today, real improvement may be slow in coming. The National Cancer Institute now has literature that it sends to those who fear they stand a risk of developing asbestos-related diseases. It also has designed posters to warn the public of the risks involved. Other government agencies have begun to provide information, chest X rays, or, occasionally, inspections of possibly contaminated areas.*

Much effort has been expended in trying to limit the number of fibers permissible in the air. While such controls are important, it is necessary to point out that even if fibers are tightly regulated, the problem may not end. Each fiber can—and does—break up into a multitude of smaller fibrils, so small that one million of them, side by side, measure an inch (Brodeur, 1974).

These fibrils can be detected only by electron microscope, which few industrial hygiene laboratories possess. Little research has been done on the fibril problem, but it is known that an asbestos worker in a supposedly safe plant, whose air contains only two fibers per cubic centimeter, can still inhale from 800 million to 8 billion fibers and fibrils in an eight-hour day (ibid.:30).

For the consumer the problem of controlling asbestos exposure may be even more difficult. Asbestos is in the environment—millions of indestructible tons of it.

Given the past history of underestimating the danger of asbestos, several important and disturbing questions remain. How much of this asbestos poses an immediate danger to the public? How much is a time bomb that will explode each time an old building is demolished without proper safeguards or falls into disrepair? Does the asbestos have to be removed, or can it be contained? Who is going to pay for this cleanup? Are there any ways to remove asbestos once it is entrapped in the body? Are there any really safe substitutes for this "miracle fiber"?

Answering such questions will certainly take a great deal more research. But while the scientists deliberated, asbestos continued to pour into the environment virtually unchecked—over 750,000 short tons in 1976 alone (Standard and Poor's, 1977).

The asbestos industry tried to sidestep its heavy responsibility for this situation. The companies even requested the government to pay for whatever losses they would incur in over $2 billion in lawsuits that asbestos workers filed against them. This bailout was discussed at a 1978 meeting of Con-

*The White Lung Association, 12 Warren Street, New York, N.Y. 10007, a nonprofit organization, provides asbestos inspections for private and commercial buildings. It also provides counselling in asbestos liability cases and information to the general public.

gressman George Miller's (D.-Calif.) House Committee on Education and Labor. A large Johns-Manville plant operated in Congressman Miller's Martinez district, according to the *Guardian*, a New York-based radical newspaper (*Guardian*, December 20, 1978).

An even more questionable plan involved the exporting of asbestos to populations either unaware of its danger, desperate for work, or unable to do anything about the threat because of political repression. As regulations tightened in the United States, the asbestos industry began to move its factories to countries such as Taiwan, South Korea, Brazil, and India (ibid.).

This migration of so-called runaway hazardous shops began in the late 1960s. Taiwan, South Korea, and Brazil became large exporters of asbestos products to the United States: actually, they themselves imported the raw asbestos from American companies, such as Johns-Manville, and shipped their finished products back to the United States and other industrialized countries. The favorite spot for such relocation was Mexico.

In 1967, for example, Amatex, a Pennsylvania asbestos firm, closed its Milford Square plant, although it was quite new, and opened an asbestos yarn mill in Agua Prieta, a small town across the border from El Paso, Texas. It also operates a plant in Juarez, Mexico. According to Barry Castleman, a consultant to the Environmental Defense Fund and an expert on asbestos:

> In December 1974 Amatex began to import asbestos textiles into the U.S. from the Juarez plant. Amatex "imported" about 2 million pounds of asbestos textiles from its Mexican border plants in 1975, about one-fourth of U.S. imports from the entire world that year (ibid.).

U.S. journalists who visited the two Amatex plants in 1977 found "clumps of asbestos clinging to nearby bushes and fences where neighborhood children play. Inside the plants, the air was filled with the deadly white fibers" (ibid.).

The U.S. government has aided the asbestos industry in moving its hazardous plants out of the country—in effect, exporting asbestos and cancer to foreign workers. For example, most of the imports came from so-called beneficiary countries. These countries were allowed to export their goods duty-free to the United States.

Some foreign asbestos plants were even subsidized directly by the United States. According to Castleman, a plant in Madras, India, "was covered by $1 million in political risk insurance by the Overseas Private Investment Corporation," a U.S. government agency (ibid.).

As knowledge of the asbestos peril spread, however, foreign workers have fought back against the threat. In Cork, Ireland, for example, asbestos workers and the community delayed the opening of a newly completed asbestos manufacturing plant, owned and operated by Raybestos-Manhattan. The $8 million plant was unable to open for many months, and did so only at reduced capacity after the Irish government imposed safety regulations on the owners (ibid.).

In the United States a series of struggles has been waged over asbestos in schools and other public buildings. This began in April 1972 when an elementary school in Lander, Wyoming, was ordered closed after it was found that children were breathing, according to a government report, "an unhealthy mixture of air and asbestos dust" (Bourne, 1978).

According to a Public Interest Research Group study, the school librarian had become suspicious of a layer of dust covering furniture throughout the school. The dust turned out to be asbestos, falling from deteriorating ceilings that had been sprayed with an asbestos insulation eleven years before. Such sprayed-on insulation was common all over the country from the 1950s to the 1970s. The school had to be closed until the hazardous material could be replaced.

In January 1977 six elementary schools in Howell Township, New Jersey, were closed when excessive levels of asbestos were found there. One child appeared to be sick from an asbestos-related disease, and dozens of other children complained of unexplainable headaches, sore throats, and respiratory congestion. The problems of Howell Township may have been aggravated by children scraping the ceilings with sticks and grabbing at the insulation. Children played with pieces of the insulation, which looked to them like cotton candy, and threw it in each others' faces (*New York Times*, January 4, 1977).

In late 1978 Harlem parents shut down two adjacent New York City schools, P.S. 208 and P.S. 185, when they discovered asbestos flaking from a fourth-floor ceiling. The Board of Education attempted a "cosmetic cover-up," said Helen Brathwaite, head of the Parents' Association (*Second Opinion*, December 1978). They tried to put up a new ceiling and leave the asbestos in place. In doing so, they raised such a storm of asbestos that the children, teachers, and parents could hardly see their hands in front of their faces. So the parents shut the schools down. In some places, such as the auditorium, the asbestos had been exposed, behind a grille, since the school opened in 1967.

The Harlem parents demanded—and got—a secret Board of Education report which showed that at least 189 of the City's 1,000 public schools were contaminated with asbestos. This figure was later revised to about 500,

384

ASBESTOS

although no one knew for sure how bad the situation really was. Even some school officials seem to think the Board of Education was underestimating the numbers involved (ibid.).

Although using asbestos to insulate buildings has been banned since the mid-1970s, millions of office workers still work in asbestos-laden buildings, including Madison Square Garden, the World Trade Center, and about half of the country's skyscrapers. Fresh-air systems often circulate right over the sprayed-on asbestos, picking up fibers and fibrils into the air current. In the furor that followed the Harlem exposures, many workers in New York suspected that they, too, were working or living in asbestos-contaminated buildings. It was very difficult for them to find out if they were in danger. Mount Sinai maintained the only electron microscope in all of New York City that could detect asbestos in the air. Using this machine, it took a full day to test one building. When the head of the laboratory was asked what was being done to uncover the asbestos hazard, he replied—with unusual directness—, "Nothing" (*New York Post,* November 17, 1978).

In an interview at the school Helene Brathwaite voiced her frustration over this situation:

> Industry has bombarded us with different kinds of substances that are harmful to our health, without asking us if we wanted them or not, without testing properly, and then telling us *we* have a problem. This has to do with capitalism and the Almighty Dollar. That's the basic problem (*Second Opinion,* December 1978).

Postscript

On August 26, 1982, the Manville Corporation filed for protection under chapter 11 of the Bankruptcy Code in order to allow it to reorganize itself in the face of a massive assault by workers and consumers. At the time the company was facing 16,500 asbestos-related lawsuits, with 500 more coming in every month (*New York Times,* February 7, 1989). The company established a personal-injury settlement trust, based in Washington, as well as a smaller, second trust to pay property damage claims to schools, hospitals, and businesses forced to remove asbestos (*New York Times,* April 2, 1989).

The personal injury trust was initially funded with $530 million from insurers, with an additional $155 million in cash from the company itself. The trust eventually totalled $2.5 billion. The trust fund controls a majority of Manville's stock and has access, if necessary, to 20 percent of its future

385

profits. All claims have to be filed against the trust. As many as 200,000 claims might ultimately be filed. The company is no longer officially in bankruptcy (ibid.). Claims continue to come in at a rate of 1,000 a month, and each claim can represent from one to thousands of individual claimants.

Other asbestos companies have tried to follow Manville's lead. Raytech, the successor to Raybestos-Manhattan, has also filed for bankruptcy. Claimants and their lawyers regard this as an attempt to evade costly lawsuits. Raymark in the past has offered *a maximum of $452* to settle cases involving death from lung cancer, although judgments in lawsuits have often come to $1 million or more (ibid.).

The Manville trust has already paid out about $570 million in settlements to victims as well as another $95 million in other liabilities. But in early 1989 lawyers reported that the trust fund was in trouble. They said that it would run out of funds by the end of the year if settlements continued at the current rate (*New York Times*, February 7, 1989).

Meanwhile, asbestos continues its dirty work. Scientists estimate that about 10,000 deaths per year and tens of thousands of cases of disabling lung diseases are caused by residues of the mineral. This will not abate for twenty years (*New York Times*, April 2, 1989).

"As the years pass," it is stated, "the shipyard workers who dominated the original claimants are being replaced by workers in the construction, petrochemical, steel and tire industries" (ibid.).

Meanwhile, the Herculean cleanup task continues. The Asbestos Hazard Emergency Response Act became law on October 22, 1986. It provides timetables and standards for dealing with the asbestos present in over 30,000 schools, which may pose a health hazard to 50 million children (*Science News*, October 25, 1986). The bill also added $100 million to an already existing $600 million school asbestos hazard-abatement loan program (ibid.).

Although schools are the most emotionally laden sites, asbestos is practically everywhere in our environment. (Industry salesmen did their job well!) About two thirds of all the buildings in New York City have been found to contain some form of asbestos. In 1988, 19 percent of this asbestos was in poor condition and considered likely to pose a health risk. Sixty-eight percent was in fair condition, constituting a mid-level risk; only 13 percent was safely in place. The cost of repairing city-owned buildings alone was put at $100 million (*New York Times*, November 6, 1988).

In the United States as a whole it has been estimated that there are 733,000 buildings containing the deadly friable asbestos and that 43 percent of these are "significantly damaged" (*Science News*, November 15, 1986).

PART FOUR

The Cancer Business

« 17 »

The Cancer
Establishment

In the United States today, the direction of cancer management appears to be shaped by those forces financially interested in the outcome of the problem. Distinct circles of power have formed which, while differing among themselves on many issues, are sufficiently cohesive and interlocking to form a "cancer establishment." This establishment effectively controls the shape and direction of cancer prevention, diagnosis, and therapy in the United States.

There is a common belief that the doctors who administer cancer therapy and the scientists who perform laboratory research control the cancer field. It is understandable that the public believes this, since it is the surgeon, radiologist, and chemotherapist who give treatment and who appear to pass judgment on new forms of therapy. Yet most doctors practice the kind of medicine they learned in medical school. There are numerous social and legal restraints on the kind of medicine a physician can practice. At large institutions, for instance, experiments involving humans are "increasingly being restricted by regulations and decrees" (Jukes, 1976).

Peer review committees within hospitals or medical societies are taking an increasingly active role in determining the actual course of therapy a physician can prescribe. The power of insurance companies is sometimes awesome. The role of the government is also clearly on the rise. Those who seek to use new forms of therapy must first gain the approval of the Food and Drug Administration. If they seek research funds, they must pass "site visits" and reviews by the National Institutes of Health and other funding agencies.

Many of these regulations were instituted to prevent real abuses, such as the wanton human experimentation practiced on cancer patients until the mid-1960s (Katz, 1972). A side effect of this legislation, however, appears to have been to speed the centralization of power in a few hands and a growing conservatism toward new therapies within the medical profession.

Within the cancer field it appears that the major decisions are made at the top of four or five organizations. If a doctor or scientist exercises real decision-making power, it is as a result of his or her inclusion in one of these groups, rather than through professional expertise per se.

Doctors who still believe they are free to give whatever treatment they consider best for a willing patient are, in fact, toying with "quackery," as it is defined by these leading bodies.

At the pinnacles of power, the scientists and physicians are often subordinated to the control of laypersons. For example, at Memorial Sloan-Kettering, "the control and management of the operations of [MSKCC] shall be vested in its board of trustees" and the scientific administrators are "subject . . . to the control and direction of the board."*

More often than not, these laypersons are the very people with the greatest vested interest in the outcome of the cancer problem. How such individuals, as well as their banks and corporations, attained their power in the cancer field, and why they seek such control, will be examined in the case of four of the most powerful organizations.

Memorial Sloan-Kettering Cancer Center

In the nineteenth century, when the U.S. Congress took little or no interest in health or welfare, it was only natural that hospitals would be financed by the philanthropic activities of wealthy families. Often a personal tragedy would stimulate a large donation. Thus the Astors (whose wealth was derived from fur trading and tenement properties) provided the initial funds for the New York Cancer Hospital in the 1880s. After them came other wealthy families, such as the Huntingtons (railroads) and the Douglases (copper).

With these large contributions came influence and even control of the recipient organizations. The Astors' lawyer became the first chairman of the

*In 1978 the board of trustees became known as the board of overseers. This reorganization does not appear to have altered the relationship of the doctors or scientists to the board (see Appendix A).

board of the New York Cancer Hospital. The Douglases not only held leading positions on the board of directors but had their personal physician, James Ewing, appointed medical director of the newly renamed Memorial Hospital.*

Until the beginning of the twentieth century, control of a hospital conveyed great prestige but little else. Not surprisingly, wealthy families sometimes lost all interest in a particular charity with a change of their leading members. Younger members of the Astor family abandoned all interest in Memorial, and the Harrimans, once prominent in the cancer field, lost that interest and turned instead to politics (Sugiura, 1971).

James Douglas saw an opportunity to mingle his charitable and his business interests. A miner, Douglas undertook the large-scale extraction of radium from Colorado ore. For the first time, cancer had become a topic of importance to the business community.

In this respect the Rockefeller family followed in Douglas's footsteps. Since the beginning of the century, however, this group had mingled personal, financial, and political goals under a single heading—philanthropy.

There is every indication that John D. Rockefeller's (JDR I) much-vaunted support of medical causes was the result of financial calculation as much as softheartedness toward suffering humanity (Brown, 1979). According to a biographical study, JDR I "really had no way of understanding value except in dollar terms. . . . Money was the philosophical center of his world throughout his long life" (Collier and Horowitz, 1976).

JDR I's chief adviser, Frederick T. Gates, presented the value of medical research in terms of its financial benefits:

> I pointed to the Koch Institute in Berlin and at greater length to the Pasteur Institute in Paris. . . . I pointed out . . . that the results in dollars or francs of Pasteur's discoveries had saved for the French nation a sum far in excess of the entire cost of the Franco-Prussian war (ibid.).

JDR I and his son "Junior" first showed an interest in the cancer field when they contributed to the formation of the American Society for the Control of Cancer, predecessor of the ACS (Considine, 1959). In 1927 they began systematic contributions to Memorial Hospital—cash donations that eventually totaled several million dollars, as well as a square block of land on which a new Memorial Hospital was built in the 1930s (ibid.).**

*Mrs. Percy L. Douglas continues as an overseer of MSKCC (see Appendix A).

**Actually, the Rockefeller family's involvement with cancer began in the mid-nineteenth century. JDR I's father, William Avery Rockefeller, was a celebrated, if uneducated,

These contributions gave the Rockefellers influence at Memorial greater than any other family—including the Douglases, who remained nominally in control for over a decade longer. The policy of the Rockefellers, as it had been of Douglas, was to "back Ewing" (ibid.). Backing Ewing primarily meant backing radiation therapy.

In 1927 the Rockefellers greatly expanded their interest in pharmaceuticals when Standard Oil of New Jersey (Esso), which was dominated by the Rockefeller family, signed an extensive cartel agreement with the German I. G. Farben company.

I. G. Farben was a huge trust that controlled almost the entire German chemical and drug industries. Until its dissolution by the Allies after World War II, I. G. Farben was a hated and feared part of the German war machine. It had produced poison gas for the German armies in World War I and was to produce the nerve poison Zyklon B for the concentration camps during World War II. In fact, the concentration camp at Auschwitz was built to accommodate a huge Farben synthetic rubber plant nearby (Ambruster, 1947).

Esso signed a wide-ranging cooperative agreement with I. G. Farben. Under the terms of the agreement, the Germans would not market gasoline or gasoline products outside of their own borders. In return, Esso would "stay out of the existing market in all other chemical fields" (DuBois, 1952:148). In addition, the two companies set up a new firm—the Joint American Study Corporation, or JASCO—to mutually develop new discoveries, such as in the field of synthetic rubber.*

The significance of this "marriage" or "general partnership" (as Esso executives called it) was that the Esso Rockefeller empire suddenly inherited a great interest in the worldwide pharmaceutical business.

Farben's interest in drugs dated back to the nineteenth century, when

cancer "therapist" in Cayuga County, New York. According to a standard biographical study, "he found a more promising career in patent medicines. He journeyed for hundreds of miles to camp meetings, passing out handbills that read: 'Dr. William A. Rockefeller, the Celebrated Cancer Specialist, Here for One Day Only. All Cases of Cancer Cured unless too far gone and then they can be greatly benefitted.' " He sold his remedy for $25 a bottle, the equivalent of two months' wages (Collier and Horowitz, 1976:8).

*This agreement was greatly loaded in I. G. Farben's favor, which became apparent when the Japanese cut off the United States' supply of natural rubber after Pearl Harbor. The United States had no synthetic rubber, and most of the information on how to make it was locked in Esso's vaults. Only swift action by the U.S. government prevented a disaster. The one man most responsible for this problem was Frank Howard. "Perhaps Howard's previous blocking of crucial industrial developments in the United States was unwitting; now [1939] he deliberately accepted, in friendly trust, the power to prevent the United States from seizing the Farben patents" (DuBois, 1952:283). (For a fuller explanation of Howard's role, see Borkin, 1978.)

one of its predecessor companies, Bayer, discovered aspirin. Another component of the trust, Hoechst, had produced Antipyrine, Pyramidon, Novocain, Salvarsan, and Dolantin (Bäumler, 1968:215). The shadowy company had branches all over the world, and appears to have had an interest in many foreign drug companies as well.

It is interesting to note that in 1926, one year before the Rockefellers began their systematic contributions to Memorial, Frank Howard, a vice president of Esso, paid his first visit to the I. G. Farben laboratories. He later said that he was "plunged into a world of research and development on a gigantic scale such as I had never seen" (cited in Borkin, 1978). He soon discovered that the Germans were already deeply involved in cancer research.

> In the first part of this century, Germany was the undisputed leader in the drug industry. During a visit to one of the German research laboratories in 1927,* I was mystified to find an adjoining greenhouse full of plants, bearing the most horrible-looking tumors. It was a nightmare of nature gone mad! In these greenhouses and in the connected laboratories, the German scientists were making a concerted effort to find out all they could in plants and animals (Howard, 1955).

In the 1930s Howard was invited to join Memorial Hospital's board of managers. The Standard Oil executive was made chairman of the newly organized Research Committee. By 1941 limited research on chemotherapy had begun at Memorial, but this was interrupted by the outbreak of World War II. Cornelius P. "Dusty" Rhoads, who had headed this nascent program, became chief of research for the Chemical Warfare Service of the United States.

The official purpose of this service was to carry out defensive studies on the effects of poison gas. It is somewhat surprising to learn that human experiments with poison gas–like substances were also being carried out on cancer patients. In 1976 National Cancer Institute officials revealed that

> under the mantle of military secrecy, clinical trials were initiated with HN_2 . . . which became the most widely used nitrogen mustard. By the time military restrictions were removed in 1946, a total of 160 patients had been treated by several groups of investigators (Carter and Kershner, 1976).

*The Howard document states that the visit occurred in 1927. Borkin speaks only of one visit by Howard to I. G. Farben's laboratories, in March 1926 (Borkin, 1978:47).

The limited success with nitrogen mustard as a chemotherapeutic agent stimulated interest in wide-scale research. As the war neared its end, Frank Howard and a New York banker, Reginald Coombe, then president of Memorial Hospital, drew up a Post-War Development Plan calling for a vast expansion of the hospital into a combination treatment-research center (Howard, 1955).

Such a project was clearly too vast even for the Rockefellers. Howard therefore asked two prominent executives of General Motors to join the project and provide funds for the new center. Together, Alfred P. Sloan (1875–1966) and Charles F. Kettering (1876–1958) contributed several million dollars, and the new research center, the Sloan-Kettering Institute for Cancer Research, was named in their honor in August 1945.

Until that time, Memorial Hospital had been under the control of the Rockefellers and, to a lesser degree, the Douglases. With the inclusion of Sloan and Kettering in leadership positions, members of the Rockefellers' traditional rival, the Morgan banking interests, were allowed to share power.

Sloan was president of General Motors, long associated with Morgan interests, and was also a director of Du Pont and of the Morgan Guaranty Trust Company itself. Kettering, or "Boss Kett," as he was called, was vice president of General Motors and a large shareholder in the company.*

The composition of the board of trustees at that time reveals a kind of balance of power, with the Rockefellers and their allies in overall control but with those representing the Morgan interests assuming many positions of power.

The actual personnel changed over the years, of course, and new financial and industrial groups assumed key positions, but from this period forward, the world's largest private cancer center was ruled by what looks like a consortium of Wall Street's top banks and corporations.**

By the mid-1960s, the MSKCC board had begun to take on a rather uniform appearance. What stood out was that many of its leading members

---

*In 1957 Sloan's net worth was established at $200–$400 million and Kettering's at $100–$200 million (*Fortune,* November 1957).

**Some of the leading Rockefeller-affiliated trustees of the 1940s and 1950s were James Murphy, president of Rockefeller Institute, Lewis Strauss (see chapter 4), and, of course, Coombe, Howard, and Laurance S. Rockefeller, JDR II's son, who assumed top leadership of the Center in 1949. Leading Morgan-affiliated trustees included Sloan, Kettering, George Whitney, the J. P. Morgan chairman, and possibly a number of scientists affiliated with Morgan-influenced universities such as MIT and Johns Hopkins (Lundberg, 1937:374). Some of the other corporations or institutions also represented on the board were Lazard Frères (through André Meyer), Kidder, Peabody (Albert H. Gordon), Amerada Petroleum (Alfred Jacobsen), Dillon, Read (Arthur B. Treman, Jr.) and IBM (Thomas J. Watson).

were individuals whose corporations stood to lose or gain a great deal of money, depending on the outcome of the cancer war.

Appendix A lists the members of the MSKCC board, and provides the corporate affiliations of the most influential. It is immediately apparent that representatives of large and powerful companies are well represented. These companies exercise their influence not only through their personal presence, but through often-substantial gifts that they make to the Center.

For example, in June 1978, MSKCC announced that it had received $7 million toward a $65 million fund-raising goal, which included donations from Exxon, formerly Esso ($1.5 million), General Motors ($1.5 million), IBM ($1 million), Mobil Oil ($350,000), Texaco ($300,000), Union Carbide ($200,000), Morgan Guaranty ($175,000), and others. Chairman of the fund-raising effort was Clifton C. Garvin, Jr., chairman of Exxon (MSKCC *Center News,* June 1978).

These corporations undoubtedly regard their donations as the height of philanthropy and would probably regard any questioning of their motives as unfair. However, the study *Economic Factors in the Growth of Corporation Giving* gave three reasons why corporations donate money to charitable organizations such as MSKCC.

The first is the "immediate and certain tax savings that accompany contributions." Second, "contributions serve to create a favorable public image of the corporation." The third factor may be the most important in this case: "to encourage a social and political environment conducive to [the corporation's] survival and prosperity" (Nelson, 1970).

If we look at this last-named criterion, we can see immediately that many of the corporations making donations, or whose members serve as leaders of MSKCC, have been mentioned before—as corporate polluters. The oil companies in particular, whose refineries are said by some scientists to cause 30 to 40 percent of *all* cancer (see Epstein, 1978), are conspicuous supporters of the current methods of cancer management.

A review of Appendix A will also reveal that many corporations that stand to profit from the cancer field are also deeply involved in making decisions about the direction of research and treatment at Memorial Sloan-Kettering.

In the 1980s MSKCC, as well as other cancer centers, developed particularly close links with the drug industry. Jeffrey Goodell explained it this way in a *Seven Days* cover story on the hospital: In some cases the hospital is paid to test new drugs in a restricted clinical trial. In others, the hospital will contract with a drug company to manufacture a compound that the hospital has come up with in its laboratories. "Either way, the payment for

TABLE 8
Ownership of Cancer Drug Company Securities by MSKCC–1987

Security Description	Shares	Market Value (12/31/87)	Cancer Drugs
American Home Products	1,800	$ 130,950	Cerubine
Bristol-Myers	13,500	561,938	Blenoxane, Cytoxan, etc.
IC Industries	10,000	329,877	Nolvadex
Lilly, Eli	14,600	1,138,000	Oncovin, Velban, etc.
Merck & Co.	8,700	1,378,950	Cosmagen, Mustargen, etc.
Schering Plough Corp.	8,700	408,900	Intron A
Squibb	12,500	762,500	Hydrea, Teslac

Source = MSKCC Annual Financial Report, 1987

these services is usually made by arranging to split the royalties on any patents that are developed, and if one of these drugs proves to be a breakthrough, both sides stand to profit immensely" (Goodell, 1989).

"Memorial is already one of the two or three most sought-after institutions by the pharmaceutical companies," according to Jim McCamant, editor of a biotech newsletter in California. "The presence of Dr. Vincent T. DeVita can only increase that demand" (ibid.).

Another link between MSKCC and the industry is through investments. In the year ending December 31, 1987, MSKCC had over $127.2 million invested in securities. The portfolio was spread over a diverse group of industries, but a relatively large portion was devoted to drug and health care ($9.2 million), chemicals ($5.7 million), and domestic and foreign oil companies ($2.5 and $3.8 million, respectively). An additional $1 million was invested in British, German, Japanese, and Swiss pharmaceutical companies (MSKCC, 1988b).

Some of these investments included shares in manufacturers of anti-cancer drugs, as is seen in Table 8. Thus, MSKCC has a financial stake in the health of these companies whose products it tests and employs in the treatment of cancer, and some of whose officials serve on its own board.

Memorial Sloan-Kettering was the prototype for all the comprehensive cancer centers. Its enormous influence and prestige serves as an amplification mechanism for this group, spreading their decisions, ripplelike, to cancer treatment centers around the world.

In the last decade MSKCC has undergone a series of convulsive changes. In October 1980 MSKCC president Lewis Thomas stepped down, taking the honorary title Chancellor, and Paul A. Marks, M.D., took over as president and chief executive officer. There then began a "major purge of the scientific staff," according to Philip Boffey's revealing cover story on Marks in the *New York Times Magazine* (April 26, 1987).

"We needed somebody to come in and pull this place together," said Laurance Rockefeller.

Marks was brought in by Rockefeller and Benno Schmidt to accomplish several goals:

- at Memorial Hospital, to reduce the power of the surgeons and increase that of the radiotherapists and chemotherapists;
- at Sloan-Kettering Institute, to reduce the power of the immunologists and increase that of the molecular biologists;
- to get rid of "a lot of dead wood" on the staff (Laurance Rockefeller's phrase) and to get more "efficient" in collecting payments from patients (ibid.).

According to critics—and there are many—"the purge was carried out with a brutal temper and brusque tactics. There are researchers who call Marks 'Caligula,' 'Attila the Hun' or simply 'the monster' " (ibid.). The former Memorial chairman of surgery called him "a kind of administrative Rambo." Even his sponsor, Benno Schmidt, says he tends to use "a sledgehammer where he needed a tack hammer or a pin prick" (ibid.).

Marks came to MSKCC from Columbia University, where as dean of the medical school he had already developed a formidable reputation. On one occasion, during a heated discussion in his laboratory, "as four or five startled onlookers watched, he grabbed a man by the throat and dragged him across a table" (ibid.). In the *Times* interview, Marks's wife, Joan, said "he can be brutal" (ibid.).

This was the man that Rockefeller, Schmidt, and the other board members chose to reform Memorial Sloan-Kettering, at a salary of $350,000 a year. (In addition, Rockefeller bought him a $500,000 Park Avenue apartment, and Schmidt chipped in $165,000 for remodelling). Ninety tenure-track scientists left between 1982 and mid-1986, "most of them because they were discharged, fearful of or dissatisfied with the new regime" (ibid.). The first to go was SKI president Robert A. Good. First he lost his spacious office, then much of his laboratory space and budget allocation. At the end of 1981 he negotiated a settlement agreement and left. He is now physician-in-chief at All Children's Hospital in St. Petersburg, Florida.

The operating budget is now more than $335 million, with $67 million of that spent on laboratory and clinical research. In January 1984 MSKCC launched a successful five-year campaign to raise $300 million. Much of that money is going to build a new thirteen-story research facility, the Rockefeller Research Laboratories, towards which Laurance Rockefeller himself donated $36.2 million. In 1982, Rockefeller himself stepped down and became honorary chairman. Benno Schmidt, the former head of the President's Cancer Panel, took his place.

In August 1988 Vincent T. DeVita, Jr., M.D., resigned as director of the National Cancer Institute and announced that he was taking the post of physician-in-chief at MSKCC. "If you want to fly with the eagles, you don't rot with the turkeys," DeVita said, in a parting jibe (Goodell, 1989).

At the same time, a Memorial Hospital physician, Burton J. Lee 3rd, became White House physician (*New York Times,* March 14, 1989). In all, MSKCC is well-positioned to thrive under the Bush administration. DeVita's presence will greatly increase the influence of the Center as well as its ability to negotiate the federal grants that form a major part of its funding.

A look at the Institute's annual report for 1987–88 reveals a leaner and meaner Sloan-Kettering, with research programs focused on molecular biology, cell biology and genetics, immunology and developmental therapy, and clinical investigation. Gone are the meager programs in prevention and nutrition and the flirtations with unorthodoxy that marked the Good-Old days. Sloan-Kettering intends to approach the cancer problem "with the full armamentarium of both genetic engineering and pharmacology" (SKI, 1988).

The changes in the board over the last decade have been numerous but have hardly changed the Wall Street orientation. In fact, as Appendix A reveals, drug company influence has increased. Most significant is the arrival of Richard L. Gelb, chairman of Bristol-Myers, onto the MSKCC and SKI boards, where he quickly became vice chairman. His fellow vice chairman, James D. Robinson III, became a director of Bristol-Myers. This company, as noted elsewhere, is the undisputed leader in cancer chemotherapy productions. (It also figured in the scandal over MeCCNU at NCI in 1981.) Several other new managers are also directors of major drug companies (see Appendix A).

The Center received many gifts in the course of its fund-raising appeals. Gifts over $25,000 in support of research and education in 1986–87 included those from the following: Bristol-Myers Company; Dow Chemical Company; E. I. Du Pont de Nemours & Company; Hoechst-Roussel Pharmaceuticals Inc.; Hoffmann–La Roche Inc.; Johnson and Johnson Foundation; Eli Lilly and Company; Merck & Co., Inc.; Pfizer Inc.; Sandoz Corporation; Schering-Plough Foundation, Inc.; SmithKline Beckman, and Squibb Corporation (SKI 1987). Needless to say, these are many of the same corporations that sell the drugs used to treat cancer at Memorial Hospital.

MSKCC seems poised to become an even more powerful private center of the traditional, profit-oriented attack on cancer. Perhaps some new cytotoxic solutions will emerge from all this high-powered activity. Meanwhile, to those who believe in a more humane and open-minded approach to the problem, the 1970s, ironically, are beginning to look like a Golden Age!

The American Cancer Society

The American Cancer Society (ACS) is the nation's largest volunteer health organization. In 1978 the Society brought in almost $140 million in donations and bequests, putting it ahead of its older rivals, such as the American Heart Association, the National Foundation (the March of Dimes), or the American Lung Association. This increased to more than $331 million in 1987 (ACS, 1989).

What accounts for the ACS's phenomenal success? Obviously the ACS benefits from the importance of cancer as a public-health problem. But there is more to it than that. Heart and circulatory disease is a far greater cause of death than cancer. Yet the American Heart Association receives far less in donations or research funds than the cancer establishment.

The most important element in the ACS's success story is its own skillful and sophisticated appeal to the public. "Among the numerous accomplishments of the American Cancer Society," a sympathetic student of the Society wrote some years ago, "the most profoundly important is its cultivation of cancer consciousness, a national frame of mind" (Richard Carter, 1961:139).

American awareness of cancer sometimes strikes foreign visitors as almost pathological. Hardly a day goes by without a newspaper report on cancer—usually a scary account of some new environmental chemical believed to cause the disease. One cannot listen to the radio or television for long without hearing the word *cancer*. The death from malignancy of a Hubert Humphrey, a Yul Brynner, or a Gilda Radner becomes a national drama, a struggle against seemingly invincible odds, which the public follows with fascinated horror. As Susan Sontag has pointed out, cancer has become one of the favorite metaphors of our language (Sontag, 1977). Often the disease seems imbued with a personality of its own, like an alien creature from a horror movie.

How did this cancerphobia come about? Was it a spontaneous development? Not exactly. In part at least, as Richard Carter suggests in the above quote, it was cultivated by the American Cancer Society and the other opinion-shapers in the cancer field. It has proven to be an excellent fund-raising device, although "development" experts understand it must be used sparingly or it will lose its effectiveness.

The ACS was originally founded as the American Society for the Control of Cancer (ASCC) at the New York Harvard Club in 1913. John D. Rockefeller, Jr., provided funds for its founding, and most of those present at the inception were close to the Rockefeller financial group, especially the law firm of Debevoise, Plimpton.*

For several decades the ASCC was kept small and elite, a vehicle for the charitable impulses of New York's wealthiest families. Membership rarely went above two thousand. Money for the Society's activities came from the wealthy. For example, in 1921 Laura Spelman Rockefeller donated $8,000 for the Society's first movie, *The Reward of Courage*. In the late 1920s Edward H. Harkness, a Standard Oil heir active in medical affairs, gave $100,000. J. P. Morgan and Co. contributed $50,000, and founders were expected to donate $1,000 each (Richard Carter, 1961).

From the start, the Society was conscious of its role as a shaper of public opinion. "There is beyond question a perfectly legitimate use, even for a medical man, of the publicity man and the press agent," said a founder of the organization, Dr. Howard C. Taylor. "He is constantly used in the political world and there is no reason why we should not also use him to accomplish medical ends" (ibid.).

The main goal was to urge the general public to consult their physician at the first suspicion of cancer. "What they need," said the Society's managing director, George A. Soper, Ph.D., speaking of the public, "is to see the necessity of prompt and capable medical attention" (ibid.). But how to accomplish that goal?

"From the beginning [the Society] vacillated between a fear technique and the dissemination of hope," wrote Carter (ibid.). The reason for this vacillation is fairly obvious. If the Society spoke only of the brilliant hope for cancer patients (which was far less realistic in the 1920s than it is even

_____
*For example, Thomas M. Debevoise was secretary of the ASCC, and his close friend, George C. Clark, was the first president. Mrs. Robert G. Mead, described as a "one-woman gang in civic and philanthropic work," was another prominent member. She was married to a Debevoise partner. Her father, Dr. Clement Cleveland, was a surgeon prominent in the Society (Richard Carter, 1961:144).

today) people would not feel compelled to consult their doctors. On the other hand, if the Society only stirred up fear, they would feed the fatalism that still hangs over the word *cancer* like a pall.

Typical of the Society's early propaganda efforts was a 1919 poster which proclaimed boldly: "One Out of Every Ten Persons Over Forty Dies of Cancer." A subtitle then hit the hope theme: "Cancer Is Curable If Treated Early." Then the placard ended on the fear motif, by listing four ominous "Danger Signals," forerunners of the "Seven Warning Signals" of today.*

The Society's campaign raised the ire of the organized medical profession, the American Medical Association (AMA), which accused the Society of causing mass cancerphobia. Its "signs of cancer," said the Association's *Journal,* "is so small a part of the whole truth that it is better left unsaid . . ." (ibid.).

An inherent contradiction in the Society's educational campaign was that it could urge people to consult their physicians for annual checkups or therapy, but it could not expand the medical services or pay for people to have these examinations. In response to this contradiction, in the late 1920s and 1930s, the Society began to take on a populist coloring.

For example, Dr. Soper "aroused the ready hostility of organized medicine by advocating a network of free cancer clinics, to eliminate the financial barrier to prompt diagnosis" (ibid.:147).

Soper did not last long after such remarks, and in 1929 he was replaced by Clarence Cook Little, D.Sc., former president of the University of Michigan and a well-known geneticist.

Little opposed publicizing cancer among laypersons and instead placed his emphasis on building up cancer treatment as a profession. "Superficial programs of lay publicity when adequate facilities for diagnosis, treatment, and follow-up are wanting or are scattered or uncontrolled, will be of little value," he said. Both he and Soper were confronting the same problem. But while Soper advocated the rapid extension of *free* cancer centers that could have become truly popular and effective, Little advocated increasing the number of private practitioners interested in cancer. "Nothing will scare the profession back into hiding more successfully," he said, "than a noisy lay campaign. . . ." (ibid.:151).

Even at this early date the leaders of the Society showed signs of intransigence toward unorthodox approaches to the cancer problem. In particular, Little pursued a vigorous and at times unreasonable attack on Maud

*"Cancer's Seven Warning Signals: 1. Change in bowel or bladder habits. 2. A sore that does not heal. 3. Unusual bleeding or discharge. 4. Thickening or lump in breast or elsewhere. 5. Indigestion or difficulty in swallowing. 6. Obvious changes in wart or mole. 7. Nagging cough or hoarseness. If you have a warning signal, see your doctor" (ACS, 1988).

Slye, a highly innovative geneticist at the University of Chicago (McCoy, 1977).

In the mid-1930s a spin-off organization to fight cancer was formed, which almost superseded the Society itself. This was the Women's Field Army, a kind of ladies' auxiliary of the Society. In retrospect it appears as if the temper and tensions of the 1930s were about to create a new type of health organization in the United States—a grassroots organization, tapping the energy of millions of Americans.

The Women's Field Army was almost paramilitary in its approach. Its volunteers wore perky brown uniforms, insignia with quasi-military rank, and made sure that suspected cancer victims "reported" to their physicians for diagnosis and treatment (Richard Carter, 1961:153).

The Field Army was enormously successful. In 1939 it raised $171,000 for impoverished patients, in 1942, $269,000, and in 1943—in the midst of a world war—$356,270. By 1944, at a time when the American Society for the Control of Cancer itself had 986 members, the Women's Field Army had over a million members and was already "one of the most important health organizations in the history of the United States" (ibid.:154). The blue-blooded Society members fretted over this development.

At the same time, orthodox medicine appeared to be losing ideological control of the cancer field. New and innovative treatments sprang up all over the country. Harry Hoxsey, with his Hoxide herbal cures, was drawing thousands to mass meetings across the Midwest, where he mingled unorthodox cancer theory with populist politics. Hoxsey even had his own daily radio program (ACS, 1971b).

Looking back on this period, Frank Howard of Esso complained that "the research for new cancer treatments . . . was in danger of becoming abandoned to quacks, and to pseudo-scientific frauds in the years just before the war" (Howard, 1955).

In the early 1940s a group of wealthy individuals, deeply distressed by the situation in the cancer field, began to plan a reorganization of the ASCC. The "benevolent plotters," as they sometimes called themselves, actually took control of the Society in 1944, changed its name to the catchier American Cancer Society and set about restructuring the organization.

One of the first things they did was to abolish the Women's Field Army and institute top-down control of all branches of the Society from its New York headquarters. Clarence Cook Little was also forced out. He eventually wound up as scientific spokesman for the tobacco lobby (Little, 1957).

Key figures among the new ACS leaders were: Elmer Bobst, president of the American branch of Hoffmann–La Roche and, later, of the Warner-

Lambert pharmaceutical company. Bobst was basically a drug salesman, with close connections to the medical profession and to politicians, such as Richard Nixon (Bobst, 1973).

Albert and Mary Lasker, health philanthropists and originators of the Lasker Awards, an American version of the Nobel Prize. Albert Lasker was among the most prominent advertising men of his day. Both Lasker were, at times, Memorial Sloan-Kettering trustees.

Ironically, Lasker's greatest advertising coup was for the American Tobacco Company. His slogan—"Reach for a Lucky instead of a sweet"—convinced thousands of women to start smoking in the 1930s and 1940s.

If Bobst spoke for the Society in Republican administrations, Mrs. Lasker was familiar with and at ease amid the heirs of the New Deal. She was on close terms with Hubert Humphrey and Lyndon Johnson and became a familiar figure on Capitol Hill. It has been said: "She is able to produce results for congressmen and they love it. . . . Health in the abstract is a popular ideal for politicians, ranking just behind motherhood and apple pie" (*Medical Dimensions,* March 1976). Mrs. Lasker was and remains a skilled broker; she brought the congressmen who control federal funds together with prestigious medical leaders.*

As opposed to the American Society for the Control of Cancer, the American Cancer Society was dominated by laypersons. "We realized that the Board should include the businessmen who had become interested in the Society," Mrs. Lasker later said in a statement on the Society's reorganization (ACS, 1965).

Bobst and Lasker introduced the most advanced Madison Avenue techniques into cancer fund raising. Bobst ran it "like a business with a well-planned 'sales' campaign" (Bobst, 1973). "Dollars flooded the treasurer's office," and ACS writer recollects, "finally totaling more than $280,000" from a single story in *Reader's Digest* (ACS, 1965).

Initially the ACS used the fear motif rather heavily. The theme of the 1945 fund-raising campaign was "cancer kills people." It featured pictures

*Other members of the group which took over the Society in the 1940s were Emerson Foote, an advertising associate of Albert Lasker; James Adams, a partner in the investment banking house of Lazard Frères, a director of Standard Brands, Inc., which had drug and food interests, and a former official of the Johns-Manville asbestos company; General William J. Donovan, director of the U.S. government's intelligence agency (OSS), which evolved into the Central Intelligence Agency; Howard Pew, Sun Oil executive, well-known for his espousal of ultraconservative causes; Ralph Reed, president of American Express; Harry Van Elm, president of Manufacturers Trust Co; Florence Mahoney, a personal friend of Mrs. Lasker's and a newspaper heiress; and Eric Johnston, president of the Motion Picture Association of America (Richard Carter, 1961; ACS, 1965).

of gravestones, coffins, and a terrifying "beware of cancer" message. Bobst would begin his fund-raising speeches with a dramatic "One in five of us here—every fifth person in the audience—will die of cancer" (Bobst, 1973).

Then would come the ray of hope, "We want to cure cancer in your lifetime," and an appeal for funds. Using such techniques, the ACS was not only able to raise hundreds of millions of dollars, but to enlist over two million people as unpaid volunteers in its fund-raising activities. April was officially declared "Cancer Month" by the president of the United States, and spring was ushered in with a shake of the fund raiser's can.

The press has been carefully cultivated, an art that Lasker practiced in the 1920s, when he used his clients' clout to influence stories or even, it is said, "to suppress . . . newspaper material hostile to [Lasker's] aims" (Lundberg, 1937).

About three decades ago, Patrick McGrady, Sr., the Society's science editor, initiated national tours of cancer laboratories for science writers. When these became too crowded, in 1958 he initiated the annual Science Writers' Seminar. Originally a chance for leading science writers to meet prominent researchers in a congenial setting, McGrady came to believe the seminars became a "medium of self-serving propaganda" for the ACS (cited in Chowka, 1978c). In the eyes of critic Robert A. Houston:

> Held at holiday resorts to lure and pacify reporters, it can usually be counted on to generate a barrage of breathless copy about how a mote in a scientist's lens spells imminent victory against the dread disease. Softened up by the exalted false hopes (most of which later turn out to be cul-de-sacs, or worse, bottomless pits), the public is an easy prey for the Society's volunteer army, 2.3 million strong. This year's Seminar was booked for March 25–28 at Florida's Daytona Hilton. The strike-force hits on April 1 (Houston, 1979a).*

So successful has been this media cultivation that the Associated Press once ran an ACS publicity piece as a ten-part "objective" news series on cancer, without acknowledgment of its origin within the Society.

Asked about the propriety of this, a top Associated Press executive replied, "I never considered the ACS to be a political organization. . . . That's just like saying that God is political" (Bloom, 1979).

*Even some very established science writers have begun to question the usefulness of the Science Writers' Seminar. Writing in the newsletter of the National Association of Science Writers, Ed Edelson of the *New York Daily News* and Jerry Bishop of the *Wall Street Journal* raised questions about the Society's motives for holding the seminar and about the value of attending (see *NASW Newsletter*, September and December 1978).

The Society is a power among researchers in the United States. Approximately one-quarter of its more than $300 million income is spent on research. As the number of applications has increased, the Society has been able to pick and choose among those research projects submitted. For example, in 1978, 1,912 scientists requested over $160 million in funds from the ACS. The Society awarded about $40 million to 639 of them. By 1987, the number of requests had risen to 2,385 and the Society was disbursing over $77 million to only 810 of them for research (ACS, 1988). Scientists thus must be responsive to the goals and thinking of the Society if they expect to be funded in this competitive situation. Conversely, although no strings are attached to these grants, ACS's wishes can often be translated into the direction of the research (ACS, 1979).

ACS grants go out to most of the major research institutions in the country, and many around the world. One year (1978), some of the biggest recipients included the University of California, with 54 projects totaling almost $3 million; Sloan-Kettering, with 25 grants totaling over $1.5 million; Yale University, which received 18 grants worth $1.3 million; and Yeshiva University in New York, which was given 17 grants worth in excess of $1 million. Cancer research laboratories in Switzerland, England, Scotland, and Israel spread the Society's influence abroad. In addition, the Society spent $375,000 in 1978 to support Eleanor Roosevelt-ACS International Cancer Fellowships (ibid.).

By 1987 the various branches of the University of California were receiving $7.4 million for 69 projects. The University of Texas, with 36 awards, got $3.6 million. And Memorial Sloan-Kettering (including the Walker Laboratory in Rye, New York) came in third with 29 grants and fellowships worth nearly $3 million. In addition, grants were made to laboratories in England and France and to the International Union Against Cancer (ACS, 1988).

The ACS also supports twenty-five prominent scientists around the country in what is known as its Research Professorship Program, a lifetime stipend that frees these individuals to spend their full time on cancer research (ibid.).

The Society has numerous committees and holds many seminars and panels. By incorporating leading cancer specialists into these bodies, the ACS has involved the medical profession in its administrative and fund-raising apparatus, and made many of them committed to the Society's success. Many of those who have served on ACS committees have also benefited—either personally or institutionally—from the Society's largesse (Chowka, 1978c).

Mary Lasker, the long-time honorary chairman of the ACS, who continues as an honorary life member, has been considered by some the "most powerful person in modern medicine" (*Medical Dimensions,* March 1976). Veteran science writer Barbara J. Culliton called the National Cancer Act "Mrs. Lasker's War" (*Harper's,* June 1976).

The days are gone when a cancer specialist would think of opposing the leadership of his field by businessmen, bankers, and advertising people. The Society now has tens of millions of dollars to distribute to those who favor its hegemony, and many powerful connections to disconcert those who oppose it.

The National Cancer Institute

In terms of dollars, the most powerful force in the cancer field is the National Cancer Institute, which has primary responsibility for funding the so-called war on cancer. NCI's budget in 1978 was $910 million, most of which was spent in support of scientists at various institutions. By 1988 that had increased to almost $1.5 billion. (see Table 8).

Although NCI is larger than either Memorial Sloan-Kettering or the American Cancer Society, it is not as powerful as either. In fact, historically, the smaller private organizations have interlocked with the federal giant and guide its thinking on many matters.

ACS (especially its Women's Field Army) was influential in the founding of the NCI in 1937. In the 1940s ACS lobbied for extending the appropriations for the Institute. Senator Claude Pepper (D.-Fla.) held hearings on a bill to make "a supreme endeavor to discover the means of curing and preventing cancer" (cited in Haught, 1962).

Pepper's bill did not pass into law, but Mary Lasker and her coworkers did manage to generate a great deal of favorable publicity for cancer research. NCI's budget skyrocketed from $600,000 per year in 1946 to $92 million in 1960. It was no secret that Mary Lasker and the ACS were largely responsible for this phenomenal growth (Strickland, 1971). ACS influence within NCI grew proportionally.

"The Cancer Society and the National Cancer Institute work as partners," Dr. John R. Heller, former director of NCI, declared in 1960. "The Director of the Institute is a member of the board of directors of the Cancer Society, and the scientific advisory committees of both organizations interlock" (Richard Carter, 1961:142).

In the 1970s NCI's funds quadrupled, as a result of the "war on cancer" legislation. Passage of the National Cancer Act of 1971 increased ACS (and MSKCC) influence over the Institute.

Groundwork for the National Cancer Act was laid in the late 1960s when Senator Ralph Yarborough (D.-Tex.) established a twenty-six-person National Panel of Consultants on the Conquest of Cancer. This committee ultimately recommended the war on cancer to Congress.

Chairman of the panel was Benno Schmidt, leader of the Memorial Sloan-Kettering Cancer Center (see Appendix A). Vice chairman was Dr. Sidney Farber, a former president of the American Cancer Society and a leading cancer drug researcher.

Other scientists on the panel included two other former ACS presidents (Jonathan Rhoads, M.D., and Wendell Scott, M.D.) and a prospective president, R. Lee Clark, M.D. From MSKCC came Joseph Burchenal, M.D., a chemotherapist, and Mathilde Krim, Ph.D., a researcher whose husband was prominent in Democratic party politics (*Austin American-Statesman*, April 14, 1973).*

Lay members of the panel included Laurance S. Rockefeller of MSKCC; Elmer Bobst of Warner-Lambert; Emerson Foote, a Lasker associate; G. Keith Funston, chairman of the Olin chemical company; and Mrs. Anna Rosenberg Hoffman, a colleague of Mrs. Lasker's. All of these individuals, with the exception of Rockefeller, were board members of the American Cancer Society. (Olin has held the patents on a number of anticancer drugs, including one for the purification of interferon.)

In addition, there appears to have been token representation from the labor movement and the press: I. W. Abel of the United Steelworkers and Michael O'Neill from the *New York Daily News*.

Thus, of the twenty-six panel members who framed the war on cancer, ten were officers of the American Cancer Society and four were affiliated with Memorial Sloan-Kettering. Mrs. Lasker, who was not on the panel itself, is said to have supervised the actual writing of the panel's report (*Harper's*, June 1976).

After passage of the National Cancer Act in 1971, two special committees were set up so that the administrators of the new program could bypass some of the red tape of the National Institutes of Health, to which the National Cancer Institute belongs. These committees were the National Cancer Advisory Board (NCAB) and the elite and powerful President's Cancer Panel.

Head of the President's Cancer Panel at its inception was Benno Schmidt, the "cancer czar" of the United States (*Science*, April 16, 1976). His two companions on the panel were chosen from the scientific community. Its first scientific members were R. Lee Clark, president of the M. D.

---

*Krim later left MSKCC to become founding chair of the American Foundation for AIDS Research (Johnson, 1988).

Anderson Tumor Institute and Hospital in Houston (and ACS leader), and Robert A. Good, Ph.D., M.D., the soon-to-be-appointed head of Sloan-Kettering Institute.

The larger NCAB also showed decisive ACS-MSKCC influence. Its members included Mary Lasker, Elmer Bobst, and Laurance S. Rockefeller. In 1988 the chairman of the President's Cancer Panel was Armand Hammer of the Occidental International Corporation; his two colleagues were William P. Longmire, M.D., of the Veterans Administration in Los Angeles and John A. Montgomery, Ph.D., of the Southern Research Institute in Birmingham.

The drug industry has also exerted its influence on NCI in a number of ways.

In the past, Dr. Richard S. Schreiber, vice chairman of the Upjohn Company, manufacturer of anticancer drugs (see Table 1), was a member of the National Advisory Cancer Council, predecessor of the NCAB. Dr. Alexander M. Moore of Parke-Davis was made a member of the Chemistry Panel of NCI. Dr. Andrew C. Bratton, Jr., also of Parke-Davis, was a member of the Institute's Drug Evaluation Panel, as was Dr. Karl A. Folkes of Merck Sharp & Dohme.

Today drug-company influence appears to be more subtle, but no less real. As mentioned earlier (see chapter 15), quite a few members of the NCAB have been affiliated with drug companies. Dr. Gertrude B. Elion of Burroughs Wellcome and Dr. Phillip Frost of Key Pharmaceuticals are presently members.

The importance of this can be seen when one considers the manner in which NCI grants are approved. A grant application submitted to NCI may first be subjected to a site visit by a team of outside experts appointed by the administrators. (The reader will recall that Lawrence Burton was visited by a Sloan-Kettering chemotherapist when he applied for an NCI grant.) Not all applicants are visited—according to the NCI *Fact Book,* only about 10 percent are (NCI, 1975). An established center, such as Memorial Sloan-Kettering, is far less likely to be visited than a new applicant or one suggesting a controversial research or therapy project.

After the experts have made a visit, they assign the project a priority rating. The NCAB then considers all major grants (over $50,000). Although the final determination is made by the NCI's Grants Management Office, it is very rare for this to overrule the powerhouses on the NCAB.

Decisions at the federal level are frequently colored by economic and political questions. For example, a major medical debate on breast cancer treatment in 1989 sheds light on the politics of the National Cancer Institute and its relationship to the pharmaceutical approach to cancer.

There are 70,000 women in the United States each year who have localized breast cancer not involving their lymph nodes. The survival rate in such women is high—approximately 70 percent—and few doctors have shown a willingness to subject them to further rigors after surgery. The general attitude seems to be, let well enough alone.

In fact, only 2 percent of these women go on to have chemotherapy (DeVita, 1989). Getting them to enroll in various drug programs has been a major thrust of the NCI, especially during Dr. Vincent T. DeVita's long tenure.

In 1989 the *New England Journal of Medicine* published the results of four such testing programs as well as several contrasting editorials on the subject. Women without any visible signs of cancer (node-negative) were enrolled in one of four different treatment trials. The point of the studies was to see if various combinations of drugs and/or antihormones could affect their postoperative survival. The drugs generally increased the disease-free interval by a few percentage points. In the international study, headquartered in Switzerland, 77 percent of the chemotherapy group was alive and *disease-free* after four years, compared with 73 percent in the controls (Blume, 1989). Some special categories showed greater benefit—up to 15 percent. But an important point is that drug therapy did *not* give any *overall* survival advantage during four years of follow-up (Fisher et al., 1989). The same percentage of women were alive in one group as in the other at the end of the four-year study. That alone would seem to throw doubt on the value of chemotherapy.

In addition, there was substantial toxicity in three of the four studies. Although tamoxifen was generally well-tolerated, one patient did die from complications. In the international study three patients died as a result of the treatment (Ludwig, 1989). In another, one patient died and 33 percent encountered what the researchers themselves called "severe or life-threatening hematologic toxicity" (Mansour et al., 1989).

Furthermore, in an accompanying editorial, William L. McGuire, M.D., of the University of Texas Health Sciences Center at San Antonio, revealed the not inconsiderable costs associated with adjuvant chemotherapy:

1. The international study, with its combination of cyclophosphamide, methotrexate, fluorouracil, and leucovorin, had total direct costs (including drugs, extra office visits, and laboratory work, but without the extra expenses incurred by treatment of toxic side effects) estimated at $398 per patient.

2. The Fisher study, using methotrexate and fluorouracil followed by leucovorin, cost $5,920 per patient.

3. The Mansour study, with treatment by cyclophosphamide, methotrexate, fluorouracil, and predisone, ran to $1,829 per patient.

4. The trial of tamoxifen, an anti-estrogen manufactured by ICI under the brand name Nolvadex, cost $4,745 per patient (McGuire, 1989).

If all potential patients were enrolled in such programs, based on these figures, Dr. McGuire calculates that the total cost of adjuvant chemotherapy for node-negative breast cancer would be $338,174,200 per year.

"This analysis," he adds, with quiet understatement, "does not consider the clinical toxicity and perhaps as many as 50 to 100 treatment-related deaths" per year. "I would argue," wrote McGuire, "that the cost considerably outweighs the benefits of treating all node-negative patients, especially in the absence of a proved survival benefit" (ibid.).

Despite the limited success of this approach, its toxicity, and its high cost, the National Cancer Institute, which sponsored three of these studies, has continued to push adjuvant chemotherapy. In May 1988 it even sent out an extraordinary Clinical Alert to 13,000 physicians, in advance of the publication of this data in peer-reviewed journals, because of the alleged urgency of the findings (Blume, 1989).

"The alert and resulting publicity angered some doctors who began receiving calls from distraught breast cancer patients who hadn't received chemotherapy," according to a report in the *Wall Street Journal* (February 22, 1989).

In the 1989 editorial in the *New England Journal of Medicine*, Dr. Vincent T. DeVita, Jr., former director of NCI, claims that the tests show "an impressive reduction in the risk of recurrence among patients with node-negative disease."

Appropriating the rhetoric of the freedom-of-choice movement, DeVita tells his fellow doctors that "women with breast cancer need to make a choice, and they should be given that option. . . ." These studies, he says, "provide these women with an option" (DeVita, 1989). He brushes off the fact that the women in the treated and nontreated categories showed the same survival time with the comment that it "is almost certainly a matter of timing." In other words, he hopes and expects that some survival difference will become apparent with time.

DeVita also deals with the question of toxicity in a remarkable way. He refers to the "minimal toxicity of two of the chemotherapy programs" and claims that "short-term side effects were not excessive, and the risk of long-term adverse effects seems minimal" (ibid.). One wonders what the families of the five women who died in this trial would say to that.

And what about the one third of women in the Mansour trial who encountered "severe and life-threatening" blood disorders? No mention; apparently that is what DeVita considers a not excessive effect. And in the National Cancer Institute press release accompanying the announcement of the studies, these life-threatening situations are similarly downgraded to a mere "low blood cell count in 33 percent of treated patients" (Blume, 1989).

It is not a favorable sign that Dr. Samuel Broder, who succeeded Dr. DeVita as director of NCI, has associated himself with this drug-oriented approach. Broder came on board promising a greater emphasis on prevention. Yet he now says that "adjuvant therapy is becoming an integral part of everyday medical care" and that "increasing use of this form of therapy . . . is going to make a difference in the lives of thousands of patients" (Blume, 1989).

Reading between the lines, one may find a lack of enthusiasm here. Broder is simply describing a development, not extolling it. But Dr. Broder, who proudly proclaimed that he was not a politician, is beginning to sound like one. It is a far cry from the promise of a new and bold orientation for the nation's billion-and-a-half-dollar cancer center.

The Food and Drug Administration

Like the National Cancer Institute, the Food and Drug Administration (FDA) is a government agency, staffed by civil servants and political appointees. But whereas the NCI is a source of largesse to scientists, the FDA is generally a source of aggravation. The FDA's role is theoretically to prevent harmful or useless methods of treating cancer from entering the marketplace.

How well or equitably the FDA succeeds is a matter of dispute.

On August 15, 1974, eleven FDA scientists appeared before Senator Edward Kennedy's (D.-Mass.) Subcommittee on Health and Scientific Research and charged their own agency with being a virtual pawn of the industries it is supposed to control. Appearing without the foreknowledge of the FDA commissioner, the eleven "testified before the Senate that they were harassed by agency officials—allegedly pro-industry—whenever they recommended against approval of marketing some new drug" (Science, June 11, 1976).

Then–Secretary of Health, Education and Welfare Caspar Weinberger announced that he was going to hold a public investigation of the matter. Weinberger also announced that this "open inquiry" would be headed by an aide to former FDA commissioner Charles C. Edwards. The eleven FDA dissidents refused to participate in the investigation (*Science and Government Report*, April 1, 1975).

Meanwhile, FDA commissioner Alexander M. Schmidt (no relation to Benno Schmidt) spent almost $200,000 preparing a 900-page report that vindicated him and the agency of any wrongdoing. The HEW chief simultaneously appointed a blue-ribbon panel to investigate the FDA investigation. They countered with a $140,000, 525-page "Assessment of the Commissioner's Report of October 1975." Dan Greenberg characterized the latter group as "a bickering lot of hairsplitting metaphysicians." If the secretary of HEW chose "to sweep them all out," he added, "it [would] be no loss to the Republic or drug safety and efficacy" (*New England Journal of Medicine*, June 24, 1976).

The net result of these reports was to cover the original charges of the eleven with an avalanche of verbiage. *Science* wondered aloud:

> Who is running the Food and Drug Administration? The agency or the drug industry it is supposed to regulate? No one knows for sure, and if the latest in an endless series of FDA investigations is any indication, no one is going to find out very soon (*Science*, June 11, 1976).

However, these metaphysical exercises hardly succeeded in killing the issue. Soon afterward, the government's General Accounting Office (GAO) issued its own report, which found widespread conflict of interest within the FDA. In particular, the auditing arm of Congress found that 150 FDA employees were owners of stock in twenty-seven FDA-regulated companies. In addition, 203 FDA employees simply had not filed financial disclosure statements, while several had ignored FDA requests that they divest themselves of their personal investments in drug companies (*New York Times*, January 20, 1976).

Improper and illegal stockholding is one of the ways in which the drug industry may influence policy decision making at FDA. Another is the "revolving door"—the process by which government officials are recruited by industry or sent from industrial positions into regulatory posts. For example, Surgeon General of the United States Leonard Scheele became president of Warner-Lambert's research laboratories. FDA commissioner Charles C. Edwards later became senior vice president for research at Becton Dickinson, a medical supply company. Another former FDA commissioner, James L. Goddard, became chairman of the board of Ormont Drug & Chemical Co. The FDA's top physician, Joseph Sawdusk, later became president of Parke-Davis.

The disorganization at this vital agency has been so great as to strain credulity. Yet according to testimony offered to an HEW panel by Dr. J. Richard Crout, director of the FDA's Bureau of Drugs, the agency has been crippled by "what some people called the worst personnel in government" (cited in Pharmaceutical Manufacturers' Association, 1976). Crout then added:

> There was open drunkenness by several employees which went on for months. There was intimidation internally by people. . . . [In] '72, '73 going to certain kinds of meetings was an extraordinarily peculiar kind of exercise. People, I'm talking about division directors and their staff, would engage in a kind of behavior that invited . . . insubordination—people tittering in corners, throwing spitballs; I am describing physicians, people who would . . . slouch down in a chair, not respond to questions, moan and groan with sweeping gestures, a kind of behavior I have not seen in any other institution as a grown man (cited in *New England Journal of Medicine*, May 27, 1976).

This behavior seems more characteristic of an insane asylum than of a top government agency—yet we have the uncontradicted testimony of Dr. Crout that his bureau was "full of unhappy, uprooted people"—at least in the early 1970s.

This anarchy may help explain some of the more bizarre episodes in the treatment of unorthodox cancer therapies; for example, the FDA's approval of Andrew McNaughton's request for permission to test laetrile clinically on April 27, 1970, only to revoke this permission a few days later (see chapter 8). It also throws light on a previously described episode in which Dr. Linus Pauling was invited to Washington to discuss vitamin C with the FDA commissioner only to have that invitation abruptly withdrawn shortly thereafter (see chapter 11).

Similarly, it may explain the failure of the agency to prevent some potentially harmful drugs from entering the medical marketplace. In 1975, for example, government investigators found that two widely prescribed drugs, Aldactone and Flagyl, produced by G. D. Searle & Co., caused cancer in test animals. Searle was then the tenth-largest drug company in the nation; its sales of these two items alone totaled $17.3 million.

How was it possible that these commonly used items, employed in the treatment of high blood pressure and trichomonas infections, respectively, had been approved for sale by the FDA? Further investigation revealed that Searle had known about the tumor-producing potential of these items but had simply given the FDA fraudulent data. For example, the company destroyed the records of mice which developed tumors, or it operated on some mice to remove their tumors and then reported them as cancer-free in the test records.

At a hearing of Senator Kennedy's subcommittee, FDA officials presented evidence that at least three other companies similarly withheld information on their products or fed the agency false data. These three were Ciba-Geigy, Ayerst Laboratories, and Lederle Laboratories. In these cases the FDA began investigations that could have ended in criminal prosecution or at least strong administrative sanctions against the companies. Instead these investigations simply disappeared. "The cases somehow went into some mysterious bottomless pit that we have not been able to identify," FDA commissioner Alexander M. Schmidt told the senators (*New York Times*, July 10, 1976).

At the same time, the FDA bureaucracy slowed the number of new drugs being introduced in the United States. In 1962 it cost an average of $1.2 million to develop a new drug in the United States (Walter S. Ross, 1973). By 1976, according to the Pharmaceutical Manufacturers Association (PMA), it cost $11.5 million (*Nature*, March 11, 1976). By 1979 some business analysts claimed that it cost $50 million to develop a new drug (Standard and Poor's, 1979). The paperwork has increased proportionally. In 1948 Parke-Davis had to submit 73 pages of evidence to secure the licensing of a new drug. Twenty years later, it had to submit 72,200 pages of data in support of an anesthetic application. The documents had to be moved to the FDA by van (Ross, 1973).

By 1988 the price tag had reached $125 million. It can take 10 years from the start of development to marketing, and two or three of those years are often spent waiting for the FDA to approve the new substance (*New York Times*, February 9, 1988). It is obvious that the difficulties involved in new-drug development have become extraordinary.

While these hurdles apply equally to both big and small companies, it is obvious that the big companies are able to overcome them with greater ease. In fact, the entire bureaucratic maze at FDA greatly favors the largest companies, which are represented by a powerful Washington-based lobby, the PMA.

George Schwartz, a spokesman for the smaller drug companies, explained the situation succinctly: "These regulations favor companies with greater financial strength. They're eliminating competition" (*Business Week*, January 17, 1977). *Fortune* has called the FDA the drug industry's "unwitting ally" (*Fortune*, March 1976). Some critics would say it is not so unwitting.

The existence of a bureaucratic maze at FDA is consonant with the interests of the biggest food and drug manufacturers. The influence of these companies appears to be deep and to be exercised in numerous and diverse ways. This may explain the agency's generally poor record in controlling environmental carcinogens whose usual source is big business (see chapter 15).

It may also explain some of the agency's intransigent hostility to unorthodox approaches to cancer, or even to innovations made within established cancer centers. Such innovators, mavericks, or small companies are the antitheses of the large firms that dominate the agency. Often there is a financial conflict between the plans of the small fry and the giant companies.

The principal role of the FDA in the cancer field has been to stifle such innovators by denying, or stalling, their Investigational New Drug applications (INDs) and harrassing them when they attempt to depart from orthodox practice. In 1976 Dr. Crout told the agency's Oncology Drugs Advisory Committee, "The fact of life is, we get INDs . . . from a variety of places, not just NCI or the top research institutions. For some places you want harsh regulations backed by the full weight of the law—[we] have had INDs for laetril[e], for example, and other hoax remedies. . . . Sometimes we say it is proper to hinder research" (*Cancer Letter*, March 12, 1976). But the FDA has approved dozens of requests to market anticancer drugs from the largest companies, which have the greatest financial weight, influence at the agency, and support of other sections of the cancer establishment.

The FDA's mandate is to protect the public from the introduction of unsafe and useless drugs. Yet during the last decade the FDA's enforcement has been one-sided, at best. It has come down hard on practitioners of unconventional medicine, often unfairly branding them as quacks. At the same time it has been extraordinarily lax in the treatment of the largest companies. It is hard to escape the impression that this agency, once considered the triumph of progressive consumerism, now exists primarily to serve the interests of the "industry majors."

There is "a very lethal and dangerous partnership between the drug companies and the FDA," according to Sidney Wolfe, M.D., the Washington health advocate (Frontline, 1989).

In the last decade and a half, FDA has significantly relaxed its enforcement of the large companies' violations of the law. Between 1971 and 1975 the FDA issued sixty serious citations per year to drug companies. But between 1975 and 1987 they issued only five such citations a year (ibid.).

Nevertheless, the cost of regulation has risen to unanticipated heights. As stated, the cost of developing a new drug has risen to $125 million, two and a half times what it cost in 1976 (U.S. Department of Commerce, 1988).

Such costs encourage a conservative policy toward innovation on the part of industry: only three to four of the two dozen drugs approved in 1986 were significant advances. The rest were "me-too" drugs, slight modifications of already approved items (Frontline, 1989).

FDA has countenanced all sorts of unethical behavior on the part of the self-proclaimed ethical pharmaceutical manufacturers. Even when lives have been lost, FDA has almost never brought criminal charges. Their answer, to quote an agency official, is that "it's just a rather cutthroat world out there for the pharmaceutical industry," and "no useful purpose" would be served by prosecuting manufacturers (ibid.).

An example, already cited, was the testing of Bristol-Myers' anticancer drug MeCCNU at the National Cancer Institute. Deaths and serious illnesses resulted from side effects that were concealed from the agency and from the affected patients. One bold FDA official suggested bringing criminal charges against both the drug company and NCI for withholding information about the drug's toxicity. But FDA did not prosecute, allegedly because of "staff shortages," and the case was dropped after only one person had been interviewed (Sun, 1981).

Yet FDA has been the scourge of unorthodoxy, especially those methods of approaching cancer that are described in this book. In June, 1989 FDA agents raided Great Lakes Metabolics of Rochester, Minnesota and A-O Supply Company of Millersport, Ohio and seized their stocks of hydrazine sulfate as well as other drugs, vitamins, supplies, and books (Budd, 1989). The Burton and Burzynski chapters, in particular, show how the agency in recent years has expended an extraordinary amount of energy keeping nontoxic approaches to cancer off the market.

Admittedly the situation is now in flux, making a definitive analysis difficult. The FDA is coming under increasing attack from many quarters:

Angry AIDS patients have literally besieged the agency; the National Cancer Institute, and other treatment centers, are locked in constant battle over their freedom to do experimental chemotherapy; political conservatives, such as the Cato Institute and the *Wall Street Journal*, have called for deregulation of the drug industry; the Bush Administration, through its Lasagna Commission, has sought to streamline the drug-approval process; freedom of choice advocates have sought legislative measures that would counteract the efficacy requirements of drug testing. Finally, the majors would like the cost of new product development reduced, while maintaining a regulatory barrier to keep out small competitors.

All these attacks, while largely uncoordinated, are coming at the same time. If this opposition succeeds in getting organized, it seems unlikely that FDA will be able to withstand the strain. Already FDA Commissioner Frank Young has agreed to eliminate Phase III trials for promising drugs and to allow some unproven drugs into the country from abroad. But these maneuvers may be too little, too late.

A Grand Jury in Baltimore is said to be preparing criminal indictments against FDA and drug company officials for price-fixing of generic drugs, and a leading Congressman says the investigation is widening. As FDA approaches the 1990s, it gives the impression of an agency with its back against the wall.

Conclusion: The Cancer Establishment

Is there really a cancer establishment? The term *establishment* was first used to describe the Church of England, and later the entire English upper class. If we understand the "cancer establishment" to mean some formally organized body, such as the hierarchy of a church, then clearly there is no such organization.

Nevertheless, the leaders of the top organizations discussed in this book are certainly familiar with each other and interlock on many committees, panels, and boards. Sometimes they are friendly, and sometimes they disagree. What holds them together, however, is a community of interests and ideas. The top leaders generally see eye-to-eye on the major questions concerning cancer. They favor cure over prevention. They emphasize the use of patentable and/or synthetic chemicals over readily available or natural methods. They set the trends in research, and are careful to stay within the bounds of what is acceptable and fashionable at the moment. They are also, generally speaking, socially homogeneous—older white males predominate here.*

A union-sponsored study of the oil industry discovered a similar establishment, and described it as

> a structured pattern based on concentration of control, interlocking directorates, financial services, joint ventures, professional conformity, reciprocal fa-

---

*The existence of a "cancer establishment" does not preclude the possibility of conflicts among its constituent parts. In 1976 the FDA refused to allow NCI to distribute experimental drugs to cancer centers for the treatment of terminal cancer patients (*Cancer Letter*, January 30, 1976). The FDA cited the Flagyl-Aldactone scandal as its rationale for doing so (ibid.). The following year, it refused to allow cancer centers to *combine* approved drugs for therapy, a situation which "could put us back in the Dark Ages," according to an MSKCC official (*Staten Island Advance*, January 19, 1977). The ACS asked Congress to remove control over the testing of new anticancer drugs from the FDA to NCI (ibid.). This battle has continued. "Many factors conspire to make current regulatory procedures problematic for antineoplastic drugs," an NCI official wrote in reference to FDA procedures (Wittes, 1987). The "National Committee to Review Current Procedures for Approval of New Drugs for Cancer and AIDS" is largely concerned with NCI-FDA contradictions (Chabner, 1989).

417

vors, commonality of interests . . . long-term friendships and, at its worst, greed and arrogance (Medvin, 1974).

Not everyone accepts the existence of such an establishment. Dr. Robert C. Eyerly, chairman of the Committee on Unproven Methods of Cancer Management of the American Cancer Society, ridiculed this view:

> We, the "medical monopoly," the "cancer establishment," are purportedly involved in the "cover-up" and "suppression" of material. . . . In this time of public suspicion, such accusations are unfortunately given attention. It is difficult to respond to such an irrational statement (Eyerly, 1976).

On the other hand, certain representatives of the far right, who tend to see conspiracy in many areas of American life, have claimed that there is a conscious conspiracy to suppress laetrile. At the July 1977 hearings of the Subcommittee on Health and Scientific Research, Senator Edward Kennedy asked Dr. John Richardson, a laetrile-using physician, "Do you really think there is a conspiracy?" Richardson answered:

> Well, I've thought so for quite some time, Senator Kennedy. And it was always a ludicrous thought that while I was trying to tell people about a conspiracy, that I was caught up in a conspiracy indictment [to import laetrile] myself.
> But I definitely feel that there is; yes. Conspiracy is not unusual in any time in history, and particularly in this time. And it may be unwitting on the part of many people (U.S. Senate, 1977).

"Who is involved in the conspiracy?" Kennedy asked, obviously sensing a weak spot. Richardson went on to name various organizations interested in the cancer field: the American Cancer Society, the Food and Drug Administration, the American Medical Association and Sloan-Kettering Institute. The only major group which Richardson explicitly exempted from this conspiracy was Congress, to which, as he pointed out, his friend (and fellow John Birch Society member) Larry McDonald (D.-Ga.) belonged (ibid.).*

In *World Without Cancer*, a two-volume work that Richardson cited in support of his position, G. Edward Griffin speaks of a "malicious con-

---

*This is the same Congressman McDonald who was killed when the Soviets shot down the famous Korean Airlines Flight 007 on September 1, 1983.

418

spiracy hiding behind the smiling mask of humanitarianism" and a "conscious direction behind the opposition to laetrile" (Griffin, 1975:501–02).

The dictionary defines *conspiracy* as a planning or acting together secretly for an unlawful or harmful purpose. Not only is there no hard evidence that such a conspiracy to suppress a known cure for cancer exists, but such a theory defies logic as well.

A conspiracy theory must take into account the fact that the leaders of the cancer establishment themselves die of cancer. Many prominent cancer scientists, administrators, and politicians have died of the disease, as have many wealthy people associated with the establishment, including members of the Rockefeller family. Did someone fail to tell them about the suppressed cure?

In addition, it is apparent that the cancer establishment, while hindering the development of unorthodox approaches to cancer, is strenuously attempting to develop the orthodox approaches. For example, $2 million was poured into clinical trials of interferon, and more into the development of interleukin-2. An orthodox cure for cancer would be "worth a fortune," as a drug company executive has said (see chapter 5).

The important point is that the suppression of unorthodox methods—and the promotion of the orthodox approach—takes place mainly at an objective, unconscious level. It is an outgrowth of underlying economic and social trends rather than of conscious design. This may explain the opposition of members of the establishment itself (such as Dr. Eyerly) to this explanation, since they swim in the sea of this establishment and are rarely conscious of its pressure all around them. On the other hand, representatives of the far right may prefer a simple conspiracy theory since this targets only a few "malicious" people and spares the system itself from any fundamental criticism.

Yet the evidence points to the fact that it is the system itself, rather than any particular clique of individuals, which is really to blame for failure to make progress against the cancer problem. In particular, the fact that cancer management is itself a big business means that it must function according to the rules of profit-oriented institutions.

« 18 »

Cancer and the
Suppression of Science

American business seems to be unreservedly in favor of science. Most American industries are founded upon great technological innovations and could not function without a constant input of ideas by scientists and technicians. Especially since the end of World War II, American industry has spent billions of dollars on research and development.

It seems contradictory, and downright perverse, to say that American business *suppresses* scientific development, and that because of this, an industry-led effort to find a cure for cancer has little chance of success. Yet there is another side to American science, which is little known but has great relevance to the current impasse in cancer management.

The purpose of research from the point of view of business is, and always has been, to facilitate profit making. The first capitalists to sponsor medical research—John D. Rockefeller I and his colleagues—were conscious of the monetary value of science. The modern executive, although perhaps more subtle in his or her approach, is still aware that profit is the bottom line in all research endeavors. Science can do wonders for a corporation's balance sheet, as the histories of the aerospace, electronics, or plastics industries show. But perceptive businessmen are also aware that uncontrolled, unbridled, and unrestricted research has the potential to *destroy* industry.

"Bankers regard research as most dangerous and a thing that makes

banking hazardous due to the rapid changes it brings about in industry,"
wrote no less an authority than Charles Kettering, cofounder of Sloan-Kettering Institute (quoted in Bernal, 1967).

Justice Louis Brandeis pointed out in the early part of this century that
the gas companies tried to suppress the electric light, Western Union fought
against the telephone, and then both Western Union and the telephone companies opposed the coming of radio (ibid.).

Many other instances can be, and have been, given. A government
study made in 1937 concluded that "a banker who finances a new development that will destroy his present investments is asleep at the switch" (National Resources Committee, 1937).

Some of the factors leading to the suppression of science by business,
according to Dr. S. Lilley, include

> the permanent difficulty that manufacturers found from the late nineteenth cen-
> tury on in selling their products, chronic unemployment, and the formation of
> cartels and monopolies . . . which act by restricting production; but that means
> less incentive to install the latest type of machinery, which in turn implies less
> encouragement to invent yet better. Sometimes they go further and actively
> discourage new invention (Lilley, 1965).

How can industry "actively discourage new invention?" According to
the well-known British chemist J. D. Bernal, "the process can take two
forms. The stifling of existing invention and the choking of new invention
by restricting research" (Bernal, 1967). Obviously it is easier and neater to
stop an unwanted scientific development by refusing to fund it adequately
than it is to destroy it once it has taken root.

Research into the chemical causation of cancer, for example, has been
suppressed more frequently by the simple expedient of not sponsoring research into this controversial topic. It is only in rare instances, as in Searle's
experiments with Flagyl (see chapter 17), that outright stifling of scientific
results is employed.

David E. Lilienthal, first head of the Tennessee Valley Authority and
later an atomic energy commissioner, explained how the growth of giant
corporations facilitated this sort of suppression:

> The most effective way to "suppress" new inventions or technical ideas
> is simply not to develop them. Only large enterprises are able to sink the
> formidable sums of money required to develop basic new departures; a small
> corporation is rarely able to risk those large sums, perhaps enough to wreck

the company if the gamble fails, on the success or failure of a major new project (Lilienthal, 1953:69).

In the 1930s, when social and economic problems were sharpened, this question of technological suppression received a considerable amount of attention. Some of the best research on it was done by special U.S. government commissions. Even a big businessman of those times admitted:

> I have even seen the lines of progress that were most promising for public benefit wholly neglected or positively forbidden just because they might revolutionize the industry. We have no right to expect a corporation to cut its own throat (quoted in Bernal, 1967).

Television—one of the marvels of American technology—was actually a victim of suppression. Developed in the thirties, it was and continues to be hampered for economic reasons. According to an article in *Forbes:*

> The early development of commercial television was hampered when Hollywood movie studios refused to make TV programming or sell their old movies. A workable pay-TV system was produced by Zenith as early as 1948, but pay TV didn't get off the ground until the late 1970s because of opposition from movie theater owners. More recently the fear of piracy . . . has stopped introduction of two-bay videocassette recorders, which allow a movie to be copied by a single VCR (Block, 1986).

After World War II, however, little more was said in public about the suppression of science. The very idea had become—in the words of the *Wall Street Journal*—an "old canard" (March 4, 1976).

This change in attitude and perception was due to a number of factors. First, the period immediately following the war was one of economic growth and expansion. Many new products were marketed and some that had been held back by the Depression and the war (television and inexpensive aluminum, to name only two), were now made available to the general public. Government action, in some cases, had broken scientific logjams. For example, by breaking up the Standard Oil-I. G. Farben cartel and seizing foreign patents, the government was able to wrest the secrets of artificial rubber production from the monopolies (DuBois, 1952).

In recent years, with growing economic problems and a more open

423

attitude in general on social ideas, there has been increasing attention paid to the problem of suppression.

According to "The Breakdown of U.S. Innovation," an informative article in *Business Week,* American industry began to favor "a super-cautious, no-risk management less willing to gamble on anything short of a sure thing" (*Business Week,* February 16, 1976).

"In the long march of American technology, innovation has become a giant killer," the article noted.

> By attaching a diesel engine to a generator on an electric locomotive, General Motors Corp. all but murdered the steam engine and derailed many of the old, traditional names in locomotive manufacturing. . . . In the same way, the telephone tore up the telegram, the trolley car fell victim to the automobile, and passenger trains yielded to buses and planes (ibid.).

The tiny transistor "shook the $45 billion electronics industry to its foundations" and wiped out many old, established businesses. The goal of corporate directors, *Business Week* continued, is "to get the risks of innovation under even tighter control."

"The main thing a fellow in my position can do is turn things off," an executive vice president for research and development of a large corporation admitted. "The curse of R&D is letting things go on too long." Another executive complained, "We constantly run into the attitude of 'let somebody else go first' even for processes proven overseas" (ibid.). Since the reworking of an old idea has *a ten times greater chance* of financial success than a really new idea, according to prominent management consultants, really new ideas are either not funded, are dropped in the development stage, or are actively stifled (ibid.).

Although the news about suppression has only reached the popular media through such films as *Tucker* (1988), the story of a suppressed automotive pioneer, the science and business press are not unfamiliar with the topic. They have carried articles such as "The Silent Crisis in R&D" (*Business Week,* March 8, 1976), "The State of American Science—A Touch of Anemia" (*New England Journal of Medicine,* March 25, 1976), and "Innovative Research Is Taking Back Seat as Chemical Firms Weigh Costs, Profits" (*Wall Street Journal,* June 2, 1976).

A recent, blatant example of technological suppression is DAT, or digital audio technology. DAT is a digital tape recorder developed in Japan that makes copies as good as the original master recording. This recorder promises to revolutionize the home audio market. And that is precisely why the Japanese manufacturers and the $4 billion-a-year, primarily American and European, record industry want to suppress it.

"They want consumers to keep buying standard tape recorders and compact disk machines for another couple of years before they introduce a machine that will almost certainly be an instant hit," said *Forbes* (Block, 1986).

The record industry has demanded that each machine contain a "spoiler"—an "electronic gizmo that would scramble the sound every time the machine is asked to record a compact disc"—allegedly in order to foil commercial 'pirates' (*The Economist*, December 20, 1986).

The matter is presently being considered by the United States Congress. While a few machines are being brought into the country, without warranties and at very high prices, most consumers will have to wait years before ever hearing this perfectly duplicated sound.

But what does this have to do with cancer research?

We tend to think of cancer researchers as inhabiting a different, more ethereal and idealistic world from the grubby world of Wall Street or the practical sphere of industrial research. In some senses they do, but it is clear that the ultimate power in the cancer field rests with the same gentlemen who run the major banks and corporations.

As a consumer of corporate goods and services, a repository of invested funds, and a producer of one of America's largest service industries—health care—the cancer world is in every sense part of the industrial structure. It is business, and therefore can be expected to operate under the same rules as the rest of business.

Cancer drugs are subject to the same criteria of profitability as other commodities. Given the integration of the cancer field into the corporate and banking establishments, it could not be otherwise. Depending on its nature, a new drug can be an economic boon or it can be a "giant killer."

As indicated previously, one critical question is patentability. Most of the currently available anticancer drugs are or have been patented. Others are monopolized in some other way. Almost all of them are manufactured by the major pharmaceutical firms (see Table 1 in Chapter 5). The authoritative Standard and Poor's *Industry Survey* on pharmaceuticals made this criterion quite clear:

> The key to profitability in the [drug] industry lies in the development of patent-protected new drug products, an established marketing force, and a diverse position in the world markets.
>
> Patent expirations will bring pressures on margins over the next few years, thus accentuating the need for patented new drugs (Standard and Poor's, 1977).

Any common, off-the-shelf chemical is thus unacceptable from an economic point of view, since it offers no possibility of patent protection. Anyone with a pill-making machine could market such a substance. Hydrazine sulfate, vitamin C, and vitamin A all fall into this category. Some money can be made from marketing them, but hardly the kind of high profits customary (and the companies would say necessary) in the drug industry.*

One critic put the situation succinctly:

> The production of nonpatented drugs will give only moderate profits while the production of patented drugs will give abnormally high profits. Drug manufacturers have attempted, therefore, by every conceivable means to divert the market into the sale of high-profit patented drugs (Medical Committee for Human Rights, 1972).

Other substances mentioned in this book appear to be similarly handicapped. No patents now apply to the manufacture of laetrile, for instance, and this chemical is extracted from apricot kernels and bitter almonds in small foreign factories. Since laetrile occurs naturally in approximately 1,200 different plants, it would be impossible for anyone to corner the market on laetrile-containing substances.

This seems to be contradicted by the high cost of laetrile on the market. It was said, for example, that a one dollar and twenty-five cent laetrile pill cost only two cents to manufacture and that the rest constituted exorbitant profits for the laetrile profiteers (Schultz and Lindeman, 1973). The price in 1977 came down to 85 cents per 500 mg. capsule, where it has remained for the last dozen years (Michaelis, 1989). While the charge of profiteering may have had some merit, the high markup seemed to be a function of government harassment. Illegal or semilegal drugs are always expensive. Thus, decriminalization of laetrile would have probably brought the price down dramatically. Vitamin B-15 (pangamic acid), also pioneered by Ernst T. Krebs, Jr., was a legal substance, priced at between three and five cents for a 100-milligram pill on the open market. In 1989, it had risen, but only to 12–15 cents retail (ibid.). The reason for this small markup is that vitamin B-15, like laetrile, is an unpatentable product derived from fruit kernels. Since laetrile still cannot be freely manufactured and shipped in the United States, it seems likely that it will continue to be priced far above its actual value for some time to come.

Without entering into a discussion of other noncancer controversies, it

---

*The drug companies claim to have extraordinarily high research and development costs and thus to need extraordinarily high profits. For a critique of this argument see Klass, 1975.

is worth noting that similar disputes have broken out in other fields of medicine. For example, proponents of the use of dimethyl sulfoxide (DMSO) in a wide variety of ailments claimed that it, too, was held back by its very cheapness (McGrady, Sr., 1973). (Subsequently, DMSO became a cancer treatment as well and was added to the ACS unproven methods list in the March/April 1983 issue of *Ca*.) Lithium chloride, a treatment for manic-depressives, was not accepted for several decades. According to one book on this topic:

> Lithium, being a natural element, could not be patented, and the American pharmaceutical industry thus could not see any commercial potential in the drug, unlike most other psychopharmaceuticals (Fieve, 1976).

The pattern in these and other such controversies is often remarkably similar to those in the cancer field, and may stem from the same underlying economic and social causes.

In some instances an unorthodox method is patented, or can become so, but the rights and know-how are in the hands of independent entrepreneurs, who refuse to give in to the demands of dominant firms. This was a major charge in the Krebiozen affair (Bailey, 1958). Some aspects of Livingston's work have been patented, and Burton, Gold and Burzynski have taken out many patents on their procedures.

Is there a conscious conspiracy by the drug cartel against unpatentable methods? Again, it is not necessary to postulate such a conspiracy in order to explain the suppression of cheap and readily available alternatives.

Leaving aside the fact that complicated chemicals are often more intriguing to scientists than simple ones, all researchers need money to carry out their work. Most of the funds for cancer research come from the National Cancer Institute or the American Cancer Society. But, as Laurance Rockefeller and Lewis Thomas, M.D., once wrote in an MSKCC *Annual Report*:

> There is an increasing tendency, understandable enough at a time of so much competition for a diminishing pool of federal funds, that favors the award of grant support to "safe and sound" research programs. This means that it will henceforth be much more difficult to obtain support for scientific "gambles" (MSKCC, 1977a).

Since, as they say, "major advances have been made, almost without exception, by what seemed at the time to be gambling on unlikely hypotheses," the provision of "venture capital" or "seed money" takes on a critical importance (ibid.).

Who else besides the ACS or the NCI can provide the money to start a research project on a new compound, or a new avenue of attack on the cancer problem? Some may come from individual philanthropists, such as Laurance Rockefeller himself. But the Rockefeller Brothers Fund, which he chaired, began in the late 1970s to phase out its support of Memorial Sloan-Kettering and other recipient institutions (*New York Times*, May 27, 1979). This support ended on December 31, 1986.

Thus, to an increasing degree this crucial seed money is provided either by foundations associated with profit-making businesses, or directly by the drug companies.

Such support can take many forms.

In 1975, for example, the giant chemical company Monsanto gave $23 million to Harvard University Medical School to support the work of various scientists, including some working on cancer (*Harvard University Gazette*, February 7, 1975).

Bristol-Myers had a $2.5 million grant program with cancer research centers at five universities: Baylor, Chicago, Johns Hopkins, Stanford, and Yale. The grants reputedly went for "unrestricted, innovative cancer research." In turn, grant recipients from these institutions gave out the annual Bristol-Myers Award for Distinguished Achievement in Cancer Research, a $25,000 (now $50,000) cash prize (*Immunology Tribune*, April 30, 1979).

To an outsider, this appears to be money well spent, even if it did not directly result in marketable commodities for Bristol-Myers. The company bought goodwill, displayed its earnest interest in the cancer problem, and made invaluable contacts with leading scientists.

Sometimes seed money is targeted toward a specific goal. Pharmaceutical companies routinely make what are called restricted contributions to medical centers whose research goals are carefully pinpointed in advance. This is an ongoing practice: in May 1977, for example, Ortho Pharmaceutical Corp. gave Sloan-Kettering $25,000 in a restricted contribution; Burroughs Wellcome gave $15,000; and American Hoechst Corp., Pennwalt, and Eli Lilly donated smaller amounts. In the next month Newport Pharmaceuticals International gave $19,804.95; Sandoz, a Swiss drug company, gave two gifts totaling $1,500; and Hoffmann-La Roche, Ives Lab, and E. R. Squibb & Sons all made smaller donations (MSKCC, 1977b).

The 1987–1988 "Research and Education Programs" report of Sloan-Kettering Institute lists gifts of over $25,000 from, among others, Bristol-Myers, Dow Chemical, E. I. Du Pont de Nemours, Hoechst-Roussel Pharmaceuticals, Eli Lilly, Merck & Co., Pfizer, Sandoz, Schering Plough Foundation, Smith Kline Beckman and Squibb (Sloan-Kettering, 1987).

The available Sloan-Kettering documents do not state the purpose of these grants. It is a fair assumption that some go to further research projects in which these companies have a proprietary interest. Newport Pharmaceuticals International, for example, manufactured antiviral compounds that were patented and "developed jointly with Sloan-Kettering" (*Wall Street Journal*, September 19, 1978).

Should researchers want to investigate the anticancer potential of a readily available, nonpatentable, unprofitable compound, they will find great difficulty in getting such a project started, or in continuing it once it has begun. Thus the invisible hand of the marketplace is quite sufficient to prevent the development of many innovative research projects.

In addition, we must consider the so-called human factors that certainly play a real—although secondary—role in the suppression of new cancer therapies. A Columbia University sociologist found that "the mere assertion that scientists themselves sometimes resist scientific discovery clashes, of course, with the stereotype of the scientist as 'the open-minded man' " (Barber, 1961). Nevertheless, it is a fact.

From the earliest times, innovative scientists have faced opposition simply because their ideas have been daring and new. To chronicle all the scientists who have been unfairly opposed would require writing a history of science.

Sometimes the innovator has trampled on preexisting dogmas, religious or scientific. Anaxagoras was expelled from "enlightened" Athens in the middle of the fifth century B.C. because he maintained that the sun was a red-hot disc of stone and not a god (Farrington, 1965:74).

The discoverer of antiseptics, Ignaz Semmelweis, was expelled from his hospital position in Vienna because he dared to urge doctors to wash their hands before delivering babies. Lister, who had greater success in promoting similar ideas, later spoke of the blindness to new ideas in science that he also encountered (ibid.). Even ideas that in retrospect appear to have been readily accepted sometimes faced short but fierce seasons of opposition. Lord Kelvin regarded the announcement of Roentgen's discovery of X rays as a hoax (ibid.). Einstein faced hostile opposition to his theory of relativity. According to physicist A. M. Taylor, "Indeed, physicists were sharply divided into two camps, one enthusiastically supporting the theory, the other bitterly critical" (A. M. Taylor, 1970:32).

Almost without exception, innovators in medicine have faced opposition. The strength of the opposition often appears to be proportional to the freshness of their ideas. This does *not* prove that their ideas are correct. Orthodox science will also oppose incorrect, absurd, or harmful ideas—and there is no way to know, without a thorough investigation, whether a new concept is being opposed because it is threatening to the status quo or because it is dangerous and absurd.

The history of science does prove that a new concept should not automatically be rejected simply because it is attacked by the experts. Sometimes an attack or controversy is the birth cry of a great idea.

Right or wrong, the innovators in this book are all proposing concepts and methods at variance with current beliefs. For instance, it is not generally believed that cancer is a deficiency disease; this idea is supposed to have been refuted in the 1940s. In fact, such commonly used drugs as methotrexate are literally *anti*-vitamins (Shimkin, 1977:405).

Because the medical profession in general does not believe that cancer is caused by a lack of nutrients, one could predict serious difficulty for therapies such as laetrile, vitamin C, vitamin A, or abscisic acid, which claim to restore some lost nutritional element.

Similarly, it is a dogma that cancer is not caused by a microbe. This, supposedly, was disproven many years ago. The fact that a scientist like Virginia Livingston claims to have new evidence makes little impression on doctors who were educated to believe that this theory is passé.

Chemotherapy, after struggles of its own, has now been accepted as a third modality in cancer therapy. But it is generally believed that chemotherapy must be toxic in order to work—specifically, that it must interfere with the metabolism or replication of cells and kill them by direct poisoning. Gold's hydrazine sulfate, however, is relatively nontoxic, and appears to work in a different manner—by interrupting gluconeogenesis. This idea appears to be too new to gain ready acceptance by many oncologists.

It sometimes takes many years for the establishment to acknowledge that a pioneer was right and it was wrong. Usually all the contestants in the battle have passed away before that happens. Coley was generally ignored, and his method was cited in the ACS unproven methods list. Later Coley was hailed as a "cancer-immunology pioneer" (*New York Times Magazine*, April 2, 1978) and his name was quietly removed from the ACS list, even if his promising therapy is still not being used (see chapter 7).

Coley did not know *why* the toxins had the effects he saw. In the intervening seventy-five years, however, orthodox scientists discovered, by a circuitous route, that immune-stimulating products could indeed have a beneficial effect on some animal tumors. Coley's empirical observations were thus given what appears to be scientific justification.

Mainstream science may similarly find a new justification for Burton's vaccine in "normal human globulin," or for laetrile in the "synthetic mandelonitriles" supposedly tested at Sloan-Kettering (Chowka, 1979).

More often than not, attempts are made to deprive the pioneer of all credit. For example, hundreds of articles have been written about the role of free-radical scavengers in cancer; few have acknowledged their debt to disgraced cancer pioneer William Koch and his Glyoxylide (Houston, 1987a).* Dactinomycin was marketed as an orthodox anticancer drug without any recognition of the fact that it comes from the same ray fungus as was used in the production of Krebiozen (ibid.). Emanuel Revici was exploring the relationship of a nontoxic form of selenium to cancer as early as 1955, yet this fact is never mentioned in current articles on that mineral (NCI, 1987). The discussion of vitamin A and cancer is totally devoid of any recognition of the pioneering work of Max Gerson, a pattern of neglect Albert Schweitzer already discerned in 1959.

In 1976 the author was in a private conversation with a high official of Sloan-Kettering Institute, during which the man closed the door and asked, "Do you want to know where we get all our new ideas?" This leading scientist proceeded to take down from the shelf a copy of the American Cancer Society's *Unproven Methods in Cancer Management*. "This is our Bible," he said, simply and eloquently.

At least some Sloan-Kettering scientists have had the grace and courage to acknowledge their debt to William Coley. Most pioneers have suffered twice—unwarranted persecution in their lives and unfair obscurity in their deaths.

This pattern of intellectual appropriation continues unabated. For instance, what is one to make of a favorable, front-page article on hydrazine sulfate in a National Institutes of Health publication that fails even to mention the work of Joseph Gold? (Henrikson, 1989; one paper of Gold is referenced, without comment, in a footnote.) Similarly, what of scientific papers on the role of choriogonadotropin in cancer that make no mention of the work of Virginia Livingston? (Kellen, 1982a and 1982b)

As Dr. Gerson himself so eloquently said:

> The history of medicine reveals that reformers who bring new ideas into the general thinking and practice of physicians have a difficult time. Very few physicians like to change their medical approaches. . . . This is one of the reasons why developments in culture made very slow progress all through the centuries; they were restrained forcefully (Gerson, 1958).

*A notable exception was Nobel laureate Albert Szent-Gyorgyi, who at least discussed Koch's work, although not favorably (Szent-Gyorgyi, 1976:95–96).

New methods can also be suppressed through the normal day-to-day functioning of the funding mechanisms. Most of the research funds in the United States come from the federal government, specifically from the National Cancer Institute. The government might appear to be an ideal source of funds for an innovator; it does not have to satisfy stockholders with the profitability of a research venture.

In some instances, in fact, the government has sponsored cancer projects that would not be funded by drug companies. The National Cancer Institute, for example, put up the money to gain FDA approval of the Italian anticancer agent Adriamycin (Applezweig, 1978). It did so at a time when no American drug company was willing to invest in this effective but highly toxic product (see chapter 5). In other cases NCI has undertaken in-house research into rather unusual compounds, such as maytansine, an agent derived from an African plant (*Science*, September 19, 1975) or taxol, derived from Pacific yew bark (*New York Times*, May 3, 1987). Throughout the eighties there has been a slow but steady growth in nutrition related research (NCI, 1987).

In general, however, it is very difficult for new ideas to survive the funding mechanism. For one thing, for years NCI spent only about half of its appropriation on grants to outside researchers. The remainder went to contracts whose topics had been chosen at NCI itself, or to in-house research (NCI, 1975).

In recent years that pattern has improved, but only somewhat. In the proposed 1990 By-pass Budget 62.6 percent of the total request of $2.2 million is set aside for grants. The rest goes for contracts (15.8 percent), intramural projects (16.5 percent) and NIH management funds (5.2 percent) (NCI, 1987).

For a grant to be approved it has to follow a complicated maze laid down by the National Cancer Act of 1971. This involves assignment to an institute by a National Institutes of Health division; review and evaluation by members of the Initial Review Groups, also known as "study sections," composed of 10–15 non-Federal scientists; a site visit from scientists chosen by NIH administrators; a meeting of the review group to vote and assign the project a priority number; consideration of the application by the NCAB, with its recommendations; a funding determination by the grants management officer; and negotiations and final review (NCI, 1986).

All along the line, bureaucrats and outside advisers of the agency are called upon to pass judgment on the application, and a strong negative opinion at several important junctures can severely damage the chances of success. For example, if the NCAB decides to overturn a recommendation for approval or disapproval for reasons other than scientific merit that decision is final. To win a grant, an applicant must please the recognized experts in his field, and almost by definition must be working within the accepted framework of that field.

To a certain degree, each person who approves an application has put their own reputation on the line in doing so. The safest and most politic thing to do is to give priority to those applications coming from the more conventional and established researchers at well-known institutions. As a sign of the faith placed in them by NCI, such institutions receive site visits less frequently. Should anything go wrong, the grant giver can justify his or her decision by the prestige of the recipient institution and the supposedly high probability of success.

To approve the grant application of a small research center (such as the Syracuse Cancer Research Institute or the Immuno-Augmentative Therapy Centre) is a difficult and dangerous undertaking for any bureaucrat or adviser. It is fraught with peril: if the project becomes an embarrassment, there inevitably will be inquiries to find out who approved the application in the first place.

A new grant request must therefore be approved by a wide variety of scientists, bureaucrats, and businesspeople. It must be the result of a *consensus* of opinion among these many individuals. Almost inevitably, such an application must be well within the bounds of conventional science. These "cumbersome constraints" make it difficult, if not impossible, for radically new ideas to be approved by the NCI.*

Another factor leading to the suppression of many new ideas is the mentality of those who lead the cancer establishment. These are powerful individuals, with long lists of achievements and publications. Some of them flat-footedly and categorically lay down the law in their particular field and do not appreciate being contradicted. Some dream of Nobel Prizes, or even of being immortalized for finding a cure for humanity's most dreaded disease. "Dusty" Rhoads was "absolutely determined that the cure for cancer was going to be found in his institute and nowhere else," reporter Bernard Glemser wrote admiringly. Those around Rhoads fed his ego. When the reporter suggested a book about Sloan-Kettering in general, an aide took him aside and said, "You don't want to write a book about all this. Do a book about the director. *He's* what counts here" (Glemser, 1969:35).

Robert A. Good, another director of Sloan-Kettering, was called "a

---

*The phrase "cumbersome constraints" is from the 1978 report of Lane W. Adams, executive vice president of the ACS. In November 1978 the ACS voted to decline future federal aid in order to maintain its independence of the government bureaucracy (ACS, 1978:3).

scientific Sammy Glick who occasionally lets his ego get in the way of his intellect . . ." (*Time*, March 19, 1973).

Time's reporter commented:

> Good, who often acts as if he is running for the Nobel Prize, does not deny their charges. "Of course, I'm an operator," he admits. "I'm the most self-centered person in the world. I'll use whatever there is to get things done the way I want them done. I hope I can become an effective operator when it comes to cancer" (ibid.:69).

Virginia Livingston attributed Rhoads's long-term opposition to her work to the fact that she was an "upstart" in the cancer field. Hostility to "upstarts" can apply not only to complete unknowns but also to well-known scientists who wander into someone else's preserve.

For example, Linus Pauling was not greeted with open arms by the medical establishment when he put forward his theories on vitamin C. Dr. H. L. Newbold was asked why he thought Pauling was repeatedly turned down by the National Cancer Institute:

> They're jealous of him because he's too famous. Things are done through personalities. You think of scientists as being objective, but science is full of little men doing their own little things. This is true of people who grant research funds (Newbold, 1979).

Another factor promoting closed-mindedness toward new ideas is social prejudice. Many of geneticist Maud Slye's problems in the 1920s and 1930s appear to have been related to the fact that she was a woman—and a single woman at that—almost fanatically devoted to her work.

> Even scientists who were supposed to be objective were prejudiced when it came to women in the scientific establishment. A number of them were quick to dismiss the work and findings of the few women scientists who were able to get their research published in the medical and scientific journals (McCoy, 1977).

Cornell professor Evelyn Fox Keller has pointed to the male bias inherent in the scientific establishment. From the outset these "gender stereotypes" have played a role in the "exclusion of women in science" (Keller, 1987; also 1983, 1985).

434

Although discrimination in science today is not nearly so prevalent as it was in the 1920s, women are still not fully integrated into the cancer establishment.* One wonders how much of the resistance to the bacterial theory is due to the fact that many of its advocates in this country have been women?**

Predictably, spokesmen for the cancer establishment deny that the suppression of new ideas even takes place. "As a result of the medical profession's insistence upon reliable standards of proof of cure," according to the American Cancer Society's book *Unproven Methods,* "the proponents of unproven remedies are prone to charge that they are being persecuted by the 'medical trust' or 'organized medicine' " (ACS, 1971b:18).

"A look at two of many well-known facts will serve to answer this charge," the ACS book states, and goes on to cite two of the triumphs of modern medicine: the discovery of penicillin and the polio vaccine. According to the Society:

> When Sir Alexander Fleming discovered penicillin, all that was demanded was that the new "medicine" measure up to rigid scientific and clinical tests, to determine its efficacy and its adverse effects, if any. The tests were met. Penicillin was adopted for medical use, and today is widely accepted as one of the most important means of treating infection (ibid.).

The example is poorly chosen, from the point of view of orthodox medicine, for Fleming's discovery was ridiculed and ignored for over a dozen years after his initial publication in 1928. Typical was the reaction of a distinguished colleague of the Scottish bacteriologist, who wrote in 1929:

> The penicillium moulds are pleasant enough and we are content to use them to bring our Camembert and Roquefort cheeses into a pleasant condition of ripeness, and in that respect I would not like to miss them. But beyond that, and especially with a view to therapy in medicine, these moulds are completely useless (Böttcher, 1964).

It was only with the approach of World War II, when huge casualties loomed and the Allies faced the loss of German sulfa drugs, that some Brit-

---

*As of 1987 at Memorial Sloan-Kettering Cancer Center, only two women held major administrative posts out of thirteen positions. None of the top positions was held by a woman. With one or two exceptions, all department chairs and program heads were male (MSKCC 1987).

**Virginia Livingston-Wheeler, Eleanor Alexander-Jackson, Irene Cory Diller, Eva Bordkin, and Camille Mermod.

ish scientists began a campaign to develop penicillin commercially (Bäumler, 1968). Two British scientists were brought to the United States in 1941, under the auspices of the Office of Scientific Research and Development (OSRD), to try to get private pharmaceutical companies interested in working on the project. "They had almost no luck," Richard Harris wrote in *The Real Voice*, summarizing the results of an investigation by Senator Estes Kefauver's staff (Richard Harris, 1964).

A few weeks after the Japanese attacked Pearl Harbor, Dr. Vannevar Bush, director of OSRD, personally brought a number of drug companies into the research effort. A year and a half later he wrote:

> Now, the pharmaceutical companies have cooperated in this affair after a fashion. They have not made their experimental results and their development of manufacturing processes generally available, however (cited in ibid.).

The problem, Harris remarked, "was that most firms were too busy trying to corner patents on various processes in the production of penicillin to produce much of it . . ." (ibid.). On January 19, 1944, the coordinator of the penicillin program of the War Production Board wrote that he could not "with a clear conscience assume the responsibility for coordinating this program" because of the refusal of the drug companies to exchange information, a refusal that was costing thousands of lives on the battlefield.

The deadlock was broken only when an obscure outpost of a government agency, the Department of Agriculture's laboratory in Peoria, Illinois, figured out how to mass-produce penicillin, took out a patent on the method, and then made "all of its patents . . . available to any producer without charge" (ibid.).

Even so, the drug companies never showed much enthusiasm for penicillin. "The synthesis of penicillin brought laurels to the scientists," wrote *Fortune* (March 1976), "but precious little else." For this reason, John McKeen, the president of Pfizer, said in 1950, "If you want to lose your shirt in a hurry, start making penicillin and streptomycin" (quoted in Rozental, 1961). Economics professor Alek A. Rozental commented further:

> Pfizer announced that it would henceforth concentrate on the development of new and exclusive antibiotic specialties. Other firms had the same idea. Today the few that control production of the broad-spectrum antibiotics (Achromycin, Terramycin, Aureomycin, and tetracyclines) have managed to avoid repetition of the "unhappy" penicillin experience (ibid.).

436

The ACS's second "well-known fact" supposedly demonstrating the fairness of organized medicine concerns the polio vaccine:

> When Dr. Salk discovered his polio vaccine, again it was only required that he provide clear proof that his vaccine was safe and effective. He did so under the most rigid rules, and the result was that the Salk vaccine shots became an accepted prophylactic measure against poliomyelitis (ACS, 1971b:18).

The Salk vaccine is certainly a triumph of modern medicine. But it is simply not true that it was required only that Salk prove his vaccine safe and effective for it to be automatically snapped up by the medical profession or the pharmaceutical industry.

The vaccine was the result of efforts by the National Foundation, a massive fund-raising organization, whose relations with the medical profession were often strained. Salk's intention of making a *killed* virus vaccine instead of a live one made him something of a maverick within the establishment. When the National Foundation announced the development of Salk's vaccine, the American Medical Association responded:

> The American medical profession was surprised and put in a difficult situation, so far as public relations were concerned in recent months, when a national health organization, without any official consultation with any qualified council or group of the American Medical Association, launched a nationwide comprehensive program for the use of a new vaccine which gives great theoretical promise of success in combatting a dread disease and yet which admittedly has been used a few months without sufficient time to evaluate the safety as well as the efficacy of the vaccine. . . . (cited in Wayne Martin, 1977:63).

When in May 1955 Cutter Laboratories sold batches of vaccine which accidentally included some live virus, and 204 cases of polio resulted, orthodox medicine attempted to stop *all* production of the Salk vaccine for two years. In fact, the Surgeon General of the United States withdrew the vaccine from use until a public uproar made him restore the program (ibid.:67).*

There is no doubt that the Salk vaccine was highly effective: It re-

---

*The hostility of the American medical profession also stemmed from the fact that the chairman of the National Foundation, Basil O'Connor, sought to raise $15 million to pay for *free* public vaccination of children in the United States. "The American Medical Association resisted the idea as being a step toward socialized medicine" (Wayne Martin, 1977).

duced the incidence of polio from 28,985 cases in 1955, to 3,190 in 1960, and 910 in 1962. The remaining cases were almost entirely among poor people who could not afford the cost of a private-doctor visit to obtain the vaccine (ibid.). Moreover, the Salk vaccine was quite safe when produced correctly. It was the responsibility of the U.S. government—not Salk—to make sure the drug companies complied with good production standards. Yet the "government remained passive during the massive field trials of 1954," which led to the debacle of 1955 (ibid.:68).

On the other hand, the Sabin vaccine, while effective, was potentially dangerous because it was made from live vaccine. In 1964, for example, the Surgeon General warned of a very small risk involved in taking this vaccine. Yet the American Medical Association, on the basis of Russian trials, endorsed the Sabin vaccine. The Salk vaccine was pushed into near-oblivion by the force of medical orthodoxy. "A vaccine which had come within 98 percent of eradicating polio and which would not cause polio," said Basil O'Connor, "was replaced with a new vaccine that could cause polio" (cited in ibid.:69).

Nor was the pharmaceutical industry's role in the Salk vaccine one that is likely to be pointed to with pride. The drug companies contributed very little to polio research—the American people did that by contributing $500 million to the March of Dimes, the National Foundation's fund-raising appeal. When a Winthrop Laboratories executive was asked by the National Foundation to participate in the development of the Salk vaccine, he declined, saying, "We felt it would be a socialized rat race" (quoted in Rozental, 1961). "This premonition," said Rozental, "seems to have been unwarranted," and he went on to state:

> When the Justice Department indicted the makers of the vaccine for criminal conspiracy and demanded to see their books on the pre-trial examination, the manufacturers opposed the request on the grounds that disclosure of their high profits might prejudice the jury (ibid.).

These are the *best* examples the American Cancer Society spokesman can come up with as proof that there is no suppression of innovation by the medical establishment! Nothing in the history of these innovations, nor of any of the other examples cited in this book, contradicts the view that new ideas often have a difficult time getting established and must face the indifference—and even the hostility—of vested interests.

As people become aware of this suppression, however, they are increasingly thrown into action against it. Millions of people no longer automatically believe what the leaders of the cancer establishment tell them. They are resisting the introduction of carcinogens into the environment; demanding alternative forms of therapy; suing companies; signing petitions; writing, picketing, and protesting. Scientists and doctors are pursuing independent avenues of research.

There is no need to exaggerate the scope of this rebellion: It is still embryonic. But given the current impasse in the war on cancer, it is most likely that it will gain strength and spread. Eventually it may play a decisive role in bringing the war on cancer to a successful conclusion.

« Appendix A »

Structure and Affiliation of the Memorial Sloan-Kettering Cancer Center Leadership

An analysis of the leadership of the world's largest private cancer center shows that those men and women with a vested interest in the cancer problem control the direction of research.

The board of overseers, reorganized in 1978, is composed of fifty-two individuals. Only four of these are medical doctors and three others are Ph.D's. Most of these serve ex officio as executives of MSKCC itself or of affiliated institutions. [See Table 9].

As indicated earlier, in the early eighties there was a major reorganization by the Board of the top administrators. Lewis Thomas retired as president and was replaced by Paul A. Marks, M.D., who took the additional title of Chief Executive Officer. Robert Good was replaced as president of Sloan-Kettering Institute by Richard A. Rifkind, M.D. (Good is presently a pediatrician at All Children's Hospital, St. Petersburg, Florida). This led to a major shake up of the professional staff. In 1988, Dr. Vincent T. DeVita became physician-in-chief.

The changes on the Board have been less drastic, which is understandable, since it was the board that initiated the new direction. Since 1979, however, certain familiar names have disappeared by attrition: Harold W. Fisher, James D. Landauer, Arnold Schwartz, William S. Sneath, T. F. Walkowicz, and Harper Woodward have all either retired or died.

Laurance S. Rockefeller retired from active management of the Board

441

APPENDIX A

TABLE 9
Boards of Overseers and Managers
Memorial Sloan-Kettering Cancer Center
December 31, 1988

Laurance S. Rockefeller
Honorary Chairman

Benno C. Schmidt
Chairman

James D. Robinson III *Vice Chairman*	Paul A. Marks, M.D. *President and Chief Executive Officer*	Richard L. Gelb *Vice Chairman*
Peter O. Crisp *Treasurer*		William Rockefeller *Secretary*

Frederick R. Adler*	Henry Forrest Hill	Frank H. T. Rhodes, Ph.D
Edward J. Beattie, M.D.	Samuel Hellman, M.D.	James D. Robinson, III*
Mrs. Elmer H. Bobst	Deane F. Johnson*	James S. Rockefeller
Mrs. H. Lawrence Bogert	Mrs. Virginia W. Kettering	Laurance S. Rockefeller*
Mrs. Edwin M. Burke	Richard D. Lombard*†	William Rockefeller*
Mrs. Joseph A. Califano Jr.	Mrs. John L. Marion*	Robert V. Roosa*
Joseph E. Connor, Jr.	Paul A. Marks, M.D.*	Benjamin M. Rosen*
Peter O. Crisp*	Elizabeth J. McCormack, Ph.D.*	Jack Rudin*
Mrs. Percy L. Douglas	John K. McKinley*	Fayez S. Sarofim
Richard M. Furlaud	W. Earle McLaughlin	Benno C. Schmidt*
Clifton C. Garvin Jr.*	Thomas A. Murphy	Frederick Seitz, Ph.D.
Richard L. Gelb*	James G. Niven*	H. Virgil Sherrill*
Louis V. Gerstner Jr.*	Alfred Ogden*	J. McLain Stewart*
Mrs. Bruce A. Gimbel*	Ellmore C. Patterson	Lewis Thomas, M.D.
Albert H. Gordon*	Mrs. Milton Petrie*	Carl W. Timpson Jr.
George V. Grune*	John S. Reed*	Arthur B. Treman Jr.*
John R. Gunn*	Mrs. Harmon L. Remmel	James H. Wickersham Jr.
Mrs. Enid A. Haupt		

Board of Overseers Emeriti

Mrs. Edward C. Delafield	Emanuel R. Piore, Ph.D.	John M. Walker, M.D.
Harold W. Fisher	Mrs. Arnold Schwartz	Thomas J. Watson Jr.

†Died of lung cancer, February 10, 1989.

of Overseers and Managers, in 1982 and took the title Honorary Chairman. Benno C. Schmidt, formerly MSKCC vice chairman and head of the President's Cancer Panel, became the new chairman. James D. Robinson III and a new member, Richard L. Gelb, became vice chairmen.

*Member of the Board of Managers.

There are more women on this board than on the old one. Unfortunately, most of these are society ladies, unlikely to influence policy decisions. (The practice of listing women as "Mrs." plus the name of their husband continues almost undiminished.) One notable exception to this rule is Elizabeth J. McCormack, Ph.D., a foundation executive who serves as a member of the MSKCC board of managers.

The full board of overseers has responsibility for "overseeing the direction of the Center" (MSKCC, 1978). It meets three times a year. This plenum group elects, in turn a board of managers that "sets policies" and "monitors the activities of the corporations" (ibid.). Actually, it elects three boards, virtually identical in membership, for the three corporations—Memorial Sloan-Kettering, Memorial Hospital, and Sloan-Kettering Institute.

The more select board of managers consists of twenty-five individuals, plus the president of the Society, MSKCC's fund-raising auxiliary.

In addition, there are a number of other committees appointed by these boards, which deal with particular aspects of managing the Center. The most significant, from the point of view of direction of research, appears to be the Institutional Policy Committee, composed of nine overseers.

Memorial Sloan-Kettering spokespersons repeatedly refused the author's recent requests for a list of its Institutional Policy Committee (IPC) members. The 1979 IPC showed heavy corporate involvement. The 1989 IPC would probably show equal or greater influence.

The industry that stands to gain the most from cancer research is the pharmaceutical business. This industry in particular has great influence on the MSKCC board, especially on the select Institutional Policy Committee.

TABLE 10

Institutional Policy Committee—MSKCC As of 1979

Lewis Thomas, M.D., chairman	Squibb, director
Benno C. Schmidt, vice chairman	Worthington Biochemical (interlock)
Edward J. Beattie, Jr., M.D.	[none known]
Richard M. Furlaud	Squibb, chairman and chief executive officer
Louis V. Gerstner, Jr.	[none known]
Robert A. Good, Ph.D., M.D.	Merck Sharp & Dohme, consultant
Laurance S. Rockefeller	Mallinckrodt (interlock)
Frederick Seitz, Ph.D.	Organon, director
William S. Sneath	Union Carbide, chairman of the board*

*Union Carbide, although not thought of as a drug company, has had an interest in cancer-related pharmaceuticals since the early 1950s (*Chemical Week*, July 24, 1954). In 1977, attempting to diversify, Union Carbide bought Cleon Corp., maker of a medical diagnostic machine, and signed a $10-million agreement to distribute a breast X-ray machine (*Business Week*, January 24, 1977). William Sneath joined the MSKCC board in the same year.

Influencing institutional policy toward a chemotherapeutic approach to cancer is certainly a key objective of the drug companies. In 1979, the committee was composed of nine members, listed on the preceding page with their pharmaceutical affiliations:

Thus, seven out of nine—or 78 percent—of the members of the Institutional Policy Committee were affiliated (or interlocked) with companies with a direct interest in the cancer drug (or diagnostics) market.

The banking and business community's two primary interests in cancer are the *causation* of cancer and the profitable *cure* of the disease. Thus it is instructive to look at who these individuals are, and what their connections are with polluting industries or with companies interested in profiting from a solution.

Much environmentally induced cancer comes from the petrochemical industry, the automobile industry, and various other major industries and companies. At least seventeen of the overseers are affiliated with such companies:

TABLE II
Industrial Ties of MSKCC Overseers—1988

Crisp, Peter O.	Rockefeller Family & Associates
Furlaud, Richard M.	Olin, director
Garvin, Clifton C., Jr.	Exxon, president
Gerstner, Louis V., Jr.	RJR Nabisco, Inc., chairman of the board
Gordon, Albert H.	Allen Group Inc., director (automotive parts, etc.)
McCormack, Elizabeth J., Ph.D.	Philip Morris, director
McKinley, John K.	Texaco, chairman of the board (ret.); Martin Marietta Corp., director
McLaughlin, W. Earle	Algoma Steel, director
Murphy, Thomas A.	General Motors, chairman of the board (ret.)
Patterson, Ellmore C.	Bethlehem Steel Corp., director
Reed, John S.	Philip Morris, United Technologies, director
Rockefeller, Laurance S.	Exxon, Mobil, Standard Oil of Indiana, Standard Oil of California, etc., major shareholder
Roosa, Robert V.	Owens-Corning Fiberglas, Texaco, director
Schmidt, Benno C.	Freeport-McMoRan, Inc. (gas, oil, uranium oxide, etc. production), chairman of the executive committee
Serafim, Fayez S.	Pennzoil, etc., major investor
Seitz, Frederick, Ph.D.	Ogden Corporation (waste incineration, aviation fueling, etc.), director
Sherrill, H. Virgil	Reliance Electric Co., chairman

Thus, seventeen overseers—or 32.7 percent—are rather closely tied to large polluting industries, especially those connected to oil, chemicals, and automobiles. This follows the traditional affiliation of both Memorial Hospital and Sloan-Kettering Institute, which have been dominated by oil and automotive fortunes, respectively.

The power of these individuals on the board is greater than may appear at first sight. In 1979, fully half (eleven out of twenty-two) of the *outside* board of managers were on this list (excluding ex officio and inside members), including the chairmen of all the Center's boards.

Their corporations produce a wide panoply of known or suspected carcinogens. Exxon is one of the world's major producers of benzene. Many of the products of the petroleum industry are prime suspects in the hunt for industrial carcinogens (Epstein, 1978). According to Ralph Nader, General Motors alone is responsible "for about a third of the nation's air pollution by tonnage" (Esposito and Silverman, 1970). American Cyanamid long represented by James B. Fisk, Ph.D., produces acrylonitrile, which, a government official claims, "can pose a life-threatening danger in a very brief period of exposure" (Epstein, 1978:211).*

And these are only the direct corporate links. If one looks at interlocks (boards on which MSKCC directors serve with other polluters) the list becomes far longer. For example, the Rockefeller-dominated Chase Manhattan Bank had a director on the board of Raybestos-Manhattan, the asbestos manufacturer. Ellmore C. Patterson's Morgan Guaranty Trust Co. had a director on the board of Johns-Manville. General Motors president Thomas A. Murphy sat on the GM board with the chairman of Allied Chemical, manufacturer of Red Dyes #2 and #40.

If one asks, like the Romans, *"Cui bono?"* (Who stands to gain?), it is immediately apparent that the overseers and managers of Memorial Sloan-Kettering have a large stake in the outcome of the cancer problem.

The other main vested interest of the overseers is in corporate investments. Many of these men and women are bankers, stockbrokers, and venture capitalists. Tabe 12, next page, confirms this.

In other words, eighteen out of fifty-two—or 34.6 percent—of the board of overseers are professional investors or persons closely associated with such investors (e.g., William Rockefeller, James D. Robinson). More significant is the manner in which these investors dominate the select board of managers. Fully fourteen out of twenty-two of the outside managers, or 64 percent, are investors by profession or closely involved with such investors.

*In fact, a 1979 strike at American Cyanamid's organic chemicals division in Bound Brook, New Jersey, centered largely around workers' concern about the possible cancer-causing hazard of the company's products (*New York Times,* January 14, 1979).

TABLE 12
Investment Ties of MSKCC Overseers—1988

Adler, Frederick A.	Venture capitalist
Crisp, Peter O.	Rockefeller Family & Associates, association
Furlaud, Richard M.	Shearson Lehman Hutton, director
Gordon, Albert H.	Kidder, Peabody & Co., chairman
Grune, George V.	Chemical Bank, director
McCormack, Elizabeth, Ph.D.	JDR 3d Fund, vice president
McLaughlin, W. Earle	Sun Alliance Insurance Co., chairman of the board
Patterson, Ellmore C.	Morgan Bank, director (former chairman)
Reed, John S.	Citibank, chairman
Robinson, James D., III	American Express, CEO, Shearson Lehman Hutton Holdings Corp., director
Rockefeller, Laurance S.	Rockefeller Brothers Fund, chairman
Rockefeller, William	Shearman Sterling, partner (law firm closely associated with Citibank)
Rosen, Benjamin M.	Venture capitalist
Roosa, Robert V.	Brown Brothers Harriman & Co., partner; American Express, director
Serafim, Fayez S.	Money manager
Schmidt, Benno C.	J. H. Whitney & Co., managing partner
Sherrill, H. Virgil	Prudential-Bache Securities, vice chairman
Wickersham, James H., Jr.	Morgan Guaranty Trust Co., vice president

Why would investors be attracted to these positions? Part of the reason seems to be the need of investors to understand the latest scientific and technological developments before they become generally available.

The career of the chairman of the board, Laurance S. Rockefeller, can be taken as a paradigm for the rest. He is a self-described venture capitalist who has made a career of turning science into money. "In venture capital investments," reads his official biographical handout, "the main line of Mr. Rockefeller's activities has involved new or young enterprises operating on the 'frontiers of technology' . . . with his risk capital keeping pace with scientific developments and changing technology. ("Laurance S. Rockefeller," 1971).

Since MSKCC is on the "frontiers of technology," this puts Rockefeller and his colleagues in a good position to pursue business, as well as philanthropic, interests.

Although it would be illegal for an overseer personally to sell products or services to the Center, it is not illegal for a public company with which he or she is associated to do so. In fact, according to the by-laws of the Center,

> no Trustee or other officer of the Corporation [i.e., MSKCC] shall be deemed to be personally interested, directly or indirectly, and no personal interest shall be presumed or inferred, solely because of his ownership of shares in any publicly owned corporation or solely because of his being an officer or director of any corporation which has any such contract with the Corporation (MSKCC, 1960).

There are a number of instances in which directors' companies appear to have benefited from their association with the Center or with other such research facilities.

Two companies in which Laurance S. Rockefeller is a major shareholder, Standard Oil of California and Standard Oil of Indiana, own 25 percent and 22 percent, respectively, of Cetus; this corporation, valued at $100 million, specializes in recombinant DNA techniques. The president of Rockefeller University, which is headed by Laurance's brother David, is chairman of Cetus's board of scientific advisers (*Science,* November 9, 1979). Since 1976 Sloan-Kettering has been deeply involved in such research as well.

An associate of Rockefeller's, M. Frederick Smith, was director of Mallinckrodt, a drug and chemical company that does extensive business with MSKCC and other cancer centers.* Such an affiliation would imply a substantial investment on Rockefeller's part (Collier and Horowitz, 1976:296). Rockefeller was an early investor in Airborne Instruments Laboratories, which produced one of the first automated cell analyzers (*New York Times,* August 23, 1954). Nationwide, the automated clinical laboratory instruments industry has grown to over half a billion dollars a year (*Business Week,* May 10, 1976).

Connections of this sort are difficult to discover, since the laws on disclosure of corporation ownership are more lax than an investigator might wish. Sometimes these links are made through interlocking board membership. Thus, biographical information on Benno Schmidt does not reveal any financial interest in the cancer field. Yet Don E. Ackerman, one of his partners at J. H. Whitney & Co., is a director of Worthington Biochemical Corporation, which has advertised its PHI monitoring system for cancer therapy in the medical journals (*Cancer,* April 1973).

---

*Mallinckrodt is a producer of radioactive tests and medicines. Since the 1950s it has been considered a leader in attempting to develop anticancer drugs in conjunction with Sloan-Kettering (*Chemical Week,* July 24, 1954).

447

TABLE 13
Drug Company Ties of MSKCC Overseers—1988

Adler, Frederick R.	Bio Technology General, Life Technologies, Inc., Scitex Corp., etc., director
Furlaud, Richard M.	Squibb, president; Pharmaceutical Manufacturers Association, director
Gelb, Richard L.	Bristol-Myers, chairman of the board
Gerstner, Louis V., Jr.	Squibb, director
Marks, Paul A., M.D.	Pfizer, director
McKinley, John K.	Merck & Co., director
Robinson, James D., III	Bristol-Myers, director

In 1954 Sloan-Kettering director C. P. Rhoads declared that future gains in cancer research would depend largely upon the pharmaceutical industry, and that without close cooperation between cancer researchers and industry, "we can see no possibility of achieving our goal . . ." (*Drug Trade News*, October 25, 1954).

At the time, the drug industry needed prodding to get involved in a serious way in the cancer field. Twenty-five years later, the industry appears not only to have become involved but also to have gained a decisive voice in the direction of research at MSKCC.

Table 13 shows the growing drug-company presence on the board. This is perhaps the most remarkable change since 1979, for not only are Squibb, Bristol-Myers, Pfizer, and Merck generously represented, but their officials hold top MSKCC positions: Dr. Paul Marks, the chief executive officer, is a director of Pfizer, and the two vice chairmen of the Center, Gelb and Robinson, are *both* officials of Bristol-Myers, the nation's preeminent manufacturer of anticancer drugs. Add to that the use of Bristol-Myers products and the Center's investment of over half a million dollars in B-M stock (see Table 8), and it all adds up to a very intimate relationship indeed.*

Finally, in Table 14 we have taken note of the board's direct influence on media companies. Two of the most powerful overseers (Gelb and Gerstner) are also directors of the New York Times Corporation; two are affiliated with Reader's Digest; Benno Schmidt has been associated with CBS; and the president of Warner Communications, Deane F. Johnson, has joined the board. Cancer policy today is often fought out in the court of public opinion. These connections, accidental or not, cannot hurt and might possi-

*In July 1989 Bristol-Myers and Squibb merged, consolidating their influence even further.

448

TABLE 14
Media Ties of MSKCC Overseers—1988

Gelb, Richard L.	New York Times Corp., director
Gerstner, Louis V., Jr.	New York Times Corp., director
Grune, George V.	Reader's Digest, chief exec. officer
Johnson, Deane F.	Warner Communications, president
Rockefeller, Laurance S.	Reader's Digest, director
Schmidt, Benno C.	CBS, director (ret.)

bly help to put forward MSKCC's particular point of view to millions of people.

Of particular importance is the growing presence (and one would presume influence) of the $55 billion cigarette industry. Two directors of Philip Morris (McCormack and Reed) and the new chairman of RJR Nabisco (Gerstner) are all influential members of the board of America's largest private cancer center. Gerstner's attitude toward the smoking-cancer connection became clear in the news stories about his appointment:

> Asked whether he had qualms about running a tobacco business—a concern of some other candidates contacted in the search—Mr. Gerstner said, "I'm sitting here smoking a cigar. No." (*Wall Street Journal*, March 14, 1989)

It is Philip Morris and RJR Nabisco that are responsible for the "richly financed nationwide campaign to organize opposition" to antismoking legislation (*New York Times*, December 24, 1988).*

It hardly seems surprising, then, that MSKCC favors an expensive-cure approach over that of prevention. And as noted elsewhere, a MSKCC scientist heads the antienvironmentalist American Council on Science and Health, and Sloan-Kettering does not have even a token program on environmental carcinogenesis (SKI, 1988).

The members of the MSKCC board represent many industrial interests, and not all of them are associated with the cancer field. Nor is it necessary to postulate a conspiracy to control cancer research. There are many reasons why a corporate investor would serve on the MSKCC board, not all of them suspect.

Nevertheless, it is clear that these directors can—and must—bring to their jobs as MSKCC officials the same general philosophy and interests that guide their business and financial activities. The result is the direction of

---

*Gerstner resigned from the MSKCC board in 1989.

research away from prevention, away from radical solutions and inexpensive remedies, and toward more profitable avenues.

In effect, the MSKCC board is a very exclusive club, which meets regularly to discuss and take actions that have repercussions for the majority of Americans. Meeting in private, keeping a low profile, they are accountable to no one but themselves for the policy decisions they make.

References

Abady, Samuel A., in conversation with Avis Lang: "Schneider v. Revici: A Victory for Cancer Patients and Nonconventional Physicians." *Cancer Victors Journal* 21(2), Summer 1987.

Acevedo, Hernan F. "Immunohistochemical Localization of a Choriogonadotrophin-like Protein in Bacteria Isolated from Cancer Patients." *Cancer* 41:1217–29, 1978.

*Agran, Larry. *The Cancer Connection—And What We Can Do About It*. Boston: Houghton Mifflin Company, 1977. [Interesting investigation of the chemical causes of cancer. Especially valuable for its interview with Dr. William C. Hueper.]

Ambruster, Howard Watson. *Treason's Peace: German Dyes and American Dupes*. New York: Beechhurst Press, 1947.

American Cancer Society. "A Twentieth Anniversary." In *Annual Report*. New York, 1965.

———. *Cancer Facts and Figures*. New York, 1971a.

———. *Unproven Methods of Cancer Management*. New York, 1971b. [Updated periodically. Indispensable guide to orthodox thinking on the question of "quackery." Not to be confused with a small pamphlet of the same name.]

———. *Annual Report*. New York, 1972.

———. *Cancer Facts and Figures*. New York, 1974.

———. "Plants That Cure and Cause Cancer." *Cancer News* 29(2), Fall 1975.

———. "Hydrazine Sulfate." *Ca—A Cancer Journal for Clinicians* (26)2, March–April 1976.

REFERENCES

————. *Annual Report*. New York, 1978. [N.B.: Annual reports are routinely published in the year following the date of their title. To avoid confusion, all such reports are listed by the year which they describe.]

————. *Cancer Facts and Figures*. New York, 1979. [The early series of ACS's *Cancer Facts and Figures* was routinely published in the year *before* the cover date; e.g., this volume was actually published in 1978. To avoid confusion, the fact books are listed according to the year to which they refer on the cover.]

————. "Unproven Methods of Cancer Management." New York: ACS, 1982.

————. "Unproven Methods of Cancer Management: Burzynski." *Ca—A Cancer Journal for Clinicians* 33:57–59, January/February 1983.

————. *Annual Report*, 1986.

————. "Unproven Methods of Cancer Management: The Metabolic Cancer Therapy of Harold W. Manner, Ph.D." *Ca—A Cancer Journal for Clinicians*, 36:185–189, May/June, 1986.

————. *Cancer Facts and Figures*. New York, 1988.

————. Hydrazine Sulfate and Cancer Cachexia: 1988. News service release from the ACS's Thirtieth Science Writers' Seminar, Daytona Beach, Florida, March 20–23, 1988b.

————. "Estimated New Cancer Cases By Sex for All Sites—U.S., 1989." *Ca—A Cancer Journal for Clinicians* 39:12–13, January/February 1989.

————. *Cancer Facts and Figures*, Atlanta, 1989.

Anderson, Alan, Jr. "The Politics of Cancer: How Do You Get the Medical Establishment to Listen?" *New York*, July 29, 1974.

*Annas, George. "Patients' Rights Movement." In *Encyclopedia of Bioethics*. New York: The Free Press, 1978. [A still-useful article in an excellent compendium.]

Antman, K.; Schnipper, L. E.; and Frei, Emil, III. "The Crisis in Clinical Cancer Research: Third-Party Insurance and Investigational Therapy." *New England Journal of Medicine* 319:46–48, July 7, 1988.

Applezweig, Norman. "Cancer and the Drug Industry: The Business of Cancer Chemotherapy." *Medical Marketing and Media* 13(1), January 1978.

Ashraf, A. Q.; Liau, M. C.; Mohabbat, M. O.; and Burzynski, S. R. "Preclinical Studies on Antineoplaston A10 Injections," *Drugs Under Experimental and Clinical Research* 12 (Supp. 1):37–47, 1986.

Ashraf, A. Q., and Burzynski, S. R. "Comparative Study of Antineoplaston A10 Levels in Plasma of Healthy People and Cancer Patients." *Advances in Experimental and Clinical Chemotherapy*, February 1988. [Workshop, 15th International Congress of Chemotherapy, July 1987.]

Bailar, J. C. "Mammography screening in women under age 50 years" (letter) 260–476, March 11, 1988. *Journal of the American Medical Association*, March 11, 1987.

Bailar, John C., III, and Smith, Elaine M. "Progress Against Cancer?" *New England Journal of Medicine* 314(19):1226–1232, May 8, 1986.

REFERENCES

Bailey, Herbert. *A Matter of Life and Death: The Incredible Story of Krebiozen.* New York: G. P. Putnam's Sons, 1958.

————. *Vitamin E, Your Key to a Healthy Heart.* New York: Arco Books, 1971.

————. *The Vitamin Pioneers.* New York: Pyramid Publications, 1972.

Barber, Bernard. "Resistance by Scientists to Scientific Discovery." *Science* 134:596–602, September 1, 1961.

Bard, Morton. "The Price of Survival for Cancer Victims." In *Where Medicine Fails,* edited by Anselm Strauss. New Brunswick, N.J.: Transaction Books, 1973.

Bäumler, Ernst. *A Century of Chemistry.* Translated by David Goodman. Düsseldorf: Econ Verlag, 1968.

Beard, H. H. *A New Approach to the Conquest of Cancer, Rheumatic and Heart Diseases.* Los Angeles: Cancer Book House, 1962.

Beard, John. *The Enzyme Treatment of Cancer and Its Scientific Basis.* London: Chatto and Windus, 1911. [Provides the theoretical underpinnings for much of the laetrile movement.]

Bernal, J. D. *The Social Function of Science.* Cambridge, Mass.: MIT Press, 1967.

————. *Science in History.* Cambridge, Mass.: MIT Press, 1971.

Bernheim, Bertram M. *The Story of the Johns Hopkins.* New York: Whittlesey House, 1948.

Block, Alex Ben. "Digital Dream, Digital Nightmare," *Forbes,* November 3, 1986.

Bloom, Mark. "AP Syndicates Blakeslee Cancer Series." *National Association of Science Writers Newsletter* 8(3), August 1979.

Blue Cross/Blue Shield. A Hospital Service Contract or Certificate. New York, 1988.

Blume, Elaine. Additional Treatment May Benefit Patients with Node-Negative Breast Cancer. News release from Office of Cancer Communications, National Cancer Institute, February 22, 1989.

*Bobst, Elmer H. *Bobst: Autobiography of a Pharmaceutical Pioneer.* New York: David McKay Company, 1973. [Unwitting self-revelations from a key member of the cancer establishment.]

Boesch, Mark. *The Long Search for the Truth About Cancer.* New York: G. P. Putnam's Sons, 1960.

Bohanon, Luther. *Opinion in the Case of Glen L. Rutherford vs. U.S.A. in the U.S. District Court for the Western Region of Oklahoma.* No. CIV-75-0218-B. December 5, 1977.

Boies, Elaine. Personal communication. October 19, 1988.

*Boly, William. "Cancer, Inc." *Hippocrates,* February 1989. [Excellent article on Biotherapeutics, Inc. Reprinted in Washington Post's *Health,* February 14, 1989.]

Borkin, Joseph. *The Crime and Punishment of I. G. Farben.* New York: Free Press, 1978.

Böttcher, Helmuth M. *Wonder Drugs—A History of Antibiotics.* Translated by Einhart Kawerau. Philadelphia: J. B. Lippincott Company, 1964.

REFERENCES

Bourne, Gaylord. *Asbestos Contamination in School Buildings*. Washington, D.C.: Public Interest Research Group, 1978.

*Brodeur, Paul. *Expendable Americans*. New York: Viking Press, 1974. [Excellent study of the asbestos problem by a *New Yorker* reporter.]

Brody, Jane, and Holleb, Arthur. *You Can Fight Cancer and Win*. New York: Times Books, 1977.

+ Bross, Irwin. Personal communication. June 15, 1979.

Brothwell, Don, and Brothwell, Patricia. *Food in Antiquity*. New York: Praeger Publishers, 1969.

Brown, E. Richard. *Rockefeller Medicine Men: Medicine and Capitalism in America*. Berkeley: University of California Press, 1979.

Brown University News Service. "One of Oldest Medicines May Assist Cancer Fight." Providence, R.I., February 10, 1976.

Burdick, Carl G. "William Bradley Coley, 1862–1936" (memoir). *Annals of Surgery* 105:152–155, January 1937.

Burk, Dean. "On the Cancer Metabolism of Minimal Deviation Hepatomas." *Proceedings of the American Association for Cancer Research* 6(9), 1965.

———. Letter to Congressman Lou Frey, Jr. May 30, 1972. *Cancer Control Journal* 1(5–6):1–6.

———. "New Approaches to Cancer Therapy." *New England Natural Food Association Bulletin*, Spring 1974a.

———. "See How They Lie, See How They Lie." *Cancer News Journal* 9(3), 1974b.

———. *A Brief on Foods and Vitamins*. Sausalito, Calif.: McNaughton Foundation, 1975.

+ ———. Personal communication. December 13, 1977.

Burnef, Frank MacFarlane. *Immunological Surveillance*. Oxford: Pergamon Press, 1970.

+ Burton, Lawrence. Personal communication. November 18, 1978.

———. Letter to Vincent DeVita, Jr. June 2, 1983.

———. Personal communication. October 28, 1988.

Burton, Lawrence, et al. "The Purification and Action of Tumor Factor Extracted from Mouse and Human Neoplastic Tissue." *Transactions of the New York Academy of Sciences* 21:700–707, June 1959.

Burton, Lawrence, and Friedman, Frank. "Detection of Tumor-Inducing Factors in Drosophilia." *Science* 124:220–21, August 3, 1956.

Burzynski, S. R.; Stolzman, Z.; Szopa, B.; Stolzman, E.; and Kaltenberg, O. P. "Antineoplaston A in Cancer Therapy." *Physiol. Chem. Phys.* 9:485, 1977.

Burzynski, S. R., and Kubove, E. "Initial Clinical Study with Antineoplaston A2 Injections in Cancer Patients with Five Years' Follow-up." *Drugs Under Experimental and Clinical Research* 13 (Supp. 1):37–47, 1987.

Burzynski, S. R. Memo to Dr. Schumacher. January 4, 1977.

———. Letter to Ven L. Narayanan. June 22, 1984. [Narayanan was Chief, Drug Synthesis & Chemistry Branch, Developmental Therapeutics Program, Division of Cancer Treatment, National Cancer Institute.]

REFERENCES

————. Letter to John M. Venditti. February 15, 1985. [Venditti was Chief, Drug Evaluation Branch, Developmental Therapeutics Program, Division of Cancer Treatment, National Cancer Institute.]

————. "Antineoplastons: History of the Research (1)." *Drugs Under Experimental and Clinical Research* 12(Supp. 1):1–9, 1986.

————. "Treatment of Bladder Cancer with Antineoplaston Formulations." *Advances in Experimental and Clinical Chemotherapy*, February 1988a. [Workshop, 15th International Congress of Chemotherapy, July 1987.]

————. "Treatment of Malignant Brain Tumors with Antineoplastons." *Advances in Experimental and Clinical Chemotherapy: Antineoplastons II*, June 1988.

————. Personal communication. March 15, 1989.

Burzynski Research Institute. Taiwanese to Benefit from U.S. Biotechnological Breakthrough Regarding Cancer. October 12, 1988. News release.

————. A Brief History of His IND Application to the Food and Drug Administration. February 1989a.

————. Experimental U.S. Biotechnological Cancer Treatment to be Tested by Major European Pharmaceutical Company. March 13, 1989b. News release.

*Cairns, John. "The Treatment of Diseases and the War Against Cancer." *Scientific American* 253:51–9, November 1985. [Eloquent advocacy of prevention. Indispensable.]

California Cancer Commission. "The Treatment of Cancer with 'Laetriles.' " *California Medicine* 78(4), April 1953.

Cameron, Ewan and Pauling, Linus. *Cancer and Vitamin C.* Menlo Park: Linus Pauling Institute of Science and Medicine, 1979. [Bookstore distribution by W. W. Norton & Co., New York. The basic text on theory of ascorbic acid's effect on cancer.]

Cameron/Friedlander, Inc. *Immunology Center—Cancer Release.* Fort Lauderdale, Fla., 1979.

Cancer Care, Inc. *The Impact, Costs and Consequences of Catastrophic Illness on Patients and Families.* New York, 1973.

————. Legislative Memorandum. To Hon. Lloyd Bentsen. Re: catastrophic illness in children. April 7, 1988.

Cancer Information Service. *National Cancer Institute Statement on Mammography.* New York: Memorial Sloan-Kettering Cancer Center, November 1977.

————. *National Cancer Institute Statement on Vitamin C.* New York: Memorial Sloan-Kettering Cancer Center, April 12, 1978.

Cancer Research Institute. *A Review of Progress and Hope.* New York, 1976.

————. Annual Report, 1987.

Cancer Scandal: The Policies and Politics of Failure. New York: Patient Rights Legal Action Fund, 1988. Videotape. [See Appendix B for further information.]

Cannon, Hugh C. Letter to Hon. Al Swift. September 18, 1985. [Essentially identical to Roger C. Wetherell's undated (1984?) letter to Senator Lloyd Bentsen.]

Cantor, Robert Chernin. *And a Time to Live.* New York: Harper and Row, 1978.

REFERENCES

Cantwell, Alan R., and Kelso, Dan W. "Acid-Fast Bacteria in Scleroderma and Morphea." *Archives of Dermatology* 4, June 1971.

*Caplan, Ronald L. "The Clash Over Quackery." *Health PAC Bulletin,* Winter 1987. [Sympathetic to freedom of choice.]

Carper, Jean. "Foods for Fending Off Cancer." *Washington Post Health Plus,* March 14, 1989.

Carswell, E. A., Old, L. J., Kassel, R. L., et al. "An Endotoxin-Induced Serum Factor That Causes Necrosis of Tumors." *Proceedings of the National Academy of Sciences U.S.A.* 72:3666–70, 1975. [Now-classic paper on discovery of TNF.]

Carter, Richard. *The Gentle Legions.* New York: Doubleday and Company, 1961.

+ Carter, Stephen. Meeting on Amygdalin. Bethesda, Md., March 4, 1975. Photocopy. [Minutes by co-chairman and deputy director of Division of Cancer Treatment, National Cancer Institute. Obtained under the Freedom of Information Act.]

Carter, Stephen, and Kershner, Lorraine M. "Cancer Chemotherapy: What Drugs Are Available." *Medical Times,* February 1976.

Cassileth, B. R.; Lusk, E. J.; Strouse, T. B.; and Bodenheimer, B. J. "Contemporary Unorthodox Treatments in Cancer Medicine." *Annals of Internal Medicine* 101:105–112, 1984.

Cassileth, B. R.; Trock, B. J.; Lusk, E. J.; Blake, A.; Walsh, W. P.; and Arnholz, D. Report of a survey of patients receiving immunoaugmentative therapy. Philadelphia: University of Pennsylvania Cancer Center, September, 1987. [Photocopy of prepublication draft. Report has not been published.]

Cassileth, B. R., and Brown, Helene. "Unorthodox Cancer Medicine." *Ca–A Cancer Journal for Clinicians* 38:3, May/June 1988.

Centers for Disease Control [CDC]. "Recommendations for Protection Against Viral Hepatitis," *Annals of Internal Medicine* 103:391–402, 1985. [Recommendations of the Government's Immunization Practices Advisory Committee.]

Chabner, Bruce. Statement Before the National Committee to Review Current Procedures for Approval of New Drugs for Cancer and AIDS. January 4, 1989. [Distributed by Office of Cancer Communication, National Cancer Institute.]

Chlebowski, R. T.; Heber, D.; Richardson, B.; and Block, J. B. "Influence of Hydrazine Sulfate on Abnormal Carbohydrate Metabolism in Cancer Patients with Weight Loss." *Cancer Research* 44:857–861, 1984.

Chlebowski, R. T.; Bulcavage, L.; Grosvenor, R. D.; et al. "Hydrazine Sulfate in Cancer Patients with Weight Loss, A Placebo-Controlled Clinical Experience." *Cancer* 59:406–410, 1987a.

———. "Influence of Hydrazine Sulfate on Survival in Non–Small Cell Lung Cancer: A Randomized, Placebo-Controlled Trial." *Proceedings of ASCO* 6, March 1987b.

Chlebowski, R. T. "Significance of Altered Nutritional Status in Acquired Immune Deficiency Syndrome (AIDS)." *Nutrition and Cancer* 7:85–91, 1985.

———. Personal communication. April 3, 1989.

Chowka, Peter Barry. "An Interview with Dr. Gio Gori." *East West,* January 1978a.

REFERENCES

*————. "The National Cancer Institute and the Fifty-Year Cover-Up." *East West,* January 1978b. [One in a series of provocative essays by a bright young critic of establishment medicine.]

*————. "The Cancer Charity Rip-Off." *East West,* July 1978c.

————. "U.S. to Test Laetrile." *New Age,* February 1979.

*————. "Cancer 1988." *East West,* December 1987. [Fact-filled review of 16 years of the war on cancer. Calls for a "healing peace."]

Clark, Sir George. *A History of the Royal College of Physicians of London.* Vol. I. Oxford: Oxford University Press, 1964.

Clement, R. J.; Burton, L.; Lampe, G. N. "Peritoneal Mesothelioma." *Quantum Medicine: A Journal of Comparative Therapeutics* 1(1–2):68–70, 1988.

+ Clement, R. J. Personal communication. November 18, 1978.

Cohen, Herman, and Strampp, Alice. "Bacterial Synthesis of a Substance Similar to Human Chorionic Gonadotrophin." *Proceedings of the Society for Experimental Biology and Medicines* 152(3), July 1976.

Coley, William B. "A Preliminary Note on the Treatment of Inoperable Sarcoma by the Toxic Product of Erysipelas." *Post-graduate* 8:278–86, 1893.

*————. "The Cancer Symposium at Lake Mohonk." *American Journal of Surgery* (New Series) 1:222–25, October 1926. [Coley's call for an open-minded attitude on all unorthodox approaches to the cancer problem.]

Collier, Peter, and Horowitz, David. *The Rockefellers: An American Dynasty.* New York: Holt, Rinehart and Winston, 1976.

Collins, Vincent J. *Principles of Anesthesiology.* Philadelphia: Lea and Febiger, 1966.

Committee for Freedom of Choice in Cancer Therapy, Inc. *Anatomy of a Cover-Up: Successful Sloan-Kettering Amygdalin (Laetrile) Animal Studies.* Los Altos, Calif., 1975.

*Considine, Bob. *That Many May Live.* New York: Memorial Center for Cancer and Allied Diseases, 1959. [Informative but one-sided history of Memorial Hospital from 1880s to 1950s.]

Creagan, Edward T.; Moertel, Charles G.; et al. "Failure of High-Dose Vitamin C (Ascorbic Acid) Therapy to Benefit Patients with Advanced Cancer." *New England Journal of Medicine* 301:687–90, September 27, 1979.

*Crile, George, Jr. *What Women Should Know About the Breast Cancer Controversy.* New York: Pocket Books, 1974. [Simply written but powerful argument against radical mastectomy, by a leading surgeon.]

Culbert, Michael. *Vitamin B-17: Forbidden Weapon Against Cancer.* New Rochelle, N.Y.: Arlington House, 1974. [Laetrilist "bible" by a prolific and witty advocate of unconventional ideas.]

————. *Freedom from Cancer.* Seal Beach, Calif.: '76 Press, 1976.

————. Personal communication. August 27, 1988.

Curie, Eve. *Madame Curie.* Translated by Vincent Sheean. Garden City, N.Y.: Doubleday and Company, 1943.

Curt, Gregory A., et al. "Immunoaugmentative Therapy: A Primer on the Perils of Unproved Treatments." *JAMA* 255(4), January 24/31, 1986. [See also *JAMA* 259:3457–3458, 1988.]

REFERENCES

D'Angio, Giulio J. "Pediatric Cancer in Perspective: Cure Is Not Enough." *Cancer* 35(3), March 1975.

Danova, L. A., et al. "Results of Administration of Hydrazine Sulfate to Patients with Hodgkin's Disease." *Therapeutics Archives: Questions in Hematology* (Moscow) 49:45–47, 1977.

*Davis, Michael. "Medical Freedom Fighters." *East West*, November 1988. [Contains text of the Health Care Rights Amendment proposed by CAHAH, the Coalition for Alternatives in Nutrition and Healthcare, Inc., P.O. Box B-12, Richlandtown, PA 18955.]

+ Delaney, T. Gerald. An Update on Laetrile. New York: MSKCC Department of Public Affairs, January 26, 1977a. Memorandum.

+ ———. Statement on Laetrile. New York: MSKCC Department of Public Affairs, February 1, 1977b. Memorandum.

de Haen, Paul. "New Drug Introduction 1973–74." *Journal of the American Medical Association* 234(7), November 17, 1975.

Delmotte, N., and Meiren, L. van der. "Recherches Bactériologiques et Histologiques Concernant la Sclérodermie." *International Journal of Dermatology* (Basel) 107(3), 1953.

DeVita, Vincent T. Letter to Dr. Burton. December 1, 1982.

DeVita, Vincent T., Jr. "Breast Cancer Therapy: Exercising All Our Options" (editorial). *New England Journal of Medicine* 320:527–529, February 23, 1989.

Diagnostic and Therapeutic Technology Assessment. "Immunoaugmentative Therapy." *Journal of the American Medical Association* 259:3477–3480, June 17, 1988. [See accompanying editorial by Stuart I. Nightingale of the FDA. See also Wiewel, 1988, and Houston, 1988.]

Douglas, J. F.; Huff, J.; Peters, A. C. "No Evidence of Carcinogenicity for *L*-Ascorbic Acid (Vitamin C) in Rodents." *Journal of Toxicology and Environmental Health* 14:605–609, 1984.

DuBois, Josiah E., Jr. *The Devil's Chemists*. Boston: Beacon Press, 1952.

Dumoff, Alan. Meeting Notes: National Committee to Review Current Procedures for Approval of New Drugs for Cancer and AIDS. January 4, 1989. [Distributed by Project Cure, Dothan, AL.]

Dunham, W. B.; Zuckerkandl, E.; Reynolds, R.; Willoughby, R.; Marcuson, R.; Barth, R.; and Pauling, L. "Effects of Intake of *L*-Ascorbic Acid on the Incidence of Dermal Neoplasms Induced in Mice by Ultraviolet Light." *Proceedings of the National Academy of Sciences USA* 79:7532–7536, December 1982.

Eddy, D. M., Hasselblad, V., McGivhey, W., Hendee, W. "Mammography screening in women under age 50 years" (letter). *Journal of the American Medical Association*, 260:475, March 11, 1988.

Edson, Lee. "The Cancer Rip-Off." *Science Digest*, September 1974.

Ehrenreich, Barbara, and English, Deirdre. *Complaints and Disorders: The Sexual Politics of Sickness*. Old Westbury, N.Y.: Feminist Press, 1973.

Ellison, N. M. "Special Report on Laetrile: The NCI Laetrile Review—Results of the National Cancer Institute's Retrospective Laetrile Analysis." *New England Journal of Medicine* 299:549–52, September 7, 1978.

*Epstein, Samuel S. *The Politics of Cancer.* San Francisco: Sierra Club Books, 1978 (rev. ed. Garden City, N.Y.: Anchor Press/Doubleday, 1979). [Exhaustive study of environmental carcinogens by a leading advocate of prevention.

*Epstein, Samuel S. Are We Losing the War Against Cancer? *Congressional Record.* 100th Cong. Vol. 133, no. 135, September 9, 1987. [Stirring call for a total change in cancer policy toward prevention.]

Eriguchi, N.; Hara, H.; Yoshida, H.; Nishida, H.; Nakayama, T.; Tsuda, H.; Inoue, S.; and Ikeda, I. "Chemopreventive Effect of Antineoplaston A10 on Urethane-induced Pulmonary Neoplasm in Mice." *Journal of the Japan Society for Cancer Therapy* 23 (7):1560–1565, July, 1988.

Esposito, John C., and Silverman, Larry J., eds. *Vanishing Air: The Ralph Nader Study Group Report on Air Pollution.* Foreword by Ralph Nader. New York: Grossman Publishers, 1970.

Everson, T. C., and Cole, W. H. *Spontaneous Regression of Cancer.* Philadelphia: W. B. Saunders Company, 1966.

Ewing, James. *Neoplastic Diseases.* 2nd ed. Philadelphia: W. B. Saunders and Company, 1922.

———. *Neoplastic Diseases.* 4th ed. Philadelphia: W. B. Saunders and Company, 1940.

Ewing, Kenneth P. Affidavit for Search Warrant. U.S. District Court, Southern District of Texas. Magistrate's Case No. H-85-321M. July 16, 1985.

Eyerly, Robert. "Laetrile: Focus on the Facts" (interview). *CA—A Cancer Journal for Clinicians* 26(1), January–February 1976.

Farrington, Benjamin. *Science and Politics in the Ancient World.* London: Unwin University Press, 1965.

Feuer, Lewis S., ed. *Marx and Engels, Basic Writings on Politics and Philosophy.* Garden City: Anchor Books, 1959.

Fieve, Ronald R. *Moodswing: The Third Revolution in Psychiatry.* New York: Bantam Books, 1976.

*Fink, John M. *Third Opinion: An International Directory of Alternative Therapy Centers for the Treatment and Prevention of Cancer.* Garden City Park, N.Y.: Avery Publishing Group, Inc., 1988. [Useful compendium for those seeking alternatives.]

Fisher, B.; Redmond, C.; Dimitrov, N. V.; et al. "A Randomized Clinical Trial Evaluating Sequential Methotrexate and Fluorouracil in the Treatment of Patients with Node-Negative Breast Cancer Who Have Estrogen-Receptor-Negative Tumors." *New England Journal of Medicine* 320:473–478, February 23, 1989.

Fisher, B.; Costantino, P. H.; and Redmond, C. "A Randomized Clinical Trial Evaluating Tamoxifen in the Treatment of Patients with Node-Negative Breast Cancer Who Have Estrogen-Receptor-Positive Tumors." *New England Journal of Medicine* 320:479–484, February 23, 1989.

REFERENCES

Fisher, Bernard, et al. "Surgical Adjuvant Chemotherapy in Cancer of the Breast." *Annals of Surgery* 161:339–56, 1968.

Fogg, Susan. "Laetrile Tests on Cancer Patients Delayed." *Mobile* [Ala.] *Press*, March 21, 1979.

+ Fogh, Jørgen. Personal communication. January 3, 1979.

+ Food and Drug Administration. Meeting on Laetrile. Beltsville, Md., July 2, 1974. Photocopy. [Part of these minutes, obtained under the Freedom of Information Act, are signed by H. L. Walker, M.D.]

————. *Consumer Memo: Laetrile*. DHEW Publ. No. (FDA) 75-3007. Beltsville, Md., 1975.

Frank, Irwin N., et al. "Urological and Male Genital Cancers." In *Clinical Oncology—A Multidisciplinary Approach*. 6th ed., edited by Philip Rubin. American Cancer Society, 1983.

Frank, Mark D. "A Drug to Fight Cancer's Starvation Effects." United Press International feature. New York, January 26, 1979.

Fraumeni, Joseph F., Jr., ed. *Persons at High Risk of Cancer*. New York: Academic Press, 1975.

+ Fredericks, Carleton. Personal communication. November 25, 1978.

*Frontline. "Prescriptions for Profits." WGBH-TV, Boston. Produced by David Fanning. Aired on PBS, March 28, 1989. [Transcript available for $5 from Frontline, Box 322, Boston, MA 02123. An excellent exposé of how pharmaceutical companies manipulate the public, the FDA, and the medical profession to launch new drugs—in this case, patented painkillers—into a competitive marketplace.]

+ Garfinkel, Lawrence. Personal communication. October 2, 1979. [Garfinkel was vice president for epidemiology and statistics at the American Cancer Society.]

Garrison, Omar. *Dictocrats: Our Unelected Rulers*. Chicago: Books for Today, 1970.

Gastrointestinal Tumor Study Group. "Adjuvant Therapy of Colon Cancer—Results of a Prospective Randomized Trial." *New England Journal of Medicine* 310: March 22, 1984. [Charles Moertel was one of the study participants.]

Gershanovich, M. L.; Filov, V. A. "Hydrazine Sulfate in Late Stage Cancer: Completion of Initial Clinical Trials in 225 Evaluable Patients." Abstract 969 in *Proceedings*, Seventieth Annual Meeting of the American Association for Cancer Research. Edited by S. Weinhouse. Baltimore: Cancer Research, Inc., 1979.

Gershanovich, M. L.; Danova, L. A.; Ivin, B. A.; and Filov, V. A. "Results of Clinical Study of Antitumor Action of Hydrazine Sulfate." *Nutrition and Cancer* 3:7–12, 1981.

*Gerson, Max. *A Cancer Therapy—Results of Fifty Cases*. New York: Whittier Books, 1958. [Documented presentation of Gerson's theories and cases.]

Gibbons, John. Letter to Senator Charles E. Grassley. November 2, 1988.

Gieringer, Dale H. "Compassion vs. Control: FDA Investigational Drug Regulation." *Cato Institute Policy Analysis* No. 72, May 20, 1986. [Libertarian viewpoint.]

Glasser, Ronald. *The Greatest Battle*. New York: Random House, 1979.

REFERENCES

Glemser, Bernard. *Man Against Cancer*. New York: Funk and Wagnalls, 1969.

Gold, Joseph. "Proposed Treatment of Cancer by Inhibition of Gluconeogenesis." *Oncology* 22:185–207, 1968.

———. "Inhibition of Walker 256 Intramuscular Carcinoma in Rats by Administration of Hydrazine Sulfate." *Oncology* 25:66–71, 1971a.

———. "Combination of Therapy of Hydrazine with Cytoxan and Mitomycin C on Walker 256 Intramuscular Carcinoma in Rats." *Proceedings of the American Association for Cancer Research* 12(9), 1971b.

———. "Inhibition by Hydrazine Sulfate and Various Hydrazides of In-Vivo Growth of Walker 256 Intramuscular Carcinoma, B-16 Melanoma, Murphy-Sturm Lymphosarcoma, and L-1210 Solid Leukemia." *Oncology* 27:69–80, 1973.

+———. Letter to Manuel Ochoa, M.D. April 3, 1974.

———. "Enhancement by Hydrazine Sulfate of Anti-Tumor Effectiveness of Cytoxan, Mitomycin C, Methotrexate, and Bleomycin in Walker 256 Carcinosarcoma in Rats." *Oncology* 31:44–53, 1975a.

+———. Personal communication. June 16, 1975b.

———. "Use of Hydrazine Sulfate in Terminal or Preterminal Cancer Patients: Results of Investigational New Drug (IND) Study in 84 Evaluable Patients." *Oncology* 32:1–10, 1975c.

+———. Personal Communication. June 21, 1979.

———. "Hydrazine Sulfate: A Current Perspective." *Nutrition and Cancer* 9:59–66, 1987.

———. Personal communication. November 20, 1988.

Gong, Viktor, and Rudnich, Norman. *AIDS—Facts and Issues*. New Brunswick: Rutgers University Press, 1986.

Goodell, Jeffrey. "Whose Cancer Is It Anyway?" *Seven Days*, March 29, 1989.

Green, Saul, "Cancer and Surveillance by the Immune System in Man," *Cope*, April/May, 1989.

+Grauer, Marshall Jay. Letter to Dr. Lewis Thomas. November 24, 1975.

Green, Thomas. *Gynecology*. Boston: Little, Brown and Company, 1971.

Greenberg, Daniel S. "A Critical Look at Cancer Coverage." *Columbia Journalism Review*, January–February 1975.

Greenberg, David M. "The Vitamin Fraud in Cancer Quackery." *The Western Journal of Medicine* 122:345–48, April 1975.

Greenberg, E. R., et al. "Social and Economic Factors in the Choice of Lung Cancer Treatment." *The New England Journal of Medicine* 318(10):612 ff., March 10, 1988.

Griffin, G. Edward. *World Without Cancer: The Story of Vitamin B-17*. Thousand Oaks, Calif.: American Media, 1975.

Grossman, John, "Quackbuster," *Hippocrates*, November/December, 1988.

Gunther, John. *Death Be Not Proud: A Memoir*. New York: Harper and Brothers, 1949.

Gyarfas, William J. Letter to S. R. Burzynski. May 31, 1983.

Halstead, Bruce. *Amygdalin (Laetrile) Therapy*. Los Altos, Calif.: Committee for Freedom of Choice in Cancer Therapy, 1977.

REFERENCES

Harper, Harold W. and Culbert, Michael L. *How You Can Beat the Killer Diseases.* New Rochelle, N.Y.: Arlington House, 1977.

+ Harris, Mrs. Bertha. Personal communication. November 4, 1979.

Harris, Richard. *The Real Voice.* New York: Macmillan Publishing Company, 1964.

Harris, H. Seale. *Woman's Surgeon: The Life Story of J. Marion Sims.* New York: Macmillan Publishing Company, 1950.

Haught, S. J. *Has Max Gerson a True Cancer Cure?* Canoga Park, Calif.: Major Books, 1962.

Hecht, Annabel. "DES Update." *FDA Consumer,* April 1986.

Henney, Jane E. "Unproven Methods of Cancer Treatment," in DeVita, Vincent T., et al.

Henriksen, Ole. "Cachexia of Malignancy Treated with New Drug or Enteral Nutrition." *Research Resources Reporter,* 13(2), February, 1989. [An article by Gold is mentioned in the "Additional Reading" section.]

Hile, Joseph P. Letter to Dr. S. R. Burzynski. April 17, 1986. [From the associate commissioner for regulatory affairs, Food and Drug Administration.]

———. Letter to H. Tsuda. April 17, 1986. [*Practices of Oncology,* Philadelphia-Lippincott, 1985.]

Hixson, Joseph. *The Patchwork Mouse.* Garden City, N.Y.: Doubleday and Company, 1976a.

———. "Vitamin A and the Forces That Be." *Harper's,* June 1976b.

Hoefer-Amidei Public Relations. Linus Pauling Rebuts New Mayo Study on Vitamin C. San Francisco, September 28, 1979. Press release.

Hoffman, Frederick L. *Cancer and Diet.* Baltimore: Williams and Wilkins Company, 1937.

Hoffman, Mark S., ed. *The World Almanac and Book of Facts—1988.* New York: 1987.

Holcomb, Terry Lee. Personal communication. November 27, 1988.

Holleb, Arthur I. "Risks vs. Benefits in Breast Cancer Diagnosis" (editorial). *CA—A Cancer Journal for Clinicians* 26(1), January–February 1976.

Houston, Robert. "Dietary Nitriloside and Sickle Cell Anemia in Africa." *American Journal of Clinical Nutrition* 27:766, August 1974.

*———. "Food for Peace?" *Our Town,* December 24, 1978. [One in a series of iconoclastic pieces on cancer in a New York community newspaper.]

*———. "Contributing to Cancer." *Our town,* April 1, 1979a.

*———. "The Burton Syndrome." *Our Town,* April 22, 1979b.

———. "Reply to Letter." *Our Town,* June 24, 1979c.

*———. *Repression and Reform in the Evaluation of Alternative Cancer Therapies.* Otho, IA: IATPA, 1987a. (Reprinted in the *Townsend Letter for Doctors* 58–65, May–December 1988.) [An excellent study of the current impasse in the evaluation of alternatives, with explicit suggestions for change.]

———. "Statistics, Data and Evidence in Medicine: Tools for Suppression." *The Null Report* 299, April 4, 1987b.

———. Analysis of a Survey of Patients on Immuno-Augmentative Therapy. Photocopy, [Available through IATPA.] 1988, See Appendix B.

REFERENCES

————. Letter to the Editor. *Journal of the American Medical Association* 260:3435, December 16, 1988. [Articulate response to the negative DATTA survey of IAT by a science writer sympathetic to Burton's approach. See also Wiewel (1988).]

Houston, Robert, and Null, Gary. "War on Cancer: A Long Day's Dying." *Our Town*, October 29, 1978.

+ Howard, Frank. Speech at Sloan-Kettering Institute dinner. New York, October 18, 1955.

+ ————. Organizing for Technical Progress. Speech delivered in the Engineering Administration Program of George Washington University. Washington, D.C., December 5, 1956. Privately printed.

+ ————. Industrial Cooperation in Cancer Chemotherapy Research. Paper delivered at the 8th International Cancer Congress, Moscow, July 25, 1962. Privately printed.

*Huebner, Albert L. "The No-Win War on Cancer." *East West*, December 1987. [An excellent review of developments in cancer from the alternative-dietary point of view.]

Huffman, J. D. *Gynecology and Obstetrics*. Philadelphia: W. B. Saunders Company, 1962.

Hunt, Charles W. "AIDS and Capitalist Medicine." *Monthly Review*, January 1988. [See also Layon and D'Amico, below.]

————. "AIDS-Systemic and Individual Analysis." Monthly Review, April 1989.

Hunter, Beatrice Trum. "The Significance of Form." *Consumers' Research*, June 1987.

*Hunter, Donald. *The Diseases of Occupations*. 6th ed. Boston: Little, Brown and Company, 1978.

IAT Clinic. IAT: Immuno-Augmentative Therapy, Cancer Research and Treatment. Freeport, Grand Bahama. Patient brochure. n.d. [Internally dated to 1987.]

IATPA. Resolution to the Congress. June, 1986.

————. History of the IAT Patients' Association. May 1988.

Immunology Researching Centre, Ltd. Current Fee Schedule. Freeport, Bahamas, 1979.

Inosemtzeff, F. J. "Histoire de Deux Cas de Fongus Médullaire, Traités avec Succès par l'Emploi des Narcotiques." *Gazette Medicale de Paris* 37:577–82, 1845.

Institute of Medicine, National Academy of Sciences. *Mobilizing Against AIDS: The Unfinished Story of a Virus*. Cambridge: Harvard University Press, 1986. [Eve K. Nichols, writer. Based on presentations at the annual meeting of the Institute of Medicine, National Academy of Sciences.]

International Workshop on Interferon in the Treatment of Cancer. *Report*. New York: Memorial Sloan-Kettering Cancer Center, March 31, April 1, and April 2, 1975.

Israël, Lucien. *Conquering Cancer*. New York: Random House, 1978.

Issels, J. *Cancer: A Second Opinion*. London: Hodder and Stoughton, 1975.

James, M., Smith, R. L., and Williams R. T. "Conjugates of phenylacetic Acid

REFERENCES

with Taurine and other Amino Acids in various species," *Biochemical Journal* 124-15P, May, 1971.

*Johnston, Barbara. "Clinical Effects of Coley's Toxin. 1. A Controlled Study. 2. A Seven-Year Study." *Cancer Chemotherapy Reports* 21:19–68, August 1962. [One of the few controlled double-blind studies ever conducted on an "unproven method of cancer management." Remarkable photographs of regressions.]

+ ———. Personal communication. December 27, 1976.

Johnson, George. "Dr. Krim's Crusade." *New York Times Magazine*, February 14, 1988.

Johnson, Millard A. Letter to Dr. S. R. Burzynski. February 22, 1989. [Johnson is attorney for Mr. Billy W. Brown.]

Jones, Hardin B. "A Report on Cancer." Speech delivered to the ACS 11th Annual Science Writers' Conference. New Orleans, La., March 7, 1969. (Reprinted in *The Choice*, May 1977.)

———. *Transactions of the New York Academy of Sciences* (Series 2) 18:298–333, February 1956.

Judis, John B. "Mission: Impossible." *New York Times Magazine*, September 25, 1988.

Jukes, Thomas H. "Human Testing." *Nature* 261:451, June 10, 1976.

Kampalath, B. N.; Liau, M. C.; Burzynski, B.; and Burzynski, S. R. "Chemoprevention by Antineoplaston A10 of Benzo(a)pyrene-induced Pulmonary Neoplasia." *Drugs Under Experimental and Clinical Research* 13 (Supp. 1):51–55, 1987.

Karnofsky, David A. "Cancer Quackery: Its Causes, Recognition and Prevention." *The American Journal of Nursing*, April 1959.

Kassel, Robert, et al. "Complement in Cancer." In *Biological Amplification Systems in Immunology*, edited by Noorbibi K. Day and Robert A. Good. New York: Plenum Publishing Corporation, 1977.

Kassel, Robert; Burton, Lawrence; and Friedman, Frank. "Utilization of an Induced *Drosophila* Melanoma in the Study of Mammalian Neoplasms." *Annals of the New York Academy of Sciences* 100:791–816, February 15, 1963.

Kassel, Robert; Burton, Lawrence; Friedman, Frank; and Harris, J. J. "Synergistic Action of Two Refined Leukemic Tissue Extracts in Oncolysis of Spontaneous Tumors." *Transactions of the New York Academy of Sciences* 25:39–44, November 1962.

Katz, Jay. *Experimentation with Human Beings.* New York: Russell Sage Foundation, 1972.

Kellen, J. A.; Kolin, A.; and Acevedo, H. F. "Effects of Antibodies to Choriogonadotropin in Malignant Growth *I:* Rat 3230 AC Mammary Adenocarcinoma." *Cancer* 49-2300-2304, June 1, 1982a.

Kellen, J. A.; Kolin, A.; Mirakian, A.; and Acevedo, H. F. "Effects of Antibodies to Choriogonadotropin in Malignant Growth *II:* Solid Transplantable Rat Tumors." *Cancer Immunology and Immunotherapy.* Heidelberg: Springer-Verlag, 1982b.

REFERENCES

Keller, Evelyn Fox. *A Feeling for the Organism: The Life and Work of Barbara McClintlock.* New York: Freeman, 1983.

———. *Reflections on Gender and Science.* New Haven: Yale University Press, 1985.

———. "Women in Science" (letter). *Science* 236-507, May 1, 1987.

+ Kisner, Daniel L. Letter to Joseph Gold. November 7, 1978.

Klass, Alan. *There's Gold in Them Thar Pills.* Baltimore: Penguin Books, 1975.

+ Kline, Tim. Personal communication. November 7, 1979.

Knauer, Virginia. Speech to the National Health Fraud Conference. National Press Club. Washington, D.C., September 11, 1985. Photocopy.

Kohler, Robert E. *From Medical Chemistry to Biochemistry: The Making of a Biomedical Discipline.* Cambridge: Cambridge University Press, 1982.

+ Koide, Samuel. Personal communication. July 20, 1979.

*Kotelchuck, David. "Asbestos Research: Winning the Battle But Losing the War." *Health/PAC Bulletin* 61, November–December 1974. [Thorough investigation of the role of the scientific profession in the asbestos problem.]

Krebs, Ernst T., Jr. "The Nitrilosides (Vitamin B-17): Their Nature, Occurrence, and Metabolic Significance." *Journal of Applied Nutrition* 22:3–4, 1970.

———. *The Extraction, Identification, and Packaging of Therapeutically Effective Amygdalin.* Redwood City, Calif.: Nutrisearch Foundation, 1979.

Kreig, Margaret. *Green Medicine: The Search for Plants That Heal.* Chicago: Rand McNally, 1964.

Kunst, Leonard, and Ladas, Harold. "Criterion Measures in the War on Cancer: Cure, Remission, Response and Treatment." *Cancer Victors Journal* 21(2), Summer 1987.

Kushner, Rose. *Breast Cancer: A Personal History and an Investigative Report.* New York: Harcourt Brace Jovanovich, 1975. [Now called *Alternatives*]

Land, Gail. Personal communication. March 28, 1989. [Land is "information specialist" for the Livingston-Wheeler Medical Clinic.]

Lang, Avis, ed. *On the Public Record: Cancer Patients Take the U.S. Government to Court—Excerpts from the Transcript.* New York: Patient Rights Legal Action Fund, October 1986.

———. The Disease of Information Processing. Interview with Dr. S. R. Burzynski. September 22, 1986, and January 21, 1987a. Photocopy.

———. "Cancer Patients vs. the FDA: Two-Year Legal Battle Continues." *Cancer Victors Journal* 21(2), Summer 1987b.

———. "The Covert War Against Cancer Patients: Notes from the Front." *Townsend Letter for Doctors* 66, January 1989.

Langton, H. H. *James Douglas: A Memoir.* Toronto: Privately printed, 1940.

Laszlo, John. *Understanding Cancer.* New York: Harper & Row, 1987. [Survey by senior vice president for research of American Cancer Society; takes some surprising positions.]

+ Laurence S. Rockefeller. New York, June 1971. Biographical sketch, official handout.

Layon, A. Joseph, and D'Amico, Robert. "AIDS, Capitalism and Technology: A

Reply to Charles Hunt." *Monthly Review*, December 1988. [See also Hunt, above.]

Leaf, Alexander, and Launois, John. *Youth in Old Age*. New York: McGraw-Hill, 1975.

Lee, S. S., and Burzynski, S. R. "Tissue Culture and Animal Toxicity Studies of Antineoplaston A5." *Drugs Under Experimental and Clinical Research* 13 (Supp. 1):31–35, 1987.

Lehner, A. F.; Burzynski, S. R.; and Hendry, L. B. "3-Phenylacetylamino-2,6-piperidinedione, A Naturally-occurring Analogue with Apparent Antineoplastic Activity, May Bind to DNA." *Drugs under Experimental and Clinical Research* 12(Supp. 1):57–72, 1986.

Lerner, Harvey J., and Regelson, William. "Clinical Trial of Hydrazine Sulfate in Solid Tumors." *Cancer Treatment Reports* 60:959–60, July 1976.

Lilienthal, David E. *Big Business: A New Era*. New York: Harper and Row, 1953.

Lilley, S. *Men, Machines and History—The Story of Tools and Machines in Relation to Social Progress*. London: Cobbett Press, 1965.

Linus Pauling Institute of Science and Medicine. Press release. January 26, 1985.

Little, Clarence Cook. *Report of the Scientific Director*. New York: Tobacco Industry Research Committee, 1957.

Livingston, Virginia. *Cancer: A New Breakthrough*. San Diego: Production House, 1972.

Livingston, Virginia Wuerthele-Caspe, and Livingston, Afton M. "Some Cultural, Immunological, and Biochemical Properties of *Progenitor Cryptocides*." *Transactions of the New York Academy of Sciences* (Series 2) 36:569–82, June 1974.

Livingston-Wheeler, Virginia, with Addeo, Edmond G. *The Conquest of Cancer: Vaccines and Diet*. New York: Franklin Watts, 1984. [Autobiography describing the search for *Progenitor cryptocides*.]

*Livingston-Wheeler, Virginia, and Wheeler, Owen Webster. *The Microbiology of Cancer: Compendium*. San Diego: Livingston-Wheeler Clinic, 1977a. [Collection of Livingston's articles in the field, plus confirmatory papers.]

———. *Food Alive*. San Diego: Livingston-Wheeler Clinic, 1977b.

+ ———. Personal communication. June 26, 1979.

Lou, Marjorie F., and Hamilton, Paul B. "Separation and Quantitation of Peptides and Amino Acids in Normal Human Urine." *Methods of Biochemical Analysis* 25:203–271. New York: John Wiley & Co., 1979.

Ludwig Breast Cancer Study Group, The. "Prolonged Disease-Free Survival After One Course of Perioperative Adjuvant Chemotherapy for Node-Negative Breast Cancer." *New England Journal of Medicine* 320:491–496, February 23, 1989.

Lundberg, Ferdinand. *America's Sixty Families*. New York: Vanguard Press, 1937.

McCarty, Mark. "Burying Caesar: An Analysis of the Laetrile Problem." *Triton Times* (University of California, San Diego), November 29, 1975.

*McCoy, J. J. *The Cancer Lady: Maud Slye and Her Hereditary Studies*. New York: Elsevier/Nelson Books, 1977. [A revealing look at the cancer establishment in the period between the two world wars.]

REFERENCES

+ McGill, Jane. *Annual Report.* New York: Employee Health Service, Memorial Sloan-Kettering Cancer Center, 1976.

McGrady, Patrick M., Jr. "The American Cancer Society Means Well, But the Janker Clinic Means Better." *Esquire,* April 1976.

*McGrady, Patrick, Sr. *The Savage Cell.* New York: Basic Books, 1964. [A still-useful study of cancer research from a man who was called "just about the best science public relations person there ever was."]

*————. *The Persecuted Drug: The Story of DMSO.* Garden City, N.Y.: Doubleday and Company, 1973. [How suppression may work in fields other than that of cancer research.]

*————. *The New Immunology.* Ardsley, N.Y.: Independent Citizens' Research Foundation, 1975. [Unconventional approaches to cancer immunotherapy.]

+ ————. Personal communication. January 4, 1979.

McGuire, William L. "Adjuvant Therapy of Node-Negative Breast Cancer." *New England Journal of Medicine* 320:525, February 23, 1989.

McNaughton Foundation. *The Laetriles—Nitrilosides—in the Prevention and Control of Cancer.* Sausalito, Calif., 1967.

Mallinckrodt, Inc. *Annual Report.* St. Louis, 1975.

Manner, Harold, et al. *The Death of Cancer.* Chicago: Advanced Century Publishing Corporation, 1978a.

————. "Amygdalin, Vitamin A, and Enzyme-Induced Regression of Murine Mammary Adenocarcinomas." *Journal of Manipulative and Physiological Therapeutics* (Chicago), December 1978b.

Mansour, E. G.; Gray, R.; Shatila, A. H.; et al. "Efficacy of Adjuvant Chemotherapy in High-Risk Node-Negative Breast Cancer." *New England Journal of Medicine* 320:485–490, February 23, 1989.

Markle, Gerald E., and Petersen, James C. Laetrile and Cancer: The Limits of Science. Presented at the annual meeting of the Midwest Sociological Society. Kalamazoo, Mich.: Center for Sociological Research, Western Michigan University, 1977.

Martin, Daniel S. "Laetrile—A Dangerous Drug." *CA—A Cancer Journal for Clinicians,* September–October 1977.

Martin, Daniel S., et al. "Solid Tumor Animal Model Therapeutically Predictive for Human Breast Cancer." *Cancer Chemotherapy Reports* (Part 2) 5(1), December 1975.

Martin, Wayne. *Medical Heroes and Heretics.* Old Greenwich, Conn.: Devin-Adair Company, 1977.

Marx, Jean. "Burst of Publicity Follows Cancer Report." *Science* 230:1367–68, December 20, 1985.

Maugh, Thomas H., and Marx, Jean L. *Seeds of Destruction: The Science Report on Cancer Research.* New York: Plenum Publishing Corporation, 1975.

Medawar, Sir Peter B. "The Strange Case of the Spotted Mice." *New York Review of Books,* April 15, 1976.

Medical Committee for Human Rights. *Billions for Band-Aids.* San Francisco, 1972.

Medvin, Norman. *The Energy Cartel: Who Runs the American Oil Industry.* New York: Vintage Books, 1974.

REFERENCES

Memorial Hospital. *Annual Report.* New York, 1924.

———. *Annual Report.* New York, 1934.

+ ———. "Dependence of Medicine on Industrial Invention and Research" (press release). New York, March 8, 1940.

+ Memorial Sloan-Kettering Cancer Center. By-Laws of Memorial Sloan-Kettering Cancer Center (A New York Membership Corporation), as Amended Through September 20, 1960. New York, 1960.

———. *Annual Report.* New York, 1972.

+ ———. Official Laetrile Statement. New York, Fall 1973.

———. *Annual Report.* New York, 1976.

———. *Annual Report.* New York, 1977a.

+ ———. Contributions, Bequests, and Grants Received in Cash by Division of Support Activities. New York, May–June 1977b. [MSKCC internal memoranda.]

+ ———. Taped laetrile press conference. New York, June 15, 1977c.

+ ———. Statement on the firing of Ralph W. Moss. New York, November 21, 1977d.

+ ———. Statement on the Second Opinion Report on Laetrile. New York, November 30, 1977e.

———. *Annual Report.* New York, 1978.

———. *Annual Report.* New York, 1986.

———. *Annual Report.* New York, 1987a.

———. Annual Financial Report (Charitable Organization) for year ended December 31, 1987b. [Obtainable from the New York State Department of State, Albany, NY.]

Merigan, T. C. "Purified Interferon: Physical Properties and Species Specificity." *Science* 145:811, 1964.

Michaelis, Ken. Personal Coimmunication, June 14, 1989. [Mr. Michaelis is head of A-O Supply Co. of Millersport, Ohio, a hydrazine sulfate supplier.]

Moertel, C. G.; Fleming, T. R.; Rubin, J.; et al. "A Clinical Trial of Amygdalin (Laetrile) in the Treatment of Human Cancer." *New England Journal of Medicine* 306:201–206, January 28, 1982. [See also accompanying editorial by Relman, below.]

Moertel, C. G.; Fleming, T. R.; Creagan, E. T.; et al. "High-dose Vitamin C Versus Placebo in the Treatment of Patients with Advanced Cancer Who Have Had No Prior Chemotherapy." *New England Journal of Medicine* 312:137–141, 1985.

Moertel, Charles G. "A Trial of Laetrile Now" (editorial). *New England Journal of Medicine* 298:218–19, January 26, 1978.

———. "On Lymphokines, Cytokines, and Breakthroughs." *Journal of the American Medical Association* 256:3141, 1986.

Molinari, Guy V. A Hearing on the Immuno-Augmentative Therapy (IAT) of Dr. Lawrence Burton. Congressional public hearing before Congressman Molinari. January 15, 1986. Summary distributed by IATPA (see Appendix B).

———. On Alternative or Non-Traditional Cancer Therapies by Emanuel Revici, M.D. Congressional public hearing before Congressman Molinari. March 18, 1988. Transcript.

REFERENCES

Monaco, Grace Powers. "Alert," Memorandum on "Racketeering Action Filed by Aetna Against Burzynski Research Insitutute," January 13, 1988.

Mor, Vincent, Ph.D., et al. "An Examination of the Concrete Service Needs of Advanced Cancer Patients." *Journal of Psychosocial Oncology* 5(1), Spring 1987.

*Morris, Nat. *The Cancer Blackout*. Los Angeles: Regent House, 1977. [A history of unorthodox approaches to cancer.]

Morrone, John. A. "Chemotherapy of Inoperable Cancer." *Experimental Medicine and Surgery* 4, 1962. [Preliminary report of ten cases treated with laetrile.]

+ Moss, Ralph W. Hydrazine Sulfate. New York: MSKCC Department of Public Affairs, July 25, 1974. Memorandum. [Co-signed by Manuel Ochoa, M.D.]

+ ———. Subject: Laetrile. New York: MSKCC Department of Public Affairs, July 30, 1976. Memorandum. [Confidential report to T. Gerald Delaney.]

———. "Newly Found Tumor Necrosis Factor Under Study by Institute." MSKCC *Center News*, March 1977.

———. *The Cancer Syndrome*. New York: Grove Press, 1980. [Original version of this book.]

———. "The Promise of Hydrazine Sulfate." *Penthouse*, January 1983.

———. *A Real Choice*. New York: St. Martin's, 1984. [Study of breast cancer patients, based on the cases of surgeon Leslie Strong, M.D.]

———. *Free Radical: Albert Szent-Gyorgyi and the Battle Over Vitamin C*. New York: Paragon House, 1988.

Muldoon, T. G.; Copland, J. A.; and Hendry, L. B. "Actions of Antineoplaston A10 on the Genesis and Maintenance of Specific Subpopulations of Rodent Mammary Tumor Cells." *Advances in Experimental and Clinical Chemotherapy*, February 1988.

Muldoon, T. G.; Copland, J. A.; Lehner, A. F.; and Hendry, L. B. "Inhibition of Spontaneous Mouse Mammary Tumour Development by Antineoplaston A10." *Drugs Under Experimental and Clinical Research* 13 (supp. 1), 1987.

National Cancer Institute. *Fact Book*. DHEW Publication No. (NIH) 75-512. Bethesda, Md., 1975.

———. *Special Communication: Accomplishments of Benefit to People Since 1971.* Bethesda, Md.: National Cancer Program, June 9, 1976a.

———. *Cancer Patient Survival, Report No. 5*. Bethesda, Md., 1976b. [A report from the Cancer Surveillance, Epidemiology and End Results (SEER) Program.]

———. Statement on Dr. Lawrence Burton/Immunology Research Foundation. Bethesda, Md., April 1978.

———. "Clinical Study of Laetrile in Cancer Patients, Investigators' Report: A Summary." April 30, 1981. [Distributed by NCI.]

———. *Investigational Drugs—Pharmaceutical Data, 1987*. NIH Pub. No. 88-2141. Revised November 1987.

———. Grants Process. 1986.

———. *Fact Book*. Bethesda, Md.: NCI, 1987.

———. Statement on Antineoplastons. 1987.

REFERENCES

————. *1990 Budget Estimate*. Bethesda, 1988. [Despite the limiting title, this is a comprehensive publication about the NCI's war on cancer.]

National Institutes of Health. *Guide for Grants and Contracts*. Bethesda, Md., September 25, 1978.

————. *NIH Public Advisory Groups*. DHEW Publication No. (NIH) 79-11. Washington, D.C., January 1, 1979.

National Resources Committee. *Technology and Planning*. Washington, D.C., 1937.

Nauts, Helen Coley. Immunotherapy of Cancer by Bacterial Vaccines. Paper read at International Symposium on Detection and Prevention of Cancer. New York, April 25–May 1, 1976a.

+ ————. Personal communication. December 20, 1976b.

————. Bacterial Products in the Treatment of Cancer: Past, Present and Future. Paper read at the International Colloquium on Bacteriology and Cancer, Cologne, Federal Republic of Germany, March 16–18, 1982. [Also cited in Ward, 1988a.]

*Nauts, Helen Coley, et al. "A Review of the Influence of Bacterial Infection and Bacterial Products (Coley's Toxins) on Malignant Tumors in Man." *Acta Medica Scandinavica* 145 (Supp. 276), April 1953. [First in Mrs. Nauts's series of monographs on Coley's work.]

*Nelkin, Dorothy. *Selling Science: How the Press Covers Science and Technology*. New York: W. H. Freeman and Co., 1987. [Many insights into the relationship between science and society.]

Nelson, Ralph L. *Economic Factors in the Growth of Corporation Giving*. National Bureau of Economic Research Occasional Paper No. 111. New York: Russell Sage Foundation, 1970.

Newbold, H. L. "Design for Living." Interview by Carleton Fredericks, Ph.D. WOR-AM. New York, May 9, 1978.

+ ————. Personal communication. January 22, 1979.

Nieper, Hans. "Problems of Early Cancer Diagnosis and Therapy. 1. Nitrilosides, Particularly Amygdalin in Cancer Prophylaxis and Therapy." *Agressologie* (Paris) 11(1), 1970.

Nishida, H.; Yoshida, H.; Hoshino, K.; Kubota, H.; Hara, H.; Nakayama, T.; Oishi, K.; Koga, T.; Hashimoto, K.; Kakegawa, T.; and Tsuda, H. Inhibitory Effect of Oral Administration of Antineoplaston A10 on the Growth Curve of Human Breast Cancer Transplanted to Athymic Mice. 1988. [Preprint; submitted for publication.]

Nishida, H., et al. "Inhibitory Effect of Oral Administration of Antineoplaston A10 on the Growth Cure of Human Breast Cancer Transplanted to Athymic Mice." *J. Jpn. Ca. Therapy* (forthcoming).

Nobile, David F. "The Chemistry of Risk." *Seven Days,* June 5, 1979.

Null, Gary. "This Man Could Save Your Life, But He Can't Get the Money to Do It." *Our Town.* May 13–19, 1979.

————. "The Suppression of Cancer Cures." *Penthouse,* October 1979.

Null, Gary, and Steinman, Leonard. "The Vendetta Against Dr. Burton." *Penthouse,* March, 1986.

REFERENCES

Ochoa, Manuel. "Trial of Hydrazine Sulfate in Patients with Cancer." *Cancer Chemotherapy Reports* 59:1151–54, 1975.

Old, Lloyd J., "Tumor Necrosis Factor." *Scientific American*, May 1988.

Old, Lloyd J., and Boyse, Edward A. *Current Enigmas in Cancer Research*. The Harvey Lectures, Series 67. New York: Academic Press, 1973. [Lecture delivered April 20, 1972.]

Palmer, John F. Letter to S. R. Burzynski, February 13, 1984. [Palmer was Acting Director, Division of Oncology and Radiopharmaceutical Drug Products, Office of Drug Research and Review, National Center for Drugs and Biologics, Food and Drug Administration.]

———. Letter to S. R. Burzynski, August 5, 1988.

Passwater, Richard A. "In Defense of Laetrile." *Let's Live*, June 1977.

———. *Cancer and Its Nutritional Therapies*. New Canaan, Conn.: Keats Publishing, 1978.

*Patterson, James T. *The Dread Disease—Cancer and Modern American Culture*. Cambridge, Mass.: Harvard University Press, 1987. [Scholarly yet lively discussion of role of cancer in American social history.]

Pauling, L.; Nixon, J. C.; Stitt, F.; Marcuson, R.; Dunham, W. B.; Barth, R.; Bensch, K.; Herman, Z. S.; Blaisdell, B. E.; Tsao, C.; Prender, M.; Andrews, V.; Willoughby, R.; and Zuckerkandl, E. "Effects of Dietary Ascorbic Acid on the Incidence of Spontaneous Mammary Tumors in RIII Mice." *Proceedings of the National Academy of Sciences USA*, 82:5185–5189, August 1985.

Pauling, Linus. *No More War!* New York: Dodd, Mead and Company, 1958.

———. *Vitamin C and the Common Cold*. New York: Bantam Books, 1971.

———. *Vitamin C, the Common Cold, and the Flu*. San Francisco: W. H. Freeman and Company, 1976.

+ ———. Personal communication. June 18, 1979.

———. *How to Live Longer and Feel Better*. New York: Avon Books, 1987.

Pauling, Linus, and Cameron, Ewan. "Supplemental Ascorbate in the Supportive Treatment of Cancer." *Proceedings of the National Academy of Sciences*, 73:3685–89, October 1976.

Pharmaceutical Manufacturers' Association. *Newsletter*. Washington, D.C., April 26, 1976.

Physicians' Desk Reference. Oradell, N.J.: Medical Economics, 1978.

Prescott, Eleanor. "Mary Lasker: The Most Powerful Person in Modern Medicine." *Medical Dimensions*, March 1976.

Pressman, Gabe. Program on laetrile (in series on cancer), WNEW-TV. New York, May 16, 1979.

Regelson, William. "The 'Grand Conspiracy' Against the Cancer Cure" (Commentary). *JAMA* 243:337–339, January 25, 1980.

Reitnauer, P. G. "Prolonged Survival of Tumor-Bearing Mice Following Feeding Bitter Almonds." *Archiv Geschwulstforschung* (Dresden) 42:135, 1973.

Relman, A. "Closing the Books on Laetrile" (editorial). *New England Journal of Medicine* 306:236, 1982.

REFERENCES

————. "Adjuvant Treatment of Early Breast Cancer" (editorial). *New England Journal of Medicine* 320:525, 1989.

Richards, Evelleen. "Vitamin C Suffers a Dose of Politics." *New Scientist*, February 27, 1986.

————. "The Politics of Therapeutic Evaluation: The Vitam C and Cancer Controversy," *Social Studies* of Science, Vol. 18,653–701, 1988. [An excellent study affirming "the idea of neutral appraisal is a myth." See also forthcoming *Vitamin C and Cancer: Medicine or Politics* (Macmillan).]

*Richards, Victor. *Cancer, the Wayward Cell: Its Origins, Nature, and Treatment.* Berkeley: University of California Press, 1972. [Despite stereotyped view of unorthodox therapies, a useful account of the cancer problem for laypersons.]

Richardson, John, and Griffin, Patricia. *Laetrile Case Histories.* New York: Bantam Books, 1977.

Robertson, Wyndham. "Merck Strains to Keep the Pots Aboiling." *Fortune*, March 1976.

Roeder, Connie. Memo to S. R. Burzynski, December 15, 1976. [From administrative secretary, department of anesthesiology, Baylor College of Medicine.]

Rosenberg, S. A.; Lotze, M. T.; Muul, L. M.; et al. "Observations on the Systemic Administration of Autologous Lymphokine-Activated Killer Cells and Recombinant Interleukin-2 to Patients with Metastatic Cancer." *New England Journal of Medicine* 313:1485–1492, 1985.

*Rosenbaum, Ruth. "Cancer, Inc." *New Times*, November 25, 1977. [Acerbic critique of cancer establishment, especially the ACS.]

Ross, Joseph P. "Laetriles—Not a Vitamin and Not a Treatment" (editorial). *Western Journal of Medicine*, April 1975.

Ross, Walter S. "The Medicines We Need—But Can't Have." *Reader's Digest*, October 1973.

————. *Crusade: The Official History of the American Cancer Society.* New York: Arbor House, 1987.

Rossi, B., Guidetti, E., et al. "Clinical Trial of Chemotherapeutic Treatment of Advanced Cancers with L-Mandelonitrile-Beta-Diglucoside." In *Proceedings of the Ninth International Cancer Congress*, 1966. (Reprinted by the McNaughton Foundation, 1967, see above.)

Rorvik, David M. "Who Wrote the American Cancer Society's Denunciation of Hydrazine Sulfate?" *Alicia Patterson Foundation Newsletter* (New York), November 29, 1976.

+ Rottino, Antonio. Personal communication. December 18, 1978.

Rozental, Alek A. "The Strange Ethics of the Ethical Drug Industry." In *Crisis in American Medicine*, edited by Marion K. Sanders. New York: Harper & Row, 1961.

Rubin, Philip, ed. *Clinical Oncology for Medical Students. A Multidisciplinary Approach.* Third Edition. New York and Rochester: American Cancer Society and University of Rochester School of Medicine, 1971.

————. *Clinical Oncology for Medical Students and Physicians: A Mutlidisciplinary Approach.* 6th edition. New York and Rochester: American Cancer Society and the University of Rochester School of Medicine and Dentistry, 1983.

REFERENCES

Saftlas, Herman B. "Health Care, Hospitals, Drugs and Cosmetics: Current Analysis." *Standard & Poor's Industry Surveys*, New York, December 15, 1988 (3).

+ Schloen, Lloyd H. Notes from First Annual Convention of the International Association of Cancer Victims and Friends, Inc. New York, April 15, 1973. [Prepared for MSKCC administration.]

Schmahl, D.; Thomas, C.; and Auer, R. *Iatrogenic Carcinogenesis*. Berlin: Springer-Verlag, 1977.

Schmidt, E. S., et al. "Laetrile Toxicity Studies in Dogs." *Journal of the American Medical Association* 239:943–947, 1978.

Schumacher, L. F., Jr. Memo to S. R. Burzynski. December 3, 1976.

Schultz, Terri, and Lindeman, Bard. "The Victimization of Desperate Cancer Patients." *Today's Health*, November 1973.

Schuster, Donna. Personal communication. June 11, 1989.

+ Second International Workshop on Interferons in the Treatment of Cancer. *Report*. New York: Memorial Sloan-Kettering Cancer Center, et al., April 22–24, 1979.

Second Opinion. *Special Report: Laetrile at Sloan-Kettering*. Bronx, N.Y., 1977.

Seits, I. F., et al. "Experimental and Clinical Data of Antitumor Action of Hydrazine Sulfate." *Problems of Oncology* (Leningrad) 21:45–52, 1975.

Selikoff, Irving. Speech to the Society for Clinical Ecology. Key Biscayne, Fla., November 19, 1978.

Sherman, Brian. "The High Cost of Medical Care: Who's To Blame?" *Private Practice*, November 1988.

*Shilts, Randy. *And the Band Played On*. New York: St. Martin's Press, 1987. [Celebrated history of the politics of AIDS.]

Shimkin, Michael B. *Science and Cancer*. DHEW Pub. No. (NIH) 74-568. Bethesda, Md.: National Institutes of Health, 1973.

*———. *Contrary to Nature*. DHEW Pub. No. (NIH) 76-720. Bethesda, Md.: National Institutes of Health, 1977. [Readable, profusely illustrated account of cancer history.]

Shintomi, T.; Hashimoto, K.; Tanaka, M.; Hara, H.; and Tsuda, H. Inhibitory Effect of Antineoplaston A10 Injections on the Growth Curve of Human Breast Cancer Transplanted to Athymic Mice. 1988. [Submitted for publication.]

Shoemaker, R. H.; Wolpert–De Filippes, M. K.; and Venditti, J. M. "Application of a Human Tumor Clonogenic Assay to Screening for New Antitumor Drugs." *Proceedings of the 13th International Congress of Chemotherapy*, 2 (Cytostat Symposia 1). Vienna, August 28–September 2, 1983.

Shryock, Richard Harrison. *Medicine and Society in America: 1660–1860*. Ithaca, N.Y.: Cornell University Press, 1962.

Simonton, O. Carl, and Matthews-Simonton, Stephanie. *Getting Well Again*. Los Angeles: J. P. Tarcher, 1978.

60 Minutes. "The Establishment vs. Dr. Burton" (vol. 12, no. 36). CBS Television, Sunday, May 18, 1980.

Sloan-Kettering Institute. "Carcinogens . . . Internally Manufactured?" *Report*. New York, 1969.

REFERENCES

+ ————. Meeting on Amygdalin. New York, July 10, 1973. Minutes.

————. *Annual Report.* New York, 1974.

————. Research and Educational Programs, 1987–88. New York, 1987.

Smith, Richard D. "The Laetrile Papers." *The Sciences,* January 1978.

Sontag, Susan. *Illness as Metaphor.* New York: Farrar, Straus and Giroux, 1977.

Spykeman, Jeffrey M. Affadavit for Search Warrant. V. S. Magistrate, Minneapolis, MN. Magistrate's Case No. JEBTI. June 7, 1989.

Standard and Poor's. *Industry Survey.* New York, 1977.

————. *Industry Survey.* New York, July 1979.

*Stewart, R. B. *Tragedies from Drug Therapy.* Springfield: Charles C. Thomas, 1985. [Well-written study of medical oversight.]

+ Stock, C. Chester. A Second and Low Opinion of Second Opinion's Special Report: Laetrile at Sloan-Kettering. New York: Sloan-Kettering Institute, November 21, 1977. [Internal memorandum.]

Stock, C. Chester, et al. "Antitumor Tests of Amygdalin in Spontaneous Animal Tumor Systems." *Journal of Surgical Oncology* 10:81–88, 1978.

Stone, Irwin. *The Healing Factor—Vitamin C Against Disease.* New York: Grosset & Dunlap, 1972.

Strickland, Stephen P. "Integration of Medical Research and Health Politics." *Science,* September 17, 1971.

*————. *Politics, Science and Dread Disease.* Cambridge, Mass.: Harvard University Press, 1972. [History of United States medical research policy.]

Strong, Leslie, M.D. Personal communication. March 23, 1989.

Sugiura, Kanematsu. *The Publications of Kanematsu Sugiura: Memorial Edition.* 4 vols. Foreword by C. Chester Stock. New York: Sloan-Kettering Institute, 1965.

*————. "Reminiscence and Experience in Experimental Chemotherapy of Cancer." *Medical Clinics of North America* 55(3), May 1971. [Charming account of early cancer research.]

+ ————. Unpublished taped interview. July 1974.

+ ————. Personal communication. August 5, 1975.

+ ————. Personal communication. February 10, 1976a.

+ ————. Personal communication. July 29, 1976b.

+ ————. Personal communication. September 9, 1976c.

+ ————. Personal communication. December 20, 1976d.

+ ————. Personal communication. January 17, 1977a.

+ ————. Letter to Alec Pruchnicki. November 22, 1977b. [Pruchnicki was chairman of Second Opinion.]

+ ————. Personal communication. March 23, 1979.

Summa, Herbert M. "Amygdalin, a Physiologically Active Therapeutic Agent in Malignancies" (in German). *Krebsgeschehen Schriftenreihe* (Heidelberg) 4, 1972.

Sun, Marjorie. "Cancer Institute's Drug Program Reproved." *Science* 214:887–889, November 20, 1981.

Syracuse Cancer Research Institute. Informational brochure. Syracuse, N.Y., July 1979.

REFERENCES

Takaiwa, Masa. Personal communication. March 22, 1989. [Mr. Takaiwa is a U.S. representative of the Kureha Chemical Industry Co. of Japan, which manufactures the drug Krestin.]

Tayek, John A., et al. "Effect of Hydrazine Sulfate on Whole Body Protein Breakdown Measured by 14C-lysine Metabolism in Lung Cancer Patients." *The Lancet* 2(8553), August 18, 1987.

Taylor, A. M. *Imagination and the Growth of Science.* New York: Schocken Books, 1970.

Taylor, Renée. *Hunza Health Secrets.* New York: Award Books, 1960.

Teitelman, Robert. "The Baffling Standoff in Cancer Research." *Forbes,* July 15, 1985.

*Thomas, Patricia. "The Muddle Over Screening: Breast Ca." *Medical World News,* May 9, 1988. [Good overview of the problem.]

Thomas, Lewis. "Disease, Cancer and the Progress of Science" (interviewed by the author). MSKCC *Center News,* March 1975.

———. "Getting at the Roots of a Deep Puzzle." *Discover,* March 1986.

Thompson, Morton. *The Cry and the Covenant.* New York: New American Library, 1949. [Fictional account of the life of Ignaz Semmelweis.]

20/20 Special Report. "The War on Cancer: Cure, Profit or Politics?" (no. 137). Produced by Judith Moses. October 21, 1981. [Transcript available from Box 2020, Ansonia Station, New York, NY 10023.]

Tsuda, Hideaki. Affidavit to United States Food and Drug Administration. January 7, 1986. [Tsuda is Associate Professor, Department of Anesthesiology, Kurume University, School of Medicine, 67, Asahi-Machi, Kurume-Shi, Japan.]

United States Department of Commerce, Bureau of the Census. *Current Industry Reports: Pharmaceutical Preparations Except Biologicals.* Washington, D.C., 1977.

———. "Current Industry Reports: Pharmaceutical Preparations Except Biologicals (MA28G)." Washington, D.C., 1983–1987. [Each report issued in November of the following year.]

———. 1988 U.S. Industrial Outlook. Washington, D.C., 1988.

United States General Accounting Office. *Cancer Patient Survival: What Progress Has Been Made?* Washington, D.C., March 1987.

United States Senate. "Breast Cancer—1976." Hearing Before the Subcommittee on Health and Scientific Research, Committee on Human Resources. Washington, D.C., May 4, 1976.

———. "Banning of the Drug Laetrile from Interstate Commerce by FDA." Hearing Before the Subcommittee on Health and Scientific Research, Committee on Human Resources. Washington, D.C., July 12, 1977.

Upton, Arthur C. Letter to Lawrence Burton. August 11, 1978. [Letter in possession of Dr. Burton. Authenticity confirmed by Dr. Upton in following entry.]

+ ———. Personal communication. July 26, 1979.

Vallery-Radot, René. *The Life of Pasteur.* Translated by R. L. Devonshire. Garden City, N.Y.: Garden City Publishing Company, 1924.

Vogel, Virgil J. *American Indian Medicine.* Norman, Okla.: University of Oklahoma Press, 1970.

REFERENCES

Von Hoffman, Nicholas. "Fund Shortage Hurts Pauling Cancer Project" syndicated column. *Lawton* [Okla.] *Constitution*, November 17, 1976.

Wade, Leo. "Medical Public Relations for the Physician in Industry." *New York Medicine* 9:686–88, September 20, 1953.

———. "Why People Don't Work." *Texas State Journal of Medicine*, July 1958.

+ ———. The Environment in Relation to Cancer. New York, December 1962. Mimeograph.

+ ———. Occupation and Cancer: The George Gehrmann Memorial Lecture. New York, February 6, 1964. Mimeograph.

Walde, David. Report: Visit to the Burzynski Research Institute, Houston—April 2nd, 3rd, 4th, 5th, 1982. Report dated May 3, 1982.

*Waldholz, Michael, and Bogdanich, Walt. "Warm Bodies: Doctor-Owned Labs Earn Lavish Profits in a Captive Market." *Wall Street Journal*, March 1, 1989. [Excellent reporting on the scandalous greed of some doctors.]

Warburg, Otto. *The Metabolism of Tumors*. London: Constable and Company, 1930.

Ward, Patricia Spain. History of BCG. Contract report submitted to the Office of Technology Assessment, June 1988a. [Available from Ms. Ward at 1454 West Flournoy, Chicago, IL 60607.]

———. History of Gerson Therapy. June 1988b. [See note above.]

———. History of Hoxsey Treatment. May 1988c. [See note above.]

———. Memo to John H. Gibbons. December 2, 1988d. [A rebuttal to the Gibbons letter above.]

*Weinstein, Henry. "Did Industry Suppress Asbestos Data?" *Los Angeles Times*, October 23, 1978. [Incisive investigative journalism based on documents unearthed in the course of asbestos-related law suits.]

Wetherell, Robert C., Jr. Letter to the Honorable Lloyd Bentsen. Internally dated after October 29, 1984.

Wiener, Norbert. *The Human Use of Human Beings: Cybernetics and Society*. Garden City, N.Y.: Doubleday Anchor Books, 1954.

Wiewel, Frank. Letter to the editor. *Journal of the American Medical Association* 260:3435, December 16, 1988. [A response to the DATTA survey on IAT by the head of the IAT Patients' Association. With Houston, above, one of the few times *JAMA* has ever given space to antiestablishment critics.]

———. Personal communication. March 22, 1989.

Williams, Roger J. *Nutrition Against Disease: Environmental Protection*. New York: Plenum Publishing Corporation, 1971.

Wiscombe, Janet. "The Promise of a Cure: How Far Will People Go?" *Coping*, Summer 1988.

Wolf, Max, and Ransberger, Karl. *Enzyme Therapy*. Los Angeles: Regent House, 1972.

Wolin, Ronald G. PRLAF letter to Dear Friend. Summer 1988.

World Medical Association. *Ethics and Regulations of Clinical Research*. R. J. Levine: Urban and Schwarzenberg, 1981.

Wright, Jane Riddle. *Diagnosis: Cancer—Prognosis: Life*. Huntsville, AL: Albright and Co., 1985. [Available from P.O. Box 2011, Huntsville, AL 35804.]

REFERENCES

Wuerthele-Caspe, Virginia [later Virginia Livingston-Wheeler], et al. "Etiology of Scleroderma—A Preliminary Clinical Report." *Journal of the Medical Society of New Jersey* 44:256, July 1947.

Yarborough, Ralph. "Foreword" in *Report of the National Panel of Consultants on the Conquest of Cancer.* Prepared for the Committee on Labor and Public Welfare, U.S. Senate. Washington, D.C. 1970.

Yasgur, Steven S. "Can Cancer Be Destroyed by the Body's Own Agents?" *Modern Medicine,* January 1, 1975.

Young, Frank E. Public Statement, National Committee to Review Current Procedures for Approval of New Drugs for Cancer and AIDS. Bethesda, MD. January 4, 1989a. [Distributed by Office of Cancer Communications, National Cancer Institute.]

———. "Speeding Help and Hope to the Desperately Ill." *FDA Consumer,* February 1989b.

Young, G. "Disputed Bahamas Cancer Clinic Reopens." *Newsday,* March 11, 1986:22.

Young, James H. *The Medical Messiahs.* Princeton: Princeton University Press, 1967.

Zimmermann, Caroline A. *Laetrile: Hope—or Hoax?* New York: Zebra Books, 1977.

Index

INDEX

INDEX

Metastases, 8, 126
Methotrexate, 74, 75, 77, 86–87, 187
Metianu, T., 145
Meuli, Frances, 219
Miles Laboratories, 89
Miller, Mildred, 103
Miller, Thomas, 49
Mills, A. Ernest, 104
Mistletoe, 133–34
Mixed bacterial vaccine (MBV), 253
Mobil Oil, 344, 395
Moertel, Charles, 80, 131, 150, 151, 167, 173; vitamin C study of, 223, 226
Molinari, Guy V., 263, 266–68
Molomut, Norman, 104
Monoclonal antibodies, 16, 92
Monsanto Co., 89, 344
Montedison Group, 90
Morley, Andrew P., 17
Morris, Nat, 216
Morrone, John A., 147
Morton, Donald, 236
Moskowitz, Myron, 25
MRI (magnetic resonance imaging), 12–13, 17, 26
Múgos Company, 145
Multiple myeloma, 35
Munoz, Eric, 15
Murray, Paul A., 104
Mustargen, 74, 107

Naessens, Gaston, 104
National Cancer Institute (NCI), 406–9, 432–34; and asbestos, 382; and big business, ties with, 369; Biological Response Modifer Program, 129; Bross's grant application to, 72; and Burton's method, 241–42, 245, 249–54, 264, 267; and Burzynski, 291, 295, 299–303, 310; Cancer Chemotherapy National Service Center, 87; Cancer Nutrition Laboratory, 233; Cancer Patient

Survival Report No. 5, 30; and drug testing, 90, 93; and Ferguson Plant Products, 114; grants issued by, and the ACS unproven methods list, 98; and hydrazine sulfate, 190–91, 196, 199, 201–3, 205–6, 208–9; and insurance companies, letter of protest to, 19; and interleukin-2, 80; and laetrile, 148–49, 150–51, 172; and mammography, 23–24; and the prevention of cancer, 228, 349, 354–64; SEER program, 38; statistics, on survival, 28, 38–41; and vitamin A therapy, 229; and vitamin C therapy, 223, 226, 227–30, 233; and Warburg's fermentation theory, 188
National Institute of Health, 6, 200, 209, 390
National Radium Institute, 65, 66
Nauts, Helen Coley, 122, 123, 124, 125–26, 127, 128, 161; on Coley's toxins tests, 253
Navarro, Manuel D., 147
Neck, cancer of the, 60, 242
Necrosis, 69, 128
Neoplasms, 35
Neuroblastoma, 82
Nichols, Perry L., 104
Niehans, Paul, 104
Nieper, Hans A., 147, 149, 161
Nitrogen mustard, 74, 76, 393–94
Nitrosamines, 342
Nixon, Richard, 4, 5, 6, 41–42, 165, 403
NLO Inc., 71
Nobile, David F., 344
Nolvadex, 90
Normal human globulin (NHG), 246
Nuclear weapons, 68–71
Null, Gary, 298

Ochoa, Manuel, 192, 193
Old, Lloyd J., 122, 127, 149, 166;

INDEX